PHYSIOLOGY OF BLOOD

ENCYCLOPAEDIA OF ANIMAL PHYSIOLOGY SERIES

PHYSIOLOGY OF BLOOD

Edited by
M. PRAKASH
C.K. ARORA

ANMOL PUBLICATIONS PVT. LTD.
NEW DELHI-110 002 (INDIA)

ANMOL PUBLICATIONS PVT. LTD.
4374/4B, Ansari Road
Daryaganj, New Delhi-110 002

Physiology of Blood

First Edition, 1998

ISBN 81-7488-881-0

PRINTED IN INDIA

Published by J. L. Kumar for Anmol Publications Pvt. Ltd., New Delhi, Typeset by Chitra Computers, Delhi and Printed at Mehra Offset Press, Delhi.

Contents

Preface

The present volume has been designed for the introductory course in Physiology. It is prepared for students in biological, medical, and health oriented programs. Among the students specifically served by this volume are those aiming for a career as a nurse, medical assistant, physician's assistant, medical laboratory technologist, radiologist, inhalation therapist, dental hygienist, physical therapist, and medical record keeper.

Because the structures of the body are exquisitely designed to carry out specific functions one can best appreciate and understand anatomy and physiology when structure and function are studied together.

Accordingly the authors have integrated both anatomy and physiology as much as possible throughout the text of book. Authors have used a system rather than a regional approach, and although anatomy has not been slighted, an emphasis has been placed on physiology.

The present volume is devoted to blood with emphasis on formation and destruction of blood cells, life span of red cells, lymphocyte and their role in antibody production and macrophage.

Special care has been taken to make the reading level appropriate for today's college student. New technical terms are described separately and new concepts are thoroughly explained. Students will find the writing style easy to read and enjoyable.

Though, the authors have taken special care to present a current account, yet they are fully aware about their limitations, and the readers may come across the mistakes of various types. For all types of mistakes they extend their due apology.

The authors have freely consulted other standard books and research papers while preparing the manuscript, so the authors claim no originality of the work.

It has often been said that a man never writes a book alone and this was never more true than in the present case. In the actual compilation of the book the authors could not have done without the conscientious and enthusiastic help of their friends and colleagues, too numerous to mention individually, who influenced our approach to related subject. Some of the outstanding contributors nevertheless merit special acknowledgement. Prof. K.S. Rao, Head of the Department, School of Studies in Zoology,

Vikram University, Ujjain for making exceptional efforts as providing illustrative material and Prof. (Mrs.) R. Kaul, Department of Zoology for enriching intellectual ideas.

We are also thankful to Km. Neeru Nayar, for her help on diverse occasion during the work on the manuscript.

The authors are also thankful to Shri J.L Kumar, Managing Director, Anmol Publications Pvt. Ltd., New Delhi for bringing out a handsome print of this book in a comparatively short time.

Constructive criticisms and suggestion for improvement of the book will thankfully be acknowledged.

— **Authors**

1

The Blood

Blood, the red fluid of the blood vessels with which we are all familiar, is the transport medium of the body. As we have seen in the General Function Design of the body, it is the medium by which all living tissues are related to their external environment, that is the outside world. It is pumped to and fro between the tissues and the lungs and between the tissues and the alimentary canal to take up oxygen and nourishment respectively, while by its aid the products of oxidation and metabolism in the tissues are returned to the outside world by the lungs, the skin, and the kidney. It is also the medium by which growth and repair substances are transported to the tissues and by which the various controlling glands of the body can distribute their chemical messengers. In spite of having all these functions which are constantly tending to change its composition, this remains remarkably constant.

Blood is a somewhat viscid fluid, and in man and in all other vertebrate animals, with the exception of two, is red in colour. It consists of a yellowish fluid, called **plasma,** in which are suspended numerous **blood-corpuscles** or **cells,** the majority of which are coloured, and it is to their presence that the red colour of the blood is due. They form 45 per cent of the blood volume. It also contains smaller bodies known as platelets.

Even when examined in very thin layers, blood is *opaque,* on account of the refractive powers possessed by its two constituents, the plasma and the corpuscles. On treatment with ether, water, and other reagents, however, it becomes transparent and assumes a lake colour, in consequence of the colouring matter of the corpuscles having been discharged into the plasma. The average *specific gravity* of blood at 15° C. (60° F.) varies from 1055 to 1062. A rapid and useful method of estimating the specific gravity of blood was invented by Roy. Drops of blood are taken and allowed to fall into fluids of known specific gravity. When the drop neither rises nor sinks in the fluid it is taken to be of the same specific gravity as that of the standard fluid. In Van Slyke's (1942) method a series of appropriate solutions of copper sulphate are made up and a drop of blood added to each. With approximately normal plasma the result really depends on the haemoglobin concentration. The *taste* is saltish. Its *temperature* varies slightly, the average being 37.8° C. (100° F.). The blood stream is warmed by passing through the muscles and glands, but it is somewhat cooled on traversing the capillaries of the skin. Recently drawn blood has a distinct *odour,* which in many cases is characteristic of the animal from which it has been taken; it may be further developed by adding to blood a mixture of equal parts of sulphuric acid and water. The *reaction* of the blood is faintly alkaline and is dealt with in a later chapter.

Blood Volume.—The quantity of blood in an animal may be estimated in the following manner; a small quantity of blood is taken from an animal by venesection; it is defibrinated and measured, and used to make standard solutions of blood. As much blood as possible is removed from the animal by bleeding, and the blood-vessels washed out with saline solution until the washings are no longer coloured. The amounts of blood in the washings are then determined by reference to the standards. The application of the method to decapitated criminals has given values from 1/8 to 1/14. **In man** during life it is evident that other methods are necessary.

Those commonly in use involve the injection of dyes, usually "vital red" or "Evans blue."

The subject is of some practical interest as it is found that it may vary in disease. In talking of blood volume it should be realised that we really usually mean **plasma volume,** as the dye does not enter the corpuscles.

The following method is that now most extensively used. Two samples of blood (5 c.c.) are withdrawn and oxalated. A 1.5 per cent solution of the dye is injected into an arm vein—after five minutes, samples of blood are withdrawn and centrifuged. The colour is compared, the tint of the dye in the plasma compared with standards consisting of uncoloured plasma and dye solutions of known concentrations. This method gives a total blood volume of from 1/11 to 1/14 of body-weight. In an average man the amount is then about **6 litres,** but this may be increased as in anaemia or at high altitudes. Similar results have been obtained by studying the change in blood concentration which occurs when plasma is injected.

It is possible also to withdraw a number of the subject's blood corpuscles, to label them with radio-active phosphorus, then to reinject them and determine their dilution with a Geiger counter. This method gives a slightly lower value than the dye method.

All methods depending on the dilution of an injected substance have the disadvantage that they measure only the circulating volume of blood and not necessarily that available in the blood-depots, which may or may not be full at the time of the estimation. Any state which causes them to contract, such as excitement and some diseases, may upset results when they are most needed, but in the same individual at rest repeated examinations under uniform conditions give reasonably constant results, the experimental error being quite small. The resting blood volume is relatively much greater in children than in adults and those adults which take active exercise, but mere rest in bed is sufficient to cause a decrease.

The Regulation of Blood Volume.— The blood volume obviously depends ultimately on the water content of the body as a whole; but even when conditions arise which tend to change it, it keeps approximately constant. This is made possible by the fluid passing through the capillary walls in either direction according to requirements, while excess is lost by the kidney and skin. Thus the injection of small quantities of fluid changes the blood volume for only a short time, for a lowering of the blood pressure allows water to leave the vessels while excessive loss of water has the opposite effect. The subject is closely related to the water-balance of the body and to the formation of lymph, which are dealt with in separate sections.

The circulating blood volume is increased in a number of states, notably mental stress, muscular exercise, and high temperature. This is no doubt due in part to the constriction of the blood-depots, for there is an increase of cells as well as plasma. More rapidly moving blood also tends to sweep static corpuscles into the circulation. It has been calculated that five-sixths of the total blood is in the heart and larger blood-vessels at any one time.

A reduction of circulating blood volume is brought about by a number of conditions. It may occur in any generalised anhydraemia (*i.e.* loss of body water), in haemorrhage, or if the blood pools in the capillaries, as may occur when there is extensive damage to tissues. Prolonged standing has a similar effect from the pooling of blood and lymph in the legs (see "The Effect of Gravity on the Circulation"). A reduction is also produced by exposure to cold, apparently because of the vasoconstriction, of the skin brought about by the nervous system, for it does not occur if the spinal cord is cut (Barbour). The skin vasoconstriction, by raising capillary pressures, presumably increases the amount of tissue fluid and excretion by the kidney. It seems possible, too, that continued mental stress acting similarly may eventually reduce the blood volume, and hence the effect of a holiday in causing a subject to "look better" may be due to additional blood filling the superficial vessels more fully. There are, however, as yet no experimental data on the subject.

Functions of Blood

Mephistopheles, in Goethe's *Faust*, is biologically quite right when he exclaims: *"Blut ist ein ganz besonderer Saft!"* (Blood is a very peculiar fluid!)

In the first place it is not a lifeless fluid incapable of metabolic changes, but a *circulating tissue*, made up of detached living cells floating in a liquid plasma. The fact that it moves about marks it off distinctly from all other tissues. It is conspicuously kaleidoscopic in character, changing constantly in its intimate composition as it passes through the different parts of the body, for it is not only the common carrier *to* the various tissues of everything needful for their maintenance, but also the collector *from* the tissues of the products of metabolism, such as carbon dioxide and soluble nitrogen compounds.

In the last analysis cells of every kind within the animal body sooner or later contribute something to the blood and receive something in return, so that the blood reflects the entire metabolism of the body. In spite of this fact its component parts are normally kept at nearly a constant level. When serious deviations occur, as in the excessive loss of water from the blood during cholera, or the diminution of the number of blood cells in anaemia or hemorrhage, pathological consequences are sure to follow.

In general the following functions may be performed by the blood.

(*a*) **Equilibration of Water Content.**—Water is the fluid universal that facilitates the internal transport of materials, making good losses by evaporation and otherwise, as well as preventing the drying up of tissues. It is also the great solvent of all sorts of substances in the food and throughout the tissues. The degree of activity exhibited by any tissue is directly dependent upon the fluidity of the cytoplasm within its cellular units, which in turn is ultimately a matter of the amount of water supplied by the blood.

(*b*) **Liberation of Energy.**—Tissues "burn" in the presence of oxygen thus releasing energy, which is what constitutes "living." Certain softer tissues, like the muscles for example, lend themselves particularly to this oxidative process, while others, such as skeletal tissues, resemble more the iron girders of a "fire-proof" building, and do not burn as readily. The oxygen necessary for the release of stored energy is delivered to the tissues of vertebrates by the *haemoglobin* in the red corpuscles of the blood.

(*c*) **Distribution of Food.**—From one point of view blood is a solution or an emulsion of food substances carried in the plasma. To some extent also it transports food as solid undissolved particles engulfed in the white blood cells. It is thus the grocery delivery boy for the cellular community.

(*d*) **Regulation of Temperature.**—Body temperature, which results from the oxidation of the tissues, is equalized by means of the circulation of the blood, much as is the temperature of a building by the hot-water pipes of its heating plant. Such equalization is necessary because of the unequal production of heat-energy by different tissues of the body.

In so-called "warm-blooded" animals the body temperature is maintained at a practically constant level, regardless of the temperature of the environment, thus enhancing the animal's independence. "Cold-blooded" animals, on the other hand, owing partly to the low oxygen-carrying capacity of their blood, have a body temperature which fluctuates in response to that of the surroundings. A cold-blooded animal is consequently a thermal slave to the environment in which it finds itself.

It has been demonstrated, however, that even cold-blooded fishes when ill may show fever-like fluctuations in temperature.

(*e*) **Transmission of Chemical Substances.**—*Hormones*, the chemical messengers from endocrinal glands, frequently perform metabolic feats at some distance from their point of origin, after travelling along the blood highways. Drugs and poisons introduced into the organism likewise gain ready disposal over the body by means of the circulating blood. This is why a person with malaria, for example, feels "sick all over," since the blood carrying the organisms producing malarial poison literally goes over the whole body.

(*f*) **Defense against Parasitic Invasion.**—Troublesome foreign invaders, such as infective bacteria and protozoans, are regularly combatted by white blood cells which capture and devour them. The cures of most "catching" diseases depend upon the successful outcome of this function of the blood.

(*g*) **Disposal of Cell Wreckage.**—The blood is a continual funeral cortege, in which are being borne away the "ashes" of dead cells, foreign bodies, bacterial products, and wastes of metabolism generally.

GENERAL PROPERTIES OF THE BLOOD

Composition

If something is added to a sample of blood to keep it from clotting and it is permitted to stand—or better, because it goes faster, if the blood is centrifuged—it separates into two approximately equal fractions. The rapidly rotating centrifuge drives the heavier elements, e.g., the red blood cells, to the outer (lower) part of the tilted test tube. The upper, lighter half is the liquid portion of the blood, the blood plasma; it is pale yellow, some what vicious, and sticky. The **plasma** usually constitutes about **55 per cent** of the total, the cells **45 per cent**. The instrument used for this determination is the **hematocrit,** and the measurement is called the "hematocrit reading." Thus if a certain blood sample gave a hematocrit reading of 40, it would mean that the sample consisted of 40 per cent cells, 60 per cent plasma.

Colour

Everyone knows that blood is red, but it is not, necessarily. The color of the blood depends on the nature of the hemoglobin. Much will be said about hemoglobin later. Let

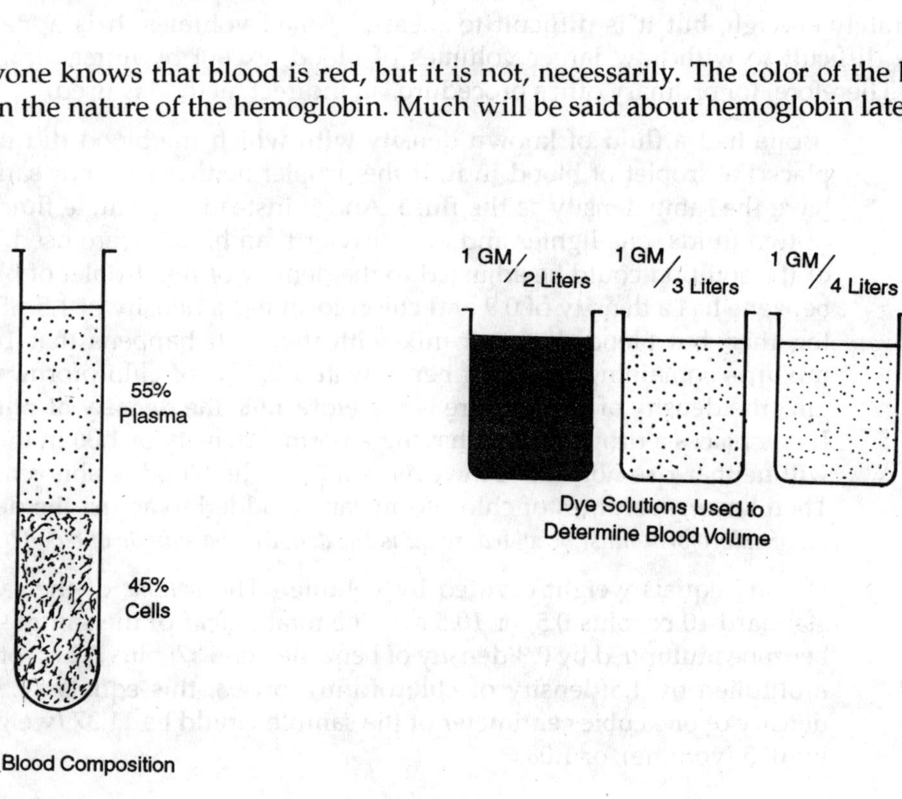

Blood Composition

Fig. 1.1

us only say now that it is the coloured pigment within the red cells of the blood, that it is the agent which transports oxygen, and that the colour of hemoglobin varies, depending on whether or not it is carrying oxygen. As the blood passes through the lungs, the hemoglobin picks up oxygen and is then called **oxyhemoglobin.** Oxyhemoglobin gives blood a bright scarlet colour. However, if the hemoglobin contains no oxygen whatever (as is the case after death), the blood is dark blue, nearly black. In passing through the living body, the blood gives up some, but by no means all, of its oxygen. Therefore blood which has passed through the tissues (**venous blood**) has less redness and more blueness than fully oxygenated (arterial) blood. As blood flows from a cut it is red, because it has not had a chance to give up much of its oxygen. Hemoglobin may take on other colours as well. For instance, in a case of carbon monoxide poisoning, it is a distinct cherry red.

Density

A moment ago we said that 6.4 kg. of blood was *roughly* 6.4 liters. It would have been *exactly* if the density of blood were 1. However, blood is not only thicker than water; it is also slightly heavier. To determine the density of blood, it is necessary to know the volume and the weight. A droplet from a skin prick would give the weight accurately enough, but it is difficult to measure small volumes. It is apparently even more difficult to withdraw larger volumes of blood, except by nurses trained for the task. Therefore, for ordinary office procedure, an indirect method is used.

> If one had a fluid of known density with which the blood did not mix and placed a droplet of blood in it, if the droplet neither rose nor sank, it would have the same density as the fluid. And if instead of a single fluid, a mixture of two fluids, one lighter and one heavier than blood, were used, the density of the solution could be adjusted to the density of the droplet of blood. Now, benzene has a density of 0.9 and chloroform has a density of 1.5. The two mix together, but blood does not mix with them. It happens that 10 cc. of the mixture, containing 7.3 cc. of benzene and 2.7 cc. of chloroform, weighs 10.6 gm.; the density of the mixture is therefore **1.06,** the **density of normal blood.** If one places a drop of blood having a normal density of 1.06 in the mixture, it will neither rise nor fall. However, suppose the blood is abnormal and falls. Then known volumes of chloroform can be added to adjust the density. *If 0.5 cc. of chloroform must be added, what is the density of a sample of blood?*
>
> Density equals weight divided by volume. The *volume* of the sample is the standard 10 cc. plus 0.5, or *10.5 cc.* The total *weight* of the sample is 7.3 cc. of benzene multiplied by 0.9(density of benzene), or 6.57; plus 3.2 cc. of chloroform multiplied by 1.5(density of chloroform), or 4.8; this equals *11.37 gm.* The density of one cubic centimeter of the sample would be 11.37 (weight) divided by 10.5 (volume), or 1.08.

Osmotic Pressure

Whole blood has practically the same osmotic pressure as that of plasma. This is not only because the red cells do not behave as molecules, being relatively much too large, but because there are so few of them compared to the number of molecules. It will be recalled that a molar solution ("one containing a molecular weight of a substance in one liter of solution") will exert an osmotic pressure of 22.4 atm. This solution will contain 6.06×10^{23} molecules. In a liter of blood there are 5,000,000 red cells per cu.mm., or 5×10^{12} red cells which is only one one-billionth as many particles as in a molar solution.

The osmotic pressure of blood is rarely determined but can be calculated from the freezing point. The freezing point of plasma is -0.56° C. A molar solution has a freezing point of -1.86° and exerts an osmotic pressure of 22.4 atm. Therefore, 0.56/1.86 X 22.4 equals 6.7 atm. This is the osmotic pressure of blood, a considerable pressure, equivalent to a column of water 69,251 mm., or 230 ft. in height.

The pH of the Blood

The term "pH" was introduced by S. P. L. Sorenson in 1909 as a handy way to express the degree of acidity or alkalinity of a solution. If a solution is neutral, i.e., neither acid nor alkaline (e.g., distilled water), it is said to have a pH of "7." Going upward on the scale, "8-9-10" indicate constantly rising **alkalinity;** going downward, "6-5-4" indicate constantly increasing **acidity.** Thus, a solution with a pH of 8.5 would

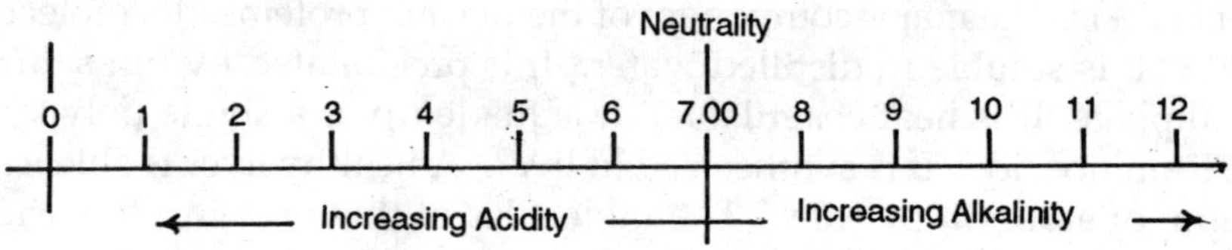

Fig. 1.2

be fairly alkaline, but one whose pH is 10.5 is more strongly alkaline. A solution whose pH is 6.3 is weakly acid; one with a pH of 2.5 is much more strongly acid. **The pH of the blood is 7.35,** which means that it is a very weak alkaline solution. The cells of the body cannot stand much departure from this figure. A pH of 8 on the one hand or much below 7 would certainly be fatal. Shifts towards the acid side occurs in diabetes, toward the alkaline side, in hyperventilation (over-breathing) and sometimes after taking large doses of sodium bicarbonate.

Choice of the number 7 to express neutrality was not because 7 is presumably a lucky number. Although ordinarily water is not thought of as ionizing-for one thing, it does not conduct the electric current-nevertheless, to a small extent it does, thus: HOH produces (H^+) plus (OH^-). The extent to which this happens is only one part hydrogen ions in 10,000,000 parts of water, or 10^7. So Sorenson chose 7, the power that expresses the ionization of water. A solution with a pH of 6 contains one part hydrogen ions per 1,000,000 parts of water, or ten times as many hydrogen ions as water. It is therefore an acid.

Measurement of the pH may be done colorimetrically. There are a large number of dyes, called "indicators," which change colour at various pH's. Or it may be done electrically by means of a meter such as "Beckman's pH meter."

Blood is a highly complex extracellular fluid which is composed of two parts-a faintly yellow transparent fluid known as the *plasma* and floating in this fluid are the *blood corpuscles.* The plasma constitutes about 55 per cent, and the cells about 45 per cent of the total volume of human blood.

Plasma

The plasma is a non-lining fluid of much more chemical complexity than appears in the test tube. It contains a constantly changing variety of substances in solution, chief among which are dissolved food materials on the way to cellular delivery, and waste products that are being collected for elimination. There are also present *enzymes* of diverse sorts which activate chemical changes: *opsonins,* that prepare trespassing bacteria for phagocytosis; *hormones,* the chemical messengers from endocrine glands on their way to the performance of tasks of internal regulation; *anti bodies,* and other problematical substances engaged in constant warfare against harmful invasion.

Plasma is made up of about 90 per cent water and 10 per cent solids. The solids include about 7 per cent proteins, and 0.9 per cent inorganic matter; the remainder is non-protein organic matter.

Albumin (4.7%) is the major component of the plasma proteins. Its molecular weight is about 69,000. It is soluble in distilled water. It is precipitated by full saturation with ammonium sulphate. It is heat coagulable. It is made up of a single polypeptide chain containing 575 aminoacids. It is synthesized in liver. A healthy liver is able to synthesize about 10-15 gm. of albumin per day. The molecules of this protein do not readily pass through vessel walls, so they aid in keeping fluid in the blood vessels by increasing the osmotic pressure of the blood. Its isoelectric pH is 4.7.

Albumin performs several functions as stated below:

(i) The albumin released from the liver is circulated to all tissues which can utilize the amino acids of albumin for the synthesis of their own proteins. Thus, it serves as a source of amino acids.

(ii) Nearly half of the calcium present in blood is loosely bound to albumin at different sites.

(iii) It helps in the transport of thyroxine and steroid hormones.

(iv) It binds the toxic products of metabolism and carries to the sites of excretion.

(v) It plays a major role in the osmotic regulation of the fluid distribution.

Globulins (1.5%). It has a molecular weight varying from 90,000 to 1,300,000. Because of the high contents of carbohydrates it is highly soluble, and is not coagulated by heat. It is a mixture of several , globulins (1) α_1 and α_2 *globulin*-mol. weight ranges from 41,000 to 200,000 with isoelectric pH 5.1. α_1 globulin is present in small amount. It is said to have an inhibitory effect on trypsin. It consists of two fractions: (a) one fraction combine with bilirubin, (b) another fraction helps in the carriage of lipids, steroids and glycoproteins. α_2 globulin consists of α_2 macroglobulins, mucoproteins, ceruloplasmin and hepatoglobulins — the latter combines with free haemoglobin in the plasma. (ii) *β-globulin.* It has molecular weight varying from 90,000 to 1,300,000. Its isoelectric pH is 5.6. The β globulin is primarily concerned with the carriage of the insoluble lipid along with fat soluble vitamins. It is also concerned with the iron transport. Prothrombin is a β-globulin. (iii) *γ globulin.* Its molecular weight ranges from 150,000 to 190,000. Its isoelectric pH is 6.0. Antibodies belong to this class.

Fibrinogens (0.3%). Fibrinogen is another glycoprotein or is globulin in nature. It has molecular weight of 340,000 daltons. It has an isoelectric pH of 5-8. It is made up of 6 peptide chains held by S-S-linkage. It is synthesized by the liver at a rate of 4 to 5 gm. per day.

Fibrinogen is primarily concerned with blood clotting during which it is converted to insoluble fibrin by the action of thrombin.

After depletion of plasma proteins, such as by severe haemorrhage or after blood donation, the plasma proteins come to the normal level in about fourteen days. Fibrinogen is regenerated first, then comes globulin and last of all serum albumin.

The inorganic material of blood includes various anions and cations such as chloride, bicarbonate, phosphate, sulphate, sodium, potassium, calcium and magnesium. Minute amounts of iron and iodine are also found. Some of these are essential for cell metabolism, and some function as buffers to maintain the pH of the blood within a normal range.

The formed elements of the blood consist of erythrocytes, leucocytes and platelets.

Erythrocytes or Red Blood Corpuscles

First described by the Duch microscopist *Leeuwenhock* in 1674 as small round globules.

Erythrocytes are found in all vertebrates except the larvae of eels ('leptocephalus' larvae) and a few antarctic fish of the family chaenichtyidae. Red corpuscles are for the most peculiar to vertebrates, although a few invertebrates, including the worms *Glycera* and *Phoronis,* the "blood clam" *Arca* and the holothurian *Thyone,* also possess red blood cells.

Shape. In all vertebrates except mammals the erythrocytes are oval shaped, biconvex and nucleated. In mammals except camel, the mature erythrocytes are circular, biconcave and non-nucleated. Camel has oval shaped erythrocytes resembling non-mammalian red blood cells in form. The biconcave shape increases the surface area, while the absence of nucleus increases the haemoglobin contents.

Size. In size erythrocytes, measured from dried smears of blood, range from 75 micra in the caudate *Amphiuma* (Salamander) to 2.5 micra in the musk deer *Tragulus.* Other measurements in micra for the largest diameter of blood corpuscles from dried smears have been reported as follows:

Proteus, 58; frog, 22; turtle, 20; carp, 17; pigeon, 14; lamprey, 13; chick, 12; conger eel, 11; elephant (biggest among mammals), 9.4; man, 7.5; dog, 7.3; rabbit, 6.9; cat, 6.5; horse, 4.6; goat, 4.1.

Human erythrocytes average 7.5 μu in diameter, 2.4 μu in thickness at the edge, but only 1 μu thick in the centre, and a volume of 90 Cu μu. One erythrocyte contains 30 μu gm. of haemoglobin which constitutes 90% of the dry weight. The erythrocytes smaller than 6 microns are called *macrocytes*. The erythrocytes of variable shape and size are called *poikilocytes*. The total area of an individual's erythrocytes amounts to about 3000 sq. m. which is 1500 times the whole surface area of the body. If all the red cells of an individual were put in a straight line, its length would almost equal one half the distance from earth to moon.

The erythrocytes are acidophilic and therefore stained with eosin. The erythrocytes are very flexible; they are able to squeeze through capillaries of only half their diameter and regain their original shape. Mammalian mature erythrocytes lack mitochondria, Golgi body, endoplasmic reticulum and other cell organelles. The human erythrocyte has a highly oriented structure of lipids, proteins and haemoglobin consisting of approximately 64% water, 28% haemoglobin (approximately 100 million haemoglobin molecules), 7% lipids or fatty materials, and the remaining 3% sugars, salts, enzymes and other proteins. Under the microscope, a single red cell seems to have a light brown or yellowish colour. But when seen in bulk, the erythrocytes appear to be red.

Number. The number of erythrocytes differs in different animals as well as the physiological state of an individual. There are about 5 million red blood cells per cubic millimeter of blood in the adult human male and 4.5 million per cubic millimeter of blood in the adult female. In infants, the count is 6 to 7 million, whereas in foetus, 7.8 million. In the first ten days of the postnatal life, a large number of red cells are destroyed. This is one cause of *jaundice* in the new born. For counting the number of R.B.C., *haemocytometer* is used.

The erythrocyte count is high in animals living at high altitudes. In lower animals, the count increases in the early stages of hibernation and thereafter decreases. The R.B.C. count decreases in human females during pregnancy and during and just after menstruation. The erythrocyte count of a normal individual may vary at least 5% during the course of a day. It is low during sleep and after meals and high during activity and high environmental temperature.

Whenever the number of erythrocytes increases much above the normal value, the stage is called *polycythemia*. The persons living at high altitude (Kashmir, Tibet etc.) have rosy cheeks.

Life Span. Within a period of 100-120 days (maximum 124 days in dog), red blood cells become very fragile. Worn out red cells are removed from circulation and destroyed by spleen and liver. In one second, there is a destruction of about 2.5 million of erythrocytes (5×10^{11} per day). This is the rate of its production. This is why the number is maintained in the body. Each red blood cell takes about 50,000 rounds of the body

Total Erythrocytes count in a Various Vertebrates

Name of animal	*Number per mm³ of blood*
Fish	
Lamprey	1,33,000
Ray	2,30,000
Flounder (Pleuronectus)	2,000,000
Amphibians	
Salamander (Amphiuma)	95,000
Frog	4,00,000
Reptiles	
Turtle	6,30,000
Birds	
Humming bird	6,500,000
Ostrich	1,600,000
Mammals	
Human being	5,000,000
Rabbit	7,000,000
Sheep	10,000,000
Llama	11,000,000

before its death. The destruction of red blood cells in healthy person produces about 250 mg. of bile salt per day.

Erythrocyte sedimentation rate. E.S.R. When blood to which an anti coagulant has been added is allowed to stand in a narrow tube the red blood corpuscles form rouleaux in which the cells are arranged face to face like a pile of coins and the aggregates gradually settle down (sediment) to leave a clear zone of plasma above. The sedimentation rate is measured as the length of the column of clear plasma above the sedimentatating erythrocytes at the end of one hour. The E.S.R. depends almost entirely on the relative concentration in the plasma of fibrinogen, and globulins. The asymmetry of the molecules promotes the aggregates of red cells into rouleaux and clumps. Almost all infections, whether acute or chronic, are accompanied by a rise in α_2- and γ-globulins and most wasting and destructive diseases by an increase in fibrinogen. The E.S.R. is thus a simple, rapid procedure for revealing such changes. It is useful in detecting the presence and activity of disease but it is quite unspecific. The sedimentation rate also varies according to the red cell count, the lower the red cell count the greater the sedimentation rate.

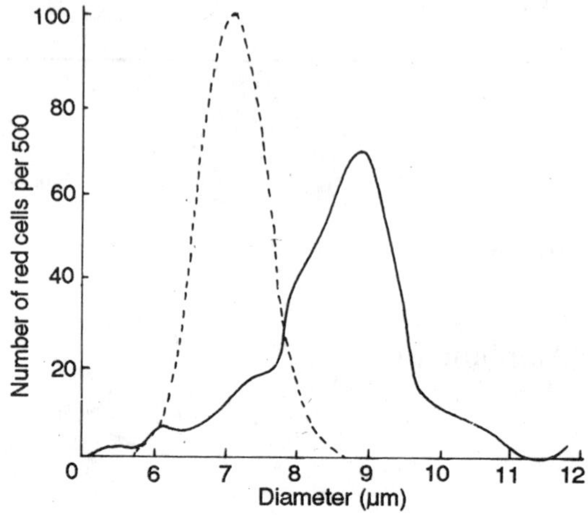

Fig. 1.3. Frequency distribution curves of diameters of healthy red cells and of cells from a case of pernicious anaemia.

The metabolism of erythrocytes. Since the red cell can be bisected without its contents escaping it seems likely that it consists of a lose network or of a jelly which is none the less flexible enough to allow the cells to assume the roughly paraboloid form in which they pass through capillaries as a succession of tiny plugs separated by plasma. The usual biconcave disc shape is regained immediately when the cells pass into a larger vessel. The elongated paraboloid form of the erythrocyte when passing through a capillary presents a much larger surface area next to the capillary wall for the transference of oxygen.

The stroma or framework of the erythrocyte consists of some 50 per cent protein and 10 per cent lipid, mainly phospholipid arranged in three layers. The outer layer of sialic acid determines the cell's electrical charge. It is traversed by pores about 0.4 mm wide which allow the passage of ions and molecules not exceeding a molecular weight of about 100.

Although erythrocytes have no nuclei and normally contain no glycogen they are metabolically quite active utilizing some 1.5 to 2.2 mmoles of glucose per litre per hour equivalent to the liberation of 100 J (25 cal). This energy is required to pump out sodium and pump in potassium against electrochemical gradients and to reduce methaemoglobin to haemoglobin.

The metabolism of glucose in the red blood cell, which is essential for its survival, takes place along the two common pathways, glycolysis and the pentose phosphate pathway, 80 per cent of the glucose being broken down by the former and 20 per cent by the latter. The red cell has no mitochondria and therefore no citric acid cycle.

In the pentose phosphate pathway, the first enzyme involved is the *glucose-6-phosphate dehydrogenase* (G-6-PD) in the operation of which large amounts of reduced NADP is utilized by the red blood cell to maintain glutathione in the reduced state.

$$\text{glucose 6-phosphate} + NADP^+ + H_2O \xrightarrow{\textit{G-6-PD}} \text{6-phosphogluconic acid} + NADPH + H^+$$

$$GSSG + NADPH + H^+ \xrightarrow[\textit{reductase}]{\textit{glutathione}} 2\ GSH + NADP^+$$

The function of the reduced glutathione within the erythrocyte is not clearly understood, but it probably prevents the oxidation of haemoglobin to methaemoglobin and its sulphydryl groups play a part in maintaining the structure of the red cell and also of the globin part of the haemoglobin molecule.

In the population of many parts of the world, there is a deficiency of the (G-6-PD) in the red blood cells. This is an inherited condition which affects more than 100,000,000 people in the world at the present time. This deficiency is a common cause of jaundice in babies, it also is responsible for heamolysis after the administration of certain drugs, particularly the antimalarials such as primaquine, and certain antibacterial drugs. Haemolysis also occurs in G-6-PD-deficient persons after the consumption of the bean of *Vicia faba* which is a common foodstuff in many countries. Many enzyme deficiencies have been discovered but only a few have serious effects.

Hydrogen peroxide is formed in small amounts in normal red cells during metabolic processes and also is generated within the cells as a result of the action of certain drugs, including those which cause haemolysis in G-6-PD deficiency. If not destroyed as rapidly as it is produced, hydrogen peroxide would oxidize haemoglobin to methaemoglobin and then, irreversibly, to oxidized degradation products; it is probable that other substances essential for the integrity of the red cell would also be oxidized, and haemolysis would follow.

There are two protective mechanisms against hydrogen peroxide within the red cell. Glutathione peroxidase uses hydrogen peroxide to oxidize reduced glutathione. Normal activity of glutathione peroxidase depends on the presence of adequate amounts of reduced glutathione which requires normal functioning of the pentose phosphate pathway, including G-6-PD. The other protective agent is the enzyme catalase which decomposes hydrogen peroxide to water and oxygen. Chemically, catalase resembles haemoglobin in being an iron-containing haemoprotein. The relative importance of glutathione peroxidase and of catalase is not fully understood.

At least one hundred enzyme systems have been identified in the red cell. But because it has no nucleus it cannot synthesize proteins (including enzymes).

Hemoglobin

The most important protein of the red cell is hemoglobin. This protein finds an important place among the other proteins due to its ability to combine with oxygen reversibly. It carries oxygen from the lungs to the tissues, and Co_2 from tissues to lungs. Normally hemoglobin is solely confined to the red blood cells.

It is a conjugated protein, possessing heme as its prosthetic group and globin as its protein portion. The heme part of most of the hemoglobulins is similar but the globin portion shows considerable variations in the amino acid composition and sequence. Each molecule of hemoglobin contains four molecules of heme attached to one molecule of globin.

Heme is a chelate compound in which iron is bound to protoporphyrin nucleus. The protoporphyrin nucleus itself is made up of four pyrrole nuclei, attached to form a ring structure. Iron is found at the middle of this ring. The ring structure is designated as tetra-pyrolic ring; or protoporphyrin nucleus. The heme nucleus remains attached with the globin molecules by its coordinate valancy at the histidine residue. Since, each hemoglobin molecule contains four heme molecules, four such attachments are found in each of the hemoglobin molecule.

As regards the globin portion of hemoglobin, it is usually formed of various combinations of four different peptide chains which are called as alpha (α), Beta (β), gamma (γ), and delta (δ) chains. Sometime another chain known as epsilon (e) chain is also found in the hemoglobin molecules. Most of the human hemoglobin contain two alpha chains and two other chains. Normal adult hemoglobin which is represented as (HbA) consists of two alpha and two beta chains as is shown as α_2A β_2A or more simply as α_2 β_2. Approximately 90 per cent of the hemoglobin found in the adult man belongs to this group. Another hemoglobin known as human foetal hemoglobin which is represented as $\alpha_2\gamma_2$. A phemoglobin which forms only a mines Component of adult hemoglobin is enoun as HbA_2 and it contains two alpha chains and two gamma chains and is therefore represented as Hb. As Hb_2A and contains two alpha and two delta chains. It is represented as $\alpha_2\delta_2$. One more form of hemoglobin which is alleged to be embryonic hemoglobin contains two alpha and two epsilon chains and is represented as $\alpha_2\varepsilon_2$.

The four peptide chains of globin are believed to be held together by non-covalent forces. The structure of globin portions of hemoglobin has been well studied now. The alpha chains, are made up of 141 amino acide, the beta and gamma chains of 146 amino acids each. The δ chains are also made up of 146 amino acids. There are differences in the amino acid sequence in these chains, however, there do also exist some striking similarities in these chains. For example there exists twenty four consecutive identical amino acid in the beta and gamma chains. Also, there occurs 65 identical amino acids in the alpha and beta chains, and 108 in the beta and gamma chains. Subsequent studies have revealed that beta and delta chains are even more similar showing 138 identical amino acids. The sequences of the N-terminal and C-terminal ends of the alpha, beta and gamma chains in the globin portions has been shown below:

	N-terminal residue	C-terminal residue
Alpha chains	Val-lew-ser-	—lys-Tyr-arg
Beta chains	Val-Hist-lew	—lys-Tyr-hist
Gamma chains	Gly-Hist-Phe	—Arg-Tyr-Pha

Most of the mammalian T hemoglobins show a molecule weight of the order of 67,000 and their shape is nearly spherical.

Chemical Properties of Hemoglobins

The chemical properties of hemoglobins have been discussed as follows:

(1) *Combination with Oxygen* — Reduced hemoglobin can loosely combine with Oxygen forming Oxyhemoglobin. The attachment of oxygen, occurs at iron in the heme portion. Iron is present in the ferrous form both in hemoglobin and oxyhemoglobin. Oxygen remains attached with the unpaired electrons of iron. Each heme can bind only one molecule of oxygen. Since, each molecules of hemoglobin contains 4 molecules of heme, hence, one molecule of hemoglobin can maximally combine with four molecules of O_2. The combination of hemoglobin with oxygen is governed by partial pressure of oxygen (pO_2) and partial pressure of Co_2 (pCo_2). The former favours combination where the later favours dissociation.

$$\text{Reduced Hemoglobin} + 4o_2 \quad \uparrow\downarrow \quad \text{Oxyhemoglobin (Hb.}4o_2\text{)}$$

2. Combination with Carbon Monoxide

The heme portion of hemoglobin can also combine with carbon mono-oxide forming Carbonyl hemoglobin which is a very stable compound. Affinity of hemoglobin for carbon monoxide is approximately 210 times more as compared to oxygen. In the presence of Co_2 therefore, hemoglobin loses capacity to combine with O_2 and asphyxiation starts. In cases of Co poisioning, the patient must be removed immediately from the poisoned atmosphere to fresh air and should be given artificial respiration using a mixture of Co_2 and Oxygen. In serious cases of such poisoning, it might also become necessary to give a blood transfusion.

$$\text{Hb} + \text{Co} \longrightarrow \underset{\text{Carbonyl hemoglobin}}{\text{Hb.Co}}$$

3. Combination of Carbon Dioxide

Hemoglobin does also combine with Co_2 through its amino groups present on the globin portion forming carbamino-hemoglobin compound. Formation of this complex is a reversible process as has been shown below.

$$\text{Hb.NH}_2 + \text{Co}_2 \rightleftharpoons \text{Hb.NH.COOH} \rightleftharpoons \text{HbNH.COO-HbNHCOO}^- = \text{H}^+$$

Normally, about 10 per cent of the total CO_2 is carried by the blood in this form.

Hemoglobin cannot combine with the hydrogen cyanide, or other cyanides

Methemoglobins

Administration of certain drugs, or exposure of hemoglobin to some poisons leads to oxidation of hemoglobin to methemoglobin in which iron remains present in ferric form. Methomoglobins therefore contain one extra positive charge per heme molecule and four extra positive charge in all. Each heme can therefore bind one negatively charged OH^- ion.

The drugs which can lead to the conversion of hemoglobin to methemoglobin are various sulphonamides, sulphonals, antipyrine nitrites and nitrobenzenes.

Methemoglobin can combine with HCN without any difficulty. Advantage is therefore taken of this property of methemoglobin in removing cyanide poisoning. A small amount of hemoglobin is allowed to be converted into methemoglobin by giving a mixture of sodium nitrite and sodium thiosulphate to the patient with cyanide toxicity. Methemoglobin is formed and it readily takes up cyanide forming cynamethemoglobin which is non toxic. The residual cyanide is changed by sodium thiosulphate into thiocyanide which is also non-toxic, and can be readily excreted.

Abnormal Hemoglobins

Sometimes, due to faulty DNA formation or Mutational changes in the DNA structures abnormal hemoglobins are formed which can be separated by electrophoresis. Some of the amino acid in these hemoglobins differ with those of the normal hemoglobins. Although, most of such abnormal hemoglobins are harmless but some of them may create problems during conditions of stress. Their oxygen carrying capacity remains unaltered.

Some of the abnormal hemoglobin have been mentioned below.

In hemoglobin C, the glutanic acid in the beta chain at position 6 is replaced by lysine. In hemoglobin D sparagine at position 68 in the alpha chain is replaced by lysine. In hemoglobin E, glycine in the beta chain at position 26 is replaced by lysine. In hemoglobin-G, glumatic acid in the alpha chain at position 36 is replaced by glutamine. In hemoglobin-M, histidine in the alpha chain at position 58 is replaced by tyrosine. In hemoglobin-Q, glutamine in the beta chain at position 121 is replaced by lysine. In Hb-S glutamine in the beta chain at position 6 is replaced by valine.

Anaemias

Normally, men contain 13 to 16 g hemoglobin and women contain 12 to 15 g hemoglobin per 100 ml blood. In man, a value of 15 g per 100 ml is taken to be the average hemoglobin. In women this average is about 14 g per 100ml. In the blood hemoglobin falls below about 11.9 g per 100 ml. The consequences become undesirable. The state of an individual whose hemoglobin content is reduced below the normal range, or the number of red blood cells is reduced below the normal range is known as anemia.

There may be many factors responsible for development of anaemic conditions, for example, excessive loss of blood, increased rate of destruction of red cells defective formation of the red cells or blood loss or blood may be lost by excessive bleeding from wounds, or in women due to menstruation. The rate of destruction of the red cells may be increased by certain hemolytic agents of metabolic, drug or bacterial origin formation of hemoglobin may be reduced during the deficiency of iron, copper, vitamin B_{12} in the diet, or due to lack of intrinsic factor in the gastric juice, or due to toxic inhibition of the bone marrow. Development of tumours, or fibrous or leukemic growth in the bone marrow also lead to anaemic conditions.

The classical examples of anemia are hypochronic anaemia pernicious anaemia and sickle cell anaemia. A hypochronic anaemia is that in which red cells contain less hemoglobin than the normal. It may develop due to lack of iron and copper in the diet. The proportion of hemoglobin is reduced in comparison to the number of red cells. The size of the red cells is reduced. In the prematurely born children who have low internal store of iron, such a type of anaemia is very common. In the foetus, iron is mostly stored from mother towards the latter part of gestation. In the young women too, this type of anaemia is very common due to dietary deficiency of the said elements, and due to excessive menstrual bleeding.

In pernicious anemia, the number of the red blood cells as well as haemoglobin content are reduced followed by a rise in the blood plasma iron. This type of anaemia is believed to develop due to deficiency of intrinsic factor in the gastric juice or due to deficiency of vitamin B_{12} in the diet. Vitamin B_{12} cannot be absorbed in the absence of intrinsic factor, therefore, presence of both the factors is essential for prevention of development of this type of anaemia.

In sickle cell anaemia, the red cells become crescent shaped and also abnormality is incorporated in the globin portion of hemoglobin. Such red cells become fragile & undergo destruction at a very low rate resulting into anaemic state. Sickle cell anaemia is hereditary in nature and mostly occurs in the Negro races.

Fate of Hemoglobin in the Body

After completing a life span of about 100-120 days, the red blood cells are phagocytised by the macrophages of reticulo endothelial system mostly in the liver, tissue, spleen and bone marrow. Simultaneously, hemoglobin is also broken down. Iron of hemoglobin is retained for further use. The globin portion is also separated from the protoporphyrin and metabolized in a manner analogous to other proteins. The porphyrin nucleous is cleaved and ultimately converted into bile-pigments. There is still controversy on the point whether protoporphyrin ring is separated from globin before or after the cleavage of the protoporphyrin nucleus itself. Whatever may be the case, biliverdin is the first pigment which is transformed. In the reticulo-endothelial cells, biliverdin is the first pigment which is formed. In the reticulo-endotheu at cells, biliverdin is readily reduced to bilirubin. Bilirubin thus is synthesized in the other tissues is transported to liner in the form of bilirubin albumin complex. One molecule of albumin able to bin two molecules of bilirubin. After reaching in the liver, bilirubin is conjugated with glucuronic acid in the presence of a microsomal enzyme uridine-diphosphate-glucuronyl transferase with the formation of bilirubin mono and diglucuronides. These conjugates are fairly water soluble and are readily excreted from the liver into digestive tract through bile and further reduced in the G.I.T.

Normally a small amount of bilirubin is found in circulation in the plasma. Under certain pathological conditions, however, circulatory bilirubin level is found to be raised. All these conditions leading to increased red blood cell destruction increase the bilirubin level e.g., hemolytic jaundice, pernicious anaemia and other hemolytic infections. Any obstruction in the billary passage, as in obstructive jaundice, also, increases circulatory bilirubin level. Decreased hepatic function as in atrophy of liver, typhoid fever, liver poisoning by carbon tetra-chloride, arsenic or other heavy metals and infective hepatits also lead to increased serum bilirubin level because of the decreased capacity of liver to conjugate bile pigments with glucuronic acid.

Biosynthesis of Hemoglobins

The globin portion of hemoglobin is synthesized from amino acids in a manner similar to other body proteins. Biosynthesis of hememoiety occurs in the following manner.

Succlnyl coenzyme A reacts with glycine in the presence of a microsomal enzyme delta-aminolevulinic anid synthetase and pyridoxal phosphate to give alpha-amino beta-ketoadipic acid which is decarboxylated to give delta-aminomoleculinic acid. Another enzyme delta aminolievulnic acid dehydrase brings about condensation of two molecules of delta amino levulinic acid to form prosphobilinogen. In the next step, three molecules of prophobilinogen condense to form tripyrryl-methano which is splitted in the presence of the third enzyme at position (A) and (B) to form two types of dipyrryl-methane. Subsequently, one molecule of type (A) dipyrryl-methane and another molecule of type (B) condense to form uroporphyrinogen III. These reactions are believed to be catalysed by the enzyme prophobilinogen deaminase. In the next step, uroporphyrinogen III is decarboxylated eliminating the molecules of Co_2 per molecule of uroporphyrinogen III forming Coproporphyrinogen III. This step is catalysed by the enzyme uroporphyrinogen decarboxylase coproroporphrinogen III is oxidatively dicarboxylated to protoporphyrin III. This reaction is catalyzed by two enzymes, namely coproporphyrinogenosidase and protoporphyrinogen oxidase. At this stage, iron is incorporated into the protoporphyrin nucleus forming hemenucleus. In the nucleated avian erythrocytes, synthesis of hemoglobin from apohemoglobin and heme has been shown in vitro. An enzyme heme synthetase has been shown to be involved in this coupling.

Iron for hemoglobin synthesis is supplied by transferrin or ferritin as has been shown in the bone marrow cells. Furthermore, it has also been shown in the rabbit bone marrow that heme and globin synthesis proceed at almost parallel rates, and simultaneously, these get attached to form new hemoglobin molecules. In the developing red blood cells however, the rate of protoporphyrin synthesis slightly exceeds the rate of hemoglobin synthesis. In addition to the red blood cells, all the aerobic cells can independently synthesize heme-proteins in the mitochondria. The heme synthesized by such cells can be incorporated into various types of cytochromes, myohemoglobin as well as hemoglobin.

Amount of Haemoglobin

To measure the haemoglobin contents *haemometer* is used. In average human adult, irrespective of sex, the haemoglobin is 14.5 gm. per 100 ml. of blood. Total haemoglobin can be calculated by multiplying the concentration of haemoglobin (gm./ml.) with blood volume (ml.) as follows:

$$\text{Total haemoglobin} = \text{conc. of haemoglobin (gm./ml.)} \times \text{blood volume (ml.)}$$

$$= 0.15 \times 5000 = 750 \text{ gm.}$$

Similarly the rate of its production can also be detected in a manner given below:

$$\text{Rate of production per day} = \frac{\text{Total haemoglobin}}{\text{Life span in days}}$$

$$= \frac{750}{120} = 6.25 \text{ gm.}$$

The amount of haemoglobin varies under different physiological conditions as shown in the following lines:

(i) *Age.* In the foetus the concentration is highest. At birth the average concentration is about 23 gm. per 100 ml. By the end of 3rd month it falls below normal, probably, because of deficiency of iron in milk. The gradual recovery takes place at the end of the first year.

(ii) *Sex.* In females the haemoglobin amounts from 13.5 to 14.5 per cent whereas in males from 14.5 to 15.5 per cent.

(iii) *Altitude.* At higher altitude, haemoglobin percentage rises.

(iv) Diurnal variation, exercise and adrenalin injections increase the amount of haemoglobin

Chart Showing R.B.C. Content and Haemoglobin Content in Different Animals

	Name of Animal	*R.B.C. content in million cu mm.*	*Haemoglobin contents in gm. %*
1.	*Pisces*		
	Carp	0.84	10.5
	Rock cod	1.55	5.9

(Contd.)

	Name of Animal	R.B.C. content in million cu mm.	Haemoglobin contents in gm. %
	American fresh water eel	2.48	9.0
	White cat fish	2.65	9.2
	Atlantic mackerel	3.94	14.9
2.	*Amphibians*		
	Mud puppy	0.02	4.6
	Two toed amphiuma	0.03	9.4
	Hell bender	0.07	13.3
	American bull frog	0.44	7.8
	Tiger salamander	1.63	8.6
3.	*Reptiles*		
	Turtles	0.62	7.3
	Tortoise (Testudo)	0.63	7.4
	Water snake	0.77	10.0
	Greater snake	1.18	8.5
4.	*Birds*		
	Turkey	2.3	11.2
	Crow	2.5	—
	Chicken	2.8	10.3
	Duck	2.8	14.8
	Street pigeon	3.2	12.8
5.	*Mammals*		
	Elephant	2.02	—
	Human female	4.5	14.5
	Human male	5.0	15.5
	Rhesus monkey	5.2	12.6
	Guinea pig	5.6	14.4
	European rabbit	5.7	11.9
	Dog	6.3	14.8
	Cow	6.5	9—14

(Contd.)

Name of Animal	*R.B.C. content in million cu mm.*	*Haemoglobin contents in gm. %*
Swine	6.5	10.5—16.5
Cat	8.0	11.2
Cattle	8.1	11.5
Horse	8.2	9.0—14
House mouse	9.3	14.8
Camel	10.4	13.0
Sheep	10.3	10.9
Goat	16.0	10.5

Haemoglobin is a conjugated protein, possessing haeme as its prosthetic group and globin as its protein portion. The haeme part is similar in most of the cases but the globin part shows considerable variations in the amino acid composition and sequence. Each molecule of haemoglobin contains four molecules of haeme attached to one molecule of globin.

Haeme is a protoporphyrin compound and consists essentially of four pyrrole groups joined together forming a ring structure. Iron is found at the middle of this ring. Thus haeme is a metalloporphyrin where the metal is iron. The iron content of haemoglobin is about 0.34% and about 3-4 gm. of iron is present as haemoglobin in the total amount of blood of an adult having 70 kg body weight. Small amount of iron is excreted through urine. It is about 0.5-1 mg daily in adult male. The loss in normal menstruation is about .1-2 mg. daily and it is 1.5-2.5 mg. per day in pregnant woman. Iron remains in ferrous (Fe^{++}) form.

The globin part of haemoglobin is usually made up of various combinations of four different peptide chains which are called the alpha (α), beta (β), gama(γ), and delta (δ) chains. The alpha chains are made up of 141 amino acids, the beta, gamma and delta chains of 146 amino acids each. The difference lies in the sequence of amino acids, however, they show some striking similarities. There exist twenty four consecutive identical amino acids in the beta and gamma chains, 65 identical amino acids in the alpha and beta chains, and 138 in beta and delta chains.

Most of the human haemoglobins have two alpha chains and two beta chains. This category is represented as HbA and is shown as $\alpha_2\beta_2$. This forms about 90 per cent of the human haemoglobin. HbF is another haemoglobin known as human *foetal* haemoglobin. It contains two alpha chains and two gamma chains ($\delta_2\gamma_2$). A haemoglobin which forms only a minor component of adult haemoglobin is known as HbA_2. It is made up of two alpha and two delta chains and is represented as $\alpha_2\delta_2$.

The approximate chemical formula is $(C_{712}H_{1130}O_{245}N_{214}S2Fe)_4$. The molecular weight of haemoglobin is about 68,000.

The Blood Pigments of Hæmochromes

In both the plant and animal worlds pigments play an important part in the supply of oxygen.

Haemoglobin and Oxyhaemoglobin.—Pigments are by far the most abundant and important of the constituents of the red cells. These are conjugated proteins, a compound of the protein globin with the complex iron-containing pigment **haem**, which belongs to the class of pigments known as **porphyrins** which contains also the green pigments of plants -chlorophyll-and cytochrome, the pigment which is associated with oxidation in cells. These pigments, together with the bile pigments and other animal pigments which are derived from them, are sometimes known as the **pyrrole pigments**, as they are derived chemically from the simple heteroring compound pyrrole, C_4H_4N. Some respiratory pigments, such as the green chlorocruorin of certain worms, contain iron, but the haemocyanin of molluscs and crustacea contains copper. In the invertebrate animals the haemoglobin is not in the cells but free in the plasma.

Hæmoglobin is the pigment which gives the red colour to the blood. When combined with oxygen (but not oxidised) it becomes the familiar bright red oxyhaemoglobin which has already been studied in relation to Respiration. The actual shade of red which blood assumes depends on the proportion of haemoglobin to oxyhaemoglobin, and, as we have seen, even venous blood contains a considerable amount of the latter.

Crystals of oxyhaemoglobin may be obtained with readiness from the blood of such animals as the rat, guinea-pig, or dog; with difficulty from other animals, such as man, ape, and most of the common mammals. The following methods are the best:

1. Mix a drop of defibrinated blood of the rat on a slide with a drop of water or Canada balsam; put on a cover-glass; in a few minutes the cells are rendered colourless, and then the oxyhaemoglobin crystallises out from the solution so formed.
2. On a larger scale, crystals may be obtained by mixing the blood with one-sixteenth of its volume of ether; the cells dissolve, and the blood assumes a *laky* appearance. After a period varying from a few minutes to days, abundant crystals are deposited.

The shape of the oxyhaemoglobin crystals in different animals varies somewhat, probably owing to the varying amounts of water of crystallisation they contain.

Hæm, the parent pigment chemically, is chiefly of academic interest but has the property of being very easily oxidised or reduced. It exists in both forms (see schema). The term haem usually refers to reduced haem. In nature, however, it does not seem likely that it ever occurs free from globin. The globin prevents the oxidation of the haem without interfering with its power to carry oxygen in loose combination. If the globin is thrown out of action in blood the haem becomes oxidised and methaemoglobin is formed (see below). This occurs to haemoglobin crystals if they are stored.

Hæmatin.—On adding an acid or alkali to haemoglobin, it is broken up into two parts-a brown pigment called *haematin,* which contains all the iron of the original substance, and *globin.*

Hæmoglobin disintegrating in the circulation is first split into globin and reduced haematin (ferrous) and is immediately oxidised to haematin (ferric), which in man combines with serum albumin to form methamalbumin.

Hæmatin has the formula $C_{34}H_{33}$ or $_{35}O_5N_4Fe$.It presents different spectroscopic appearances in acid and alkaline solutions (see accompaying plate). It may be reduced in alkaline solution by adding a reducing agent, and the well-marked absorption spectrum of reduced haematin or haemochromogen forms the most delicate of the spectroscopic tests for blood pigment. Haemochromogen is of red colour; haematin is brownish.

Haemochromogen in neutral solution undergoes spontaneous oxidation to the ferric state of parahaematin. It was this fact that suggested that the function of the neutral globin in haemoglobin is to prevent this oxidation. The reducing agent destroys this protective action of the globin by denaturing it.

Hæmin is of great importance, as the obtaining of this substance forms the best chemical test for blood. The test is much used in medicolegal work. Haemin crystals may be prepared for microscopical examination by boiling a fragment of dried blood with a drop of glacial acetic acid on a slide; on cooling, triclinic plates and prisms of a dark brown colour, often in star-shaped clusters and with rounded angles, separate out. In the case of an old blood stain it is necessary to add crystal of sodium chloride. Fresh blood contains sufficient sodium chloride in itself.

The action of the acetic acid is to split the haemoglobin into haematin and globin; a hydroxyl group of the haematin is then replaced by chlorine.

The structure of haemin has now been confirmed by synthesis and has been shown to consist of four pyrrole rings (dark in figure) linked together. The various haem derivatives differ in having different side-chains, while in the case of the bile pigments the iron is removed and the large ring breaks up to form a chain.

From haemin it is possible to produce the parent pigment haem.

Hæmatoporphyrin, $C_{34}H_{38}O_4N_6$, is iron-free haematin; it may be prepared by mixing blood with strong suphuric acid; the iron is taken out as ferrous sulphate. It is also found sometimes in nature; it occurs in certain invertebrate pigments, and may also be found in certain forms of pathological urine. Even normal urine contains traces of it. It is isomeric with the bilirubin of bile. It presents different spectroscopic appearances according as it is dissolved in acid or alkaline media. The absorption spectrum figure is that of acid haematoporphyrin.

Hæmopyrrol is formed by reduction from haematoporphyrin and prøves to be a mixture of several pyrrol derivatives. Similar derivatives are obtained from chlorophyll, a fact which illustrates the near relationship of the principal animal and vegetable pigments.

Hæmatoidin.— This substance is found in the form of yellowish red crystals in old blood extravasation, and is derived from the haemoglobin. Its crystalline form and the reaction it gives with fuming nitric acid show it to be closely allied to *bilirubin,* the chief colouring matter of the bile, and on analysis it is found to be identical with it. (See Bile.)

Hæmatoidin, like haematoporphyrin, is free from iron, but differs from it in showing no absorption bands in the spectrum.

Compounds of Hæmoglobin

Hæmoglobin forms at least four compounds with gases :

With oxygen	1. Oxyhaemoglobin 2. Methaemoglobin
With carbon monoxide	3. Carbon monoxide haemoglob in
With nitric oxide	4. Nitric oxide hæmoglobin

These compounds have similar crystalline forms with the exception of methaemoglobin; each consists of a molecule of haemoglobin combined with one molecule of the gas in question. They part with the combined gas somewhat readily; they are arranged in order of stability in the above list, the least stable first.

Oxyhæmoglobin is the compound that exists in arterial blood. Many of its properties have already been described in relation to Respiration.

We have seen that the oxygen may be removed by exposing the blood to a vaccum. The blood may also be reduced by passing hydrogen through it or by addition of other reducing agents, such as ammonium sulphide or Stokes' reagent (an ammoniacal solution of ferrous tartrate), or, best of all, sodium hydrosulphite. One gramme of haemoglobin will combine with I.34 c.c. of oxygen.

If any of these methods for reducing oxyhaemoglobin is used, the bright red (arterial) colour of oxyhaemoglobin changes to the darker(venous) tint of haemoglobin. On once more allowing oxygen to come into contact with the haemoglobin, as by shaking the solution with the air, the bright arterial colour returns. These colour changes may be more accurately studied with the spectroscope, and the constant position of the absorption bands seen constitutes an important test for blood pigment. It will be first necessary to describe briefly the instrument used.

The Spectroscope.—When a ray of white light is passed through a prism, it is refracted or bent at each surface of the prism; the whole ray is however, not equally bent, but it is split into its constituent colours which may be allowed to fall on a screen. The bands of colours beginning with the red, passing through orange, yellow, green, blue, and ending with violet, is called a *spectrum* : this is seen in nature in the rainbow.

The spectrum of sunlight is interrupted by numerous dark lines crossing it vertically, called Frauenhofer's lines. These are perfectly constant in position and serve as landmarks in the spectrum. The more prominent are A, B, and C, in the red; D in the yellow; E, *b*,

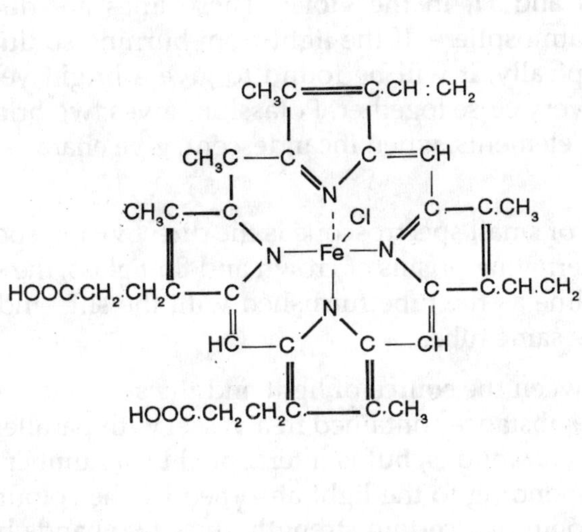

A suggested formula of hæmin (not to be memorised).

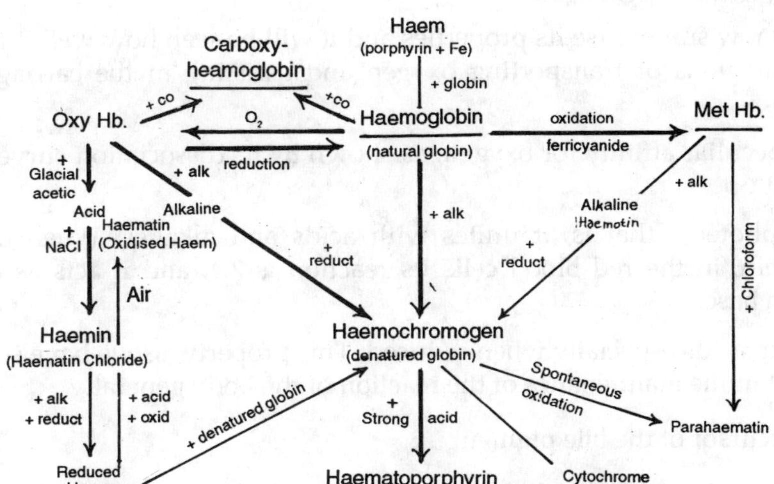

Fig. 1.4.—Derivatives of hæm related to hæmoglobin. Students are commonly expected to prepare and recognise the substances in large print. Hæm is reduced hæm and hæmoglobin is sometimes called reduced hæmoglobin.

and F, in the green; G and H, in the violet. These lines are due to certain volatile substances in the solar atmosphere. If the light from burning sodium or its compounds is examined spectroscopically, it will be found to give a bright yellow line, or, rather, two bright yellow lines very close together. Potassium gives two bright red lines and one violet line and the other elements, when incandescent, give characteristic lines, but none so simple as sodium.

A convenient form of small spectroscope is the direct vision spectroscope, in which, by an arrangement of alternating prisms of crown and flint glass, the spectrum is observed by the eye in the same line as the tube furnished with the slit—indeed, slit and prisms are both contained in the same tube.

If we interpose between the source of light and the slit a piece of coloured glass, or a solution of a coloured substance contained in a vessel with parallel sides, the spectrum is found to be no longer continuous, but is interrupted by a number of dark shadows, or absorption bands corresponding to the light absorbed by the coloured medium. Thus a solution of oxyhaemoglobin of a certain strength gives two bands between the D and E lines; reduced haemoglobin gives only one; and other red solutions, though to the naked eye similar to oxyhaemoglobin, will give characteristic bands in other positions.

The Properties of Hæmoglobin

We may now summarise its properties and it will be seen how well it is adapted to perform its functions of transporting oxygen and assisting in the carriage of carbon dioxide.

It has a peculiar affinity for oxygen, as shown by its dissociation curve, and just as readily gives it up.

It is amphoteric, that is, it unites with acids and alkalies. When oxidised, i.e. oxyhaemoglobin, in the red blood cells its reaction is 7.4, and it acts as an acid and combines with base.

It takes up acids especially when reduced. This property, as we have seen, plays an important part in the maintenance of the reaction of the body generally.

It is a precursor of the bile pigment

Methæmoglobin.—As has been said, the globin prevents the oxidation of haem by the oxygen of the air, but this occurs if the globin is thrown out of action by adding a variety of agents, especially protein precipitants or oxidising agents. Methaemoglobin, a very dark brown pigment, is thus formed. It is commonly produced by adding potassium ferricyanide or amyl nitrite to blood, and as it also may occur in certain diseased conditions and pass into the urine, it is of considerable practical importance.

Potassium ferricyanide produces another effect as well, namely it causes an evolution of oxygen, if the blood had been previously laked. In relation to respiration it will be seen that use is made of this fact in the estimation of the oxygen content of the blood. After the oxygen is discharged from oxyhaemoglobin, fresh oxygen, due to the oxidising action of the reagent added, takes its place; this new oxygen, however, is combined in some way different from that which was previously united to the haemoglobin.

This oxygen is not removable by the air-pump, nor by a stream of neutral gas such as hydrogen. It can, however, by reducing agents such as ammonium sulphide, be made to yield reduced haemoglobin. Methaemoglobin is of a brownish-red colour, and gives a characteristic absorption band in the red between the C and D lines (spectrum 7 in coloured plate). In dilute solutions other bands can be seen.

Carboxyhæmoglobin may be readily prepared by passing a stream of carbon monoxide or coal-gas through blood or through a solution of oxyhaemoglobin. It has a peculiar cherry-red colour. Its absorption spectrum is very like that of oxyhaemoglobin, but the two bands are slightly nearer the violet end of the spectrum (spectrum 4 in coloured plate). Reducing agents, such as ammonium sulphide, do not change it; the gas is more firmly combined than the oxygen in oxyhaemoglobin. CO-haemoglobin forms crystals like those of oxyhaemoglobin. It resists putrefaction for a very long time.

Carbon monoxide is given off during the imperfect combustion of carbon such as occurs in charcoal stoves or during the explosions that occurs in coal mines; it acts as a powerful poison, by combining with the haemoglobin of the blood, and thus interferes with normal respiratory processes, and a fatal anoxaemia or lack of oxygen is produced. The bright colour of the blood in both arteries and veins and its resistance to reducing agents are in such cases characteristic.

The Origin of Hæmoglobin.—As has been said, haemoglobin belongs to the class of pigments known as porphyrins and contains iron; so also does the green chlorophyll of plants. Both are widely disposed in nature but not always in a form that can be utilised; but there is no evidence of this, for the body cannot break down the chlorophyll or even the iron-containing porphyrin, haem. Articles of diet such as hare soup and black puddings made from blood are of no value as sources of iron to the body. The exact source of the pyrrole remains unknown but the globin is probably synthesised.

If animals are bled, however, and given different food stuffs we get an idea of the origin of the constituents of the blood generally, and from such studies it becomes evident that a meat diet is best for restoring haemoglobin. For this, milk and its derivatives are of little use and carbohydrates valueless. Apricots and spinach are the best foods of vegetable origin, although it is obvious that the herbivorous animals must obtain their haemoglobin from more usual sources. Most of such investigation has been carried out by Whipple and his colleagues in America on a standard anaemic dog which has had its total haemoglobin reduced to about a quarter of its normal by haemorrhage, and which is given a standard anaemic diet largely of carbohydrate to which the food under investigation is added. To a considerable extent the value of foods in this respect depends on the amount of iron they contain, although it is evident from the beneficial effect of drugs that the iron need not to be in organic form. (See Iron.) Haemoglobin formation is restricted by infections and this is one reason why if prolonged they lead to pallor of the face.

Factors affecting the Haemoglobin Content — These are the number of red blood cells and the amount of haemoglobin in each. A fall in either will obviously bring about a fall of total haemoglobin, although when there is a deficiency in cell formation, as in pernicious anaemia, there may be a compensatory rise of colour index and the fall of haemoglobin is not then so low as the cell count would lead one to expect.

By far the most important cause of low haemoglobin values is a deficiency of iron in the diet, and this is particularly liable to occur in women whose requirements are greater than those of men, because of their periodic loss of blood. Small amounts of copper are also needed.

METHODS

ENUMERATION OF THE RED BLOOD-CELLS

Several methods are employed for counting the blood-cells: most of them depend upon the same principle, *i.e.* the dilution of a minute volume of blood with a given volume of a saline solution similar in osmotic concentration to blood-plasma, so that the size and shape of the cells are altered as little as possible. A minute quantity of the well-mixed solution is then taken, examined under the microscope in a cell of known capacity, and the number of cells in a given area of the cell is counted. Having ascertained the number of cells in the diluted blood, it is easy to calculate the number in a given volume of normal blood.

The apparatus most frequently used at the present time is known as the Thoma-Zeiss hæmacytometer. It consists of a carefully graduated pipette, in which the dilution of the blood is made; this is so formed that the capillary stem has a capacity equalling one-hundredth of the bulb above it. If the blood is drawn up in the capillary tube to the line marked 0.5 the saline solution may afterwards be drawn up the stem to the line 101. This gives a dilution of 1-200 as the last I does not mix. The blood and the saline solution are well mixed by shaking the pipette. The other part of the instrument consists of a glass slide upon which is mounted a covered disc, *m*, accurately ruled so as to present one square millimetre divided into 400 squares of one-twentieth of a millimetre each. The micrometer thus made is surrounded by another annular cell, C, which has such a height as to make the cell project exactly one-tenth millimetre beyond *m*. If a drop of the diluted blood is placed upon *m*, and *c* is covered with a perfectly flat cover-glass, the volume of the diluted blood above each of the squares of the micrometer, *i.e.*, above each $\frac{1}{400}$, will be $\frac{1}{4000}$ of a cubic millimetre. Five large squares (*i.e.* 5 × 16 small) are counted and the average per small square taken by dividing by 80. This number multiplied by 4000 and again by 200 to allow for the dilution gives the number of cells in a cubic millimetre of undiluted blood, *i.e.*, where x = the number in five large squares, $\frac{x}{80} \times \frac{4000 \times 200}{I}$. In actual practice it will be noticed that no arithmetic is necessary, 0000 simply being added to the number found in the five large squares.

ENUMERATION OF THE WHITE BLOOD-CELLS

The enumeration of the colourless cells depends on the same principle, but the counting has to be carried out over the whole square millimetre. The blood is diluted (1-20) in a similar special pipette with dilute acetic acid to decolorise the red blood-cells and a stain is usually added. Since the dilution is 1-20 and the cubic capacity of the area counted 1/10 of a cubic millimetre, multiplication of the number counted by 200 gives the number of white cells in the whole cubic millimetre.

Differential Count.—The differentiation of the varieties of colourless cells (which is most important from the standpoint of disease) can be accomplished after the appropriate staining of blood-films. Five hundred white blood-cells are counted and the percentage of each variety calculated.

Estimation of Hæmoglobin

One type of haemoglobin, that of Haldane, consists of two tubes, one of which contains 20 cu. mm. of standard blood (see fig.) laked and diluted to 200. A little distilled water is placed in the other tube, which is graduated, and 20 cu. mm. of the blood (measured in a pipette) being estimated is added. This is diluted with distilled water till the colours are alike and the dilution is read off. If, for example, the colours are alike when the dilution has only been 50 (instead of the normal 100), the blood contains only 50 per cent. of the normal haemoglobin. Commonly, the standard used is a carmine jelly of the same tint as normal blood (Gowers), but since this is liable to fade, normal blood, the haemoglobin of which is converted into carboxy-haemoglobin, is used (Haldane), but in this instance carbon monoxide (coal-gas) must be mixed with the diluted blood under investigation. The blood used in the Haldane standard is capable of carrying 18.5 per cent. c.c. of oxygen per 100 c.c. of blood.

Hæmoglobin Standards.-The colour of the standard should be checked against blood capable of carrying 18.5 c.c. per cent. of oxygen or containing 14 mg. of haemoglobin per 100 c.c. of blood.

Blood Plasma

Blood plasma is a straw coloured fluid containing 90-92 per cent. water. The rest is formed by proteins, lipids, sugars, organic acids and minerals, etc. Its specific gravity varies from 1.025 to 1.035. Plasma remains in direct contact with the tissues and its various constituents are constantly interchanged with the tissues. The water of plasma has its own importance as it acts as a solvent and it can carry such substances found in the body helps in the regulation of blood pressure, osmotic pressure and body temperature. Water possesses a great deal of heat storage capacity owing to its high specific and latent heat.

Plasma proteins

Proteins constitute about 6.5 to 8.0 per cent. of plasma (w/v) of which albumin constitutes 3.2 to 5.5 per cent., globulins about 3.0 to 3.5 per cent and fibrinogen about

0.3 per cent. Other proteins found in the plasma are the enzymes responsible for blood coagulation and some of the cellular enzymes.

The normal albumin/globulin ratio (A/a ratio) varies from 1.2/1 to 1.4/1. In hepatic cirrhosis, the ratio becomes '1' or less than '1'. Also in chronic renal diseases, it is reduced.

The molecular weight of the albumin is about 68,000 and the isoelectric point is about pH. 4.64. This can be precipitated from the supernatant obtained after precipitating globulins from serum. The globulins can be precipitated by saturating the serum with ammonium sulphate by 50 per cent whereas the albumins are precipitated by saturating the supernatant obtained thereafter by 100 per cent with ammonium sulphate. The albumin fraction of serum is found to be homogenous and has been obtained in the crystalline form. Crystalline albumin has been found to contain Carbohydrates as its integral part.

The globulin fraction constitutes approximately 44-48 per cent of the total proteins. Electrophoretically, the globulin fraction has been separated into three main groups mainly, alpha-globulins beta-globulins, and gamma globulins. The approximate follows: alpha globulin-14%, beta globulin-13-13.4% and the gamma globulin-17-21%. These globulins have been further separated into more sub-groups. The alpha-beta globulins

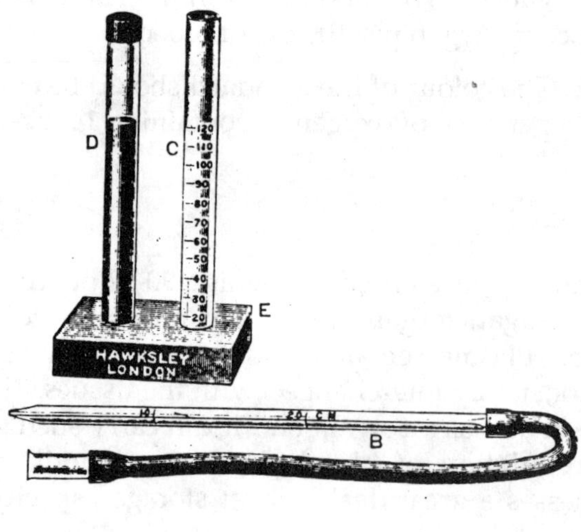

Fig. 1.5.—The Gowers-Haldane Hæmoglobinometer.

contain $beta_1$ and $beta_2$ globulins. Similarly the gamma globulin contain $gamma_1$ and $gamma_2$ globulins. Even these sub groups have not been found to be distinctly homogeneous. Furthermore, different sub groups having the same electrophoretic mobility have been shown to manifest different chemical and biological properties.

The gamma globulin fraction contains most of the circulatory anti-bodies. Some times, the terms anti-body and gamma-globulins are used synonymously but it has been definitely shown that the anti-body property is not limited only to gamma-globulins but it is also present in the $beta_1$ and even the $alpha_2$ globulin fractions. To avoid any confusion therefore, the term immuno globulin is used which covers up all the globulins possessing antibody like properties. Immunoglobulin are represented by Ig.

Immunoglobulins have been defined by the World Health Organisation (WHO) as follows -

(1) They should be proteins.

(2) They should be of the animal origin.

(3) They should have a common structure.

(4) They should function as antibodies.

Each molecule of immunoglobulin consists of two light and two heavy chains. The light chains have less number of amino acids and therefore lesser molecule weight in comparison to heavy chains. The light chains have less number of amino acids and therefore lesser molecular weight in comparison to heavy chains. These chains are connected by inter chain and interchain disulphide bridges. The heavy chains do also possess carbohydrate moiety. The whole molecule has a 'Y' shaped structure. One half of the light as well as heavy chains containing N-Terminus is called 'Variable portion and the other half is called the 'constant portion in respect of the amino acid composition and sequence. Recently, hypervariable portion' responsible for antibody action has also been reported.

The different heavy chains are known to occur so far in the antibodies. These are called as gamma (γ), alpha (α), mu (μ), delta (δ) and epsilon (ε) chains. The immunoglobulins have been classified depending upon which type of chain is present in it. Five classes of 'Ig' are known which are represented as IgG, IgA, IgM, IgD and IgE, respectively. IgG have two gamma chains. IgA have two alpha chains and so on.

Light chains of Ig may also be of two types, namely kappa (k) and lambda (λ) type. Hence each class of Ig may be subclassified into two types depending upon the type of light chains existing in them namely 'k-type' and '<-type' Hence, in all, ten types of Ig are possible which have been mentioned as below.

No.	*Class*	*Type*	*Heavy Chains*	*Light Chains*
1	IgG	K	Gamma	Kappa
2	IgG	L	Gamma	Lambda

(Contd.)

No.	Class	Type	Heavy Chains	Light Chains
3	IgA	K	Alpha	Kappa
4	IgA	L	Alpha	Lambda
5	IgM	K	Mu	Kappa
6	IgM	L	Mu	Lambda
7	IgD	K	Delta	Kappa
8	IgD	L	Delta	Lambda
9	IgE	K	Epsilon	Kappa
10	IgE	L	Epsilon	Lambda

The typical structure of Ig may be shown as follows. The molecule is about 200 A° in length and 40 A° in breadth

(1) *IgG* : These immunoglobins have got a molecular weight of the order of about 1,60,000. These constitute about 70 per cent of the total immunoglobins. These are present to the extent of 800 to 1800 mg. per 100ml. These are disturbed equally between blood and other body fluids. Most of the antibodies of the natural infections and artificial immunization with virus and bacteria and their products belong to this group. These antibodies can cross the placenta from the mother.

(2) *IgA* : These immunoglobins possess almost the same molecular weight as that of IgG. These are present in amounts 140-250 mg/100ml. These occur in the plasma and are also secreted in the saliva, intestinaljuice, respiratory secretions and colostrum. These antibodies lyse the bacteria in the presence of lysozyme which is present in the secretions containing IgA. IgA antibodies have been found to protect mucous surfaces. The Ig of diptheria, tetanus, typhoid, parathyroid B, insulin and thyroglobulin fall in this group.

(3) *IgM* : These immuniglobulins represent the polymerized forms of globulins of the molecular weight, 1,60,000 and hence have got very high molecular weight ranging from 9,00,000 to 10,00,000. Their normal concentration in plasma is about 80-110 mg/100 ml. These antibodies remain restricted in blood owing to their large molecular size and molecular weight. I gm promotes phagocytosis and cause cell lysis by digesting the cell membrane and producing holes at the site of attachment of the antigen-antibody. IgM have been found to be more effective than IgM and are more suited for destroying the bacteria on blood stream.

4. *IgD* : These have been found to be heat-labile, skin senstizing antibodies and are also called as reagins. These are responsible for anaphylatic types of hypersenstivity. These constitutes about 1 per cent of the antibodies. Very little is known at present regarding the functions of the IgD. Some anti nuclear antibodies have been found to be of IgD types.

5. *IgE* : These antibodies have been found to be fixed to the tissues when these get attached to the most cells these lead to the rupture of these cells liberating histamine. The concentration of IgE in blood is of the order of about 17 to 450 mg/ml.

IgE levels have been found to increase in tropical parasitic diseases. In such cases, defensive mechanism is shown by ejection of parasites on account of release of histamine as a result of antigen antibody action. Furthermore, IgE and eonnopluls have also been shown to provide defence against schistosomiasis. In the different Igs, the capacity to bind with antigen lies in the variable portion (N-terminal end) which is called antigen binding fragment (Fab). The constant portion crystallizable fraction (Fe) is provided with the tracts which give direction and biological activity to the Ig molecules and it determines working property.

Response to Immunization.— Antibodies are generated in the multicellular organisms when a substance, foreign to the body finds entry in the body. Infection of an antigen in some suitable form for the first time causes appearance of antibodies after a lag period of several days. The antibodies level increases gradually till a plateau is reached. This is called primary immunization. Thereafter, it starts decreasing. When a second injection (booster), is given, the response is very prompt and the antibody liter rises very quickly to a considerably higher level. Polymeric antigens cause formation of a mixture of antibodies. The antibodies interact with the antigens and nullify their effects.

The globulin fraction also include some proteins which resemble alpha and gamma globulins and have immunologic property. Examples of such proteins are mucoproteins, ossomucoid and hepatoglobulins which resemble alpha-globulins and certain metal binding proteins such as transferria, ceruloplasmin and cyroglobulins which resemble the gamma globulins.

Cyroglobulins are found in the normal plasma only in very small quantities, however in plasma of most of the patients suffering from multiple mycloma, the concentration of this protein is found to be considerably raised ocassionally the patients suffering from rheumatoid arthritis do also show elevated levels of cryoglobulins.

Fibrinogen is also a type of globulin which has a characteritic property of being coagulated on heating. Also, it has a unique property of clotting. Fibrinogen is a soluble protein and it can be converted into insoluble proteins known as fibrin or blood clot. Molecular weight of fibrinogen is approximately 4,00,000.

The plasma proteins also include the enzymes of coagulation of blood and these enzymes which come into blood stream as a result of destruction of the body tissues. Their concentration in the blood varies considerably under different conditions. Least concentration is found when all the cells are working normally, but higher concentrations are observed when damage of certain tissue occurs.

Functions of Plasma Proteins: Plasma Proteins have to perform a variety of functions which have been briefly discussed below

(1) *Regulation of Osmotic pressure and passage of water* — The colloidal osmotic pressure of blood is entirely due to proteins in plasma. This force opposes the hydrostatic pressure in the plasma is exerted by proteins, electrolytes and organic crystalloids. Since the electrolytes and organic crystalloids are diffusable across the cell memberanes and osmotic pressure exerted by these substances is equal on both the sides of memberanes.But the osmotic pressure exerted by the plasma proteins is unequal on both sides of the memberane. The protein particles are non-diffusable and their concentrateion inside the capillaries is greater. Thus, the colloidal osmotic pressure inside the capillaries remain higher as compared to the tissues. The total osmotic pressure of plasma is about 6.5 atmospheres which is almost balanced by a similar osmotic pressure of the tissue fluids which bath the capillaries. The slight differences on osmotic pressure is due to difference in the protein levels of the tissue and plasma osmotic pressure due to plasma.

Proteins - 28 mm of Hg

Osmotic pressure due to Tissue proteins - 10 mm of Hg

i.e. oncotic pressure - 18 mm of Hg.

It is evident that the oncotic pressure which may be considered to be effective is due to plasma proteins which is of the order of 18 mm of Hg. The effective hydrostatic pressure at the arterial side of the capillaries, is about 32 mm of Hg which falls to 12 mm Hg at the venous side, as a result of which at the arterial side, the hydrostatic pressure exceeds the effective colloidal osmotic pressure by about 14 mm of Hg (32-18) and therefore, the fluid passes from capillaries to exterior. At the venous side, on the other hand, the hydrostatic pressure of the capillaries is lower than the effective colloidal pressure by about 6 mm Hg (18-12) and therefore, the fluid is sucked up by the capillaries at the venous side. In other words, filteration is favoured at the arterial side and absorption at the venous side.

It has been observed that when the plasma protein content is lowered the effective colloidal pressure is also lowered. Thus, at the arterial side, more water is forced out from plasma into the tissues, and at the venous side, less water is absorbed from the tissues into the blood resulting into increased tissue water content and development of edema. Such a condition is often observed in kidney damages when plasma proteins are lost in the urine in excessive amounts.

It should be emphasized that about 80 percent of the colloidal osmotic pressure is due to albumin as it is present in greater amount than the other plasma proteins, and has a lower molecular weight as compared to globulins.

2. *Transport of Biological Substances* — Plasma proteins keep in solution many biological substances and help in their subsequent transport. Some of such substances are otherwise insoluble or sparingly soluble in water. The insoluble substances are solubelized when these combine with plasmaprotein, specially with albumin. Examples of such substances are bilirubin, sulphonomides fatty

acids, napthoquinones and their derivatives. Furthermore, phospholipids, cholesterol and fat soluble substances are carried in the plasma in the form of lipoproteins complexes. Plasma lipoproteins complexes contain 21 per cent phospholipids and 18 per cent cholesterol, and the β-lipoprotein complexes contain 27 per cent phospholipids and 30 per cent cholesterol. Fat soluble substances such as vitamin A, D, K, E and many drugs are also carried in similar combinations in the plasma.

3. *Buffering functions.* Plasma proteins do also exert buffering action. These proteins exist in circulation in the form of weak acids and their salts and their isolectric points fall in the acidic range in the physiological pH range for example, albumin at the pH of 47, globulins at pH 54 and fibrinogen in the pH range 50 to 55 are isoelectric. The buffering action due to protein is however small in comparison to overall buffering action of the body due to othe substances.

4. *Nutritive function.* The plasma proteins do not remain static. The amino acids, are constantly interchanged with the tissue proteins. On prolonged starvation, the protein level of plasma specially that of albumin falls, and it may some times reach a level to cause nutritional edema. On the basis of isotopic studies, it has been shown that at least 15g plasma proteins undergo turnover in this manner daily.

Specific functions of Plasma Proteins

1. *Metal binding function* — Some of the plasma proteins help in the binding of the metallic ions and controling their circulatory levels. Any disturbance in the protein levels of plasma leads to disturbances in the mineral level in circulation and affect their metabolism.

A β-globulion transferrin is capable of binding iron, copper, zinc. This protein constitutes approximately 3 per cent of the total plasma proteins. The most important function of this protein, however is to bind iron. Iron binding capacity of transferrin is found to be maximum at pH of 7.0 and at this pH, its copper binding capacity is reduced to half. Presence of iron further reduces its Copper binding capacity.

Another protein ceruloplasmin which binds copper has been isolated from human plasma. It is a blue protein containing 34.34 per cent copper and it binds practically all the copper of plasma. Chemically, ceruloplasma is a α-globulin of the molecular weight of about 150,000. Approximately 7.5 per cent of its weight is constituted by carbohydrates. Both the "IC" and the "ous" forms of Copper can be bound to this protein. About 50 per cent of this bound copper can be removed by dialysis against a chelating agent. In Wilson's disease which is rarely occurring disease and is inherited in most of the cases, plasma ceruloplasmin content is considerably lowered followed by rise of free Copper level in the plasma. Copper starts getting deposited in the brain tissue and liver as a result of which liver damage and neurological disorder occur. Although, the precise function of ceruloplasmin is yet to be ascertained, it cannot be denied that one of the most important role of this protein is to regulate the release of copper at different sites of the body tissues in a reversible manner.

2. *Immunological function* — The γ-globulin fraction of plasma protein which moves most slowly in the electric field during electroploresis, and to some extent α and β-globulin fractions do participate in developing immunity in the body against the action of certain foreign proteins. The foreign proteins entering in the body in the intact form are known as antigens. It is well known that when antigens find their entry in the body some newer proteins which mostly belong to the group of α-globulin and to some extent to the group of β and α_2-globulins are produced by the body which can counteract the effect of antigens. In this antagonism, antigens combine with antibody to give a visible ppt. This reaction is known as precipitin reaction. The combining sites are provided by aminoacids and the reaction is believed to be analogous to the formation of an enzyme substrate complex. It may involve electrostatic forces, hydrophobic forces and hydrogen bonding.

The antibodies produced under the influence of antigen have been named variously depending upon their nature. For example, antibodies produced under the influence of toxins are called anti toxins. If the antigens are some sort of cells and if clumping of such cells is brought about by antibodies such antibodies are known as agglutinins. If the antigen cells are lysed by the antibodies, such antibodies are known as lysins.

Antibodies are produced by the reticuloendothelial cells and lymphoid system and are transported through the body by plasma. Antibodies are normally found in the plasma of normal individuals as they are always exposed to environmental microrganisms whose proteins act as a antigens. A given antigen may induce the formation of several antibodies which can react with the induced antigen. The greater is the complexity of the antigen protein, the greater is the number of the antibodies formed.

Articial immunity may be produced by injecting non pathogenic forms of the antigens in the body such as killed bacteria of Hemophillus pertussis responsible for whooping cough, or a toxoid of tetanus or deptheria which are made by treating the antigen with formaldehyde. Temporary immunity may also be produced by giving injections of antibodies, taken from normal immune persons.

New borns of mammals usually do not produce antibodies, however the antibody producing mechanism remains present in them which gradually develops with the age. In new forms, some antibodies are found to be present in their plasma which are derived from the blood of the mother.

In some of the hereditary disease the human beings lack the ability to form globulins and consequently antibodies are found to be absent in their blood. Such individual are extremely susceptible to various types of infections.

3. *Coagulation and Fibrinolysis:* Some of the enzymic proteins of plasma are concerned with the phenomenon of blood clotting and fibrinolysis. At the site of injury, prothrombin is converted into thrombin which in turn can convert fibrinogen into fibrin. Fibrin thus formed cloggs the site of injury and prevents bleeding. Several enzymes are believed to be involved in thrombin formation. Thrombin itself has enzymitic properties. Intravascular clot, known as thrombus

whenever it is formed is digested by the enzymes of fibrinolytic system present in the plasma. This saves us from the disastrous effects of thrombosis.

Biosynthesis of Plasma Proteins

The plasma proteins are mostly synthesized in the liver. Some of the proteins are also synthesized in extra hepatic tissues such as lymphoid and reticuloendothelial system, principally that of spleen. Some of the other circulatory proteins, such as hormones are synthesized by other tissues. Albumins and fibrinogen are solely synthesized in the liver. Also, approximately 75 to 80 per cent globulins are synthesized by liver. The other plasma globulins are synthesized by extra hepatic tissues. γ-globulins are synthesized in the lymphoid tissue and reticuloendothelial system. If the liver is damaged as in hepatic cirrhosis, or is surgically removed, the level of plasma proteins falls considerably. The fall in albumin and fibrinogen level is more marked. There occurs a continuous turnover between plasma proteins and the tissue proteins. Liver and kidney tissues can utilize the circulatory proteins activity.

As regards the synthesis of antibodies or immunoglobins, it is believed that the inducer antigen is first engulfed by the macrophage-phagocytes. These phagocytes react with the small lymphocytes which actually synthesize antibodies. A soluble material is transferred from the macrophages to small lymphocytes which is effective in inducing antibody synthesis. The soluble substances is a RNA. And body formation is prevented if this material is treated with ribonuclease such an effective inducer RNA has now been isolated from immunized mice spleen. It is suggested that information is transmitted in the form of such a RNA from macrophage phagocytes to the small lymphocytes which initiates immunoglobulin biosynthesis.

The synthesis of immunoglobulins proceeds almost in a similiar manner as that of the other proteins of the body. Immunoglobulins contain in their molecular structure light (L) heavy (H) chains. Ribosomes required for the synthesis of L and H chains are different. The sedimentation rate of ribosomes responsible for synthesis of L chains is higher as compared to that of the ribosomes which synthesis H chains. During formation of immunoglobulins L chains are completed and released first as compared to the H chains. L chains then combine with the partially synthesized H chains. A prior combination of the L chains with the H chains is necessary for satisfactory release of the complete immunoglobulins. Thus, synthesis of L chains exerts the complete immunoglobulins. Thus, synthesis of L chains exerts a regulatory influence upon the biosynthesis of immunoglubulins.

Haptoglobins. The haptoglobins are a group of α_2-globulins having the distinctive property of binding haemoglobin. By starch electrophoresis three α_2-globulin bands can be identified which depend on two alternative (allelic) genes which produce three phenotypes Hp 1-1, Hp 2-2, and Hp 2-1. These are inherited in the same way as the MN blood groups. When red cells break down haemoglobin is released and up to 150 mg haemoglobin per 100 ml plasma can combine firmly with haptoglobin to be quicky picked up by the reticuloendothelial system. When the rate of destruction of red blood cells exceeds the rate of haptoglobin production heamoglobin may appear in the urine.

Normal capillary filtrates and normal lymph from the limbs contain small amounts of albumin (mol. wt. 68000) and even of globulin (mol. wt. 90000 to 175000) and fibrinogen (mol. wt. 330000). It was difficult to understand how these proteins, especially those of very high molecular weight, could pass through the capillary wall until Cohn showed that the molecules of plasma proteins are sausageshaped bodies, almost all of which have nearly the same diameter, namely 3.3 to 3.8 nm. They vary in length, however, according to their molecular weight. It appears that, although the majority of pores in the capillary walls measure from 0.7 to 2.0 nm, there are some at least 3.8 nm in diameter. All these pores allow simple salts to pass quite freely while the largest of them allow the passage of albumin and even of globulin and fibironogen provided that these large molecules strike the capillary wall in the correct orientation, that is 'end-on' to the pores. In this way we can account for the small amounts of protein which are normally found in capillary filtrates and in urine. The albumin which passes through the capillary walls returns to the circulation via the lymphatics; about half of the total plasma albumin circulates in this way every 24 hours.

Hypoproteinaemia may be said to exist when the total plasma protein concentration is less than 5.5 g per 100 ml. It may be caused by excessive protein catabolism or by loss of protein in to the urine, into the alimentary tract, or from the skin after burns or scalds. When this loss is not fully balanced by a simultaneous production of new plasma protein enter because of much reduced protein intake in the food, or as the result of liver disease, the concentration of protein in the plasma gradually falls. The colloid osmotic pressure of the plasma is diminished and the tendency for water to be attracted from the tissues into the blood is reduced. Water may therefore accumulate in the tissues; if this is excessive it may become obvious as *oedema*.

The plasma lipoproteins. The lipoproteins of blood plasma have recently attracted much attention, largely as the result of the development of the lipoprotein phenotyping system of Fredrickson and his colleagues. Their work on disorders of lipid metabolism has proved to be of great value in the study of diseases of the heart and vascular system.

The plasma lipoproteins may readily be separated by ultracentrifugation, but the simplest classification is based on paper electrophoresis which reveals four main classes of lipoproteins.

1. The *α-lipoprotien* fraction shows greatest electrophoretic mobility and consists of about 50 per cent protein, 30 per cent phospholipid and 20 per cent cholesterol (and its esters).

2. The *β-lipoproteins* have a rather lower electrophoretic mobility, and are of such low density that they float to the top of the tube upon ultracentrifugation. Their composition is about 25 per cent protein, 20 per cent phospholipid, 10 per cent triglycerides and 45 per cent cholesterol and its esters. They are, in fact, the main carriers of cholesterol in the plamsa.

3. The *pre-ß-lipoprotein* fraction migrates slightly more rapidly than the β-fraction; it is even less dense than the ß-fraction. It contains some cholesterol but its

main function is as a carrier of triglyceride of endogenous origin which may account for between 50 and 80 per cent of its composition.

4. The fourth class of 'lipoproteins' are the chylomicrons which are important in relation to fat absorption from the gut. They are large particles which do not migrate on paper and show up as a band at the origin. They consist from dietary fat together with a small amount of cholesterol.

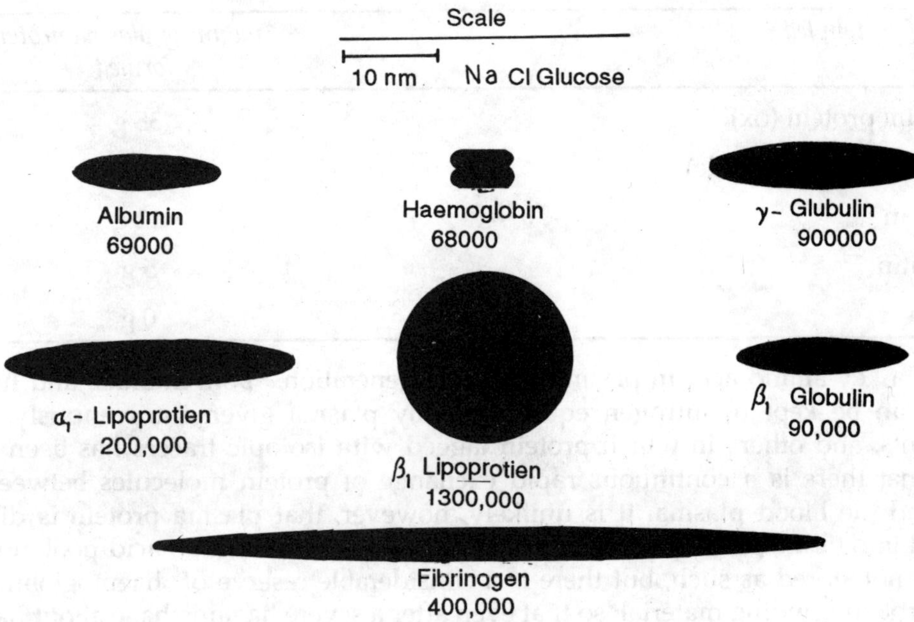

Fig. 1.6. Diagram showing relative dimensions and molecular weights of blood proteins. The molecules of albumin, globulin and fibrinogen are elongated bodies of about the same diameter but of very different lengths according to their molecular weights.

In various disorders of lipid metabolism one or more of the lipoprotein fractions may be increased, giving rise to the conditions known as *hyperlipoproteinaemias*.

The formation of plasma proteins. Experiments on dogs by Whipple have shown that the plasma proteins are formed from amino acids derived from the food. By a technique called *plasmapheresis* he has investigated some of the factors involved in the generation of plasma protein. Plasmapheresis consists in withdrawing a quantity of blood from which the red blood corpuscles, after separation by centrifugation, are washed with isotonic saline and then returned to the dog by intravenous injection. In this way the animal is deprived of plasma proteins without loss of haemoglobin. If the animal is kept on standard diet the plasma proteins can be gradually reduced by daily plasmapheresis from the normal level of 6 per cent to 4 per cent and can be kept at this lower level.

If now a protein is fed as a supplement to the standard diet without altering the amount of plasmapheresis, the percentage of protein in the plasma rises and the total amount of extra plasma protein manufactured can be estimated if the blood volume is known.

Such experiments indicate that the plasma protein is formed from amino acids derived from the food and other experiments along similar lines show further that

Table 1.1

Amount of protein fed	*Amount of plasma protein formed*
100 g serum protein (ox)	38 g
100 g meat (skeletal muscle)	18 g
100 g casein	12 g
100 g gelatin	5 g
100 g zein	0 g

cystine is a key amino acid in plasma protein regeneration. Both animals and human patients can be kept in nitrogen equilibrium by plasma given intravenously. Such experiments, and others in which protein tagged with isotopic tracers has been used, suggest that there is a continuous rapid exchange of protein molecules between the tissues and the blood plasma. It is unlikely, however, that plasma protein is directly converted into tissue protein or vice versa, except through the amino acid pool. Plasma protein is not stored as such, but there is a considerable reserve of haemoglobin- and plasma-protein-building material, so that even after a severe haemorrhage about half the amount lost can be re-formed in a day. The existence of this reserve store is clearly shown by the fact that after severe depletion by plasmapheresis, followed by a period of starvation, plasma protein is regenerated at the expense of tissue protein. An adult man synthesizes about 15 g of plasma protein per day.

White Blood Corpuscles

White blood corpuscles are nucleated non pigmented or colourless cells also known as *leucocytes*. They are described as wandering cells and are not always confined to the blood channel. Due to their amoeboid properties they can easily pass through the unruptured blood vessels by a process of *diapedesis*. These cells are attracted to areas of infection or inflammation by chemical substances released during tissue destruction. An important function of W.B.C. is *phagocytosis*. Phagocytic white blood cells protect the body by engulfing disease-producing micro-organism and digesting them with lysosomal hydrolytic enzymes.

Number. The average number of white blood cells in a healthy person ranges from 5,000 to 10,000 per cubic millimeter of whole blood. In an acute infection, such as appendicitis or pneumonia, the total leucocytes increase considerably upto 20,000 or 30,000 per cubic millimeter of blood. During pregnancy and in the new born also, the number increases above 10,000 per cubic mm. This increase is the *leucocytosis.* In contrast to this, if the number falls below 4000 the term *leucopenia* is applied. Leucopenia occurs in persons with certain diseases, such as tuberculosis. *Leukemia* is a pathological increase in number and the term is used today to denote one type of neoplastic disease.

Variations in normal count of white blood corpuscles have also been reported under following conditions.

(i) Diurnal variation

(ii) Mascular exercise

(iii) Injection of adrenalin

(iv) Emotional stress

(v) Age

(vi) Pregnancy

(vii) Cellular destruction

(viii) Asthma, hay fever, skin disease etc.

(ix) Starvation

(x) Administration of certain chemicals like benzene, sulphonamide etc.

While blood corpuscles differ from the red cells in many respects as given below:

(i) White blood cells are devoid of haemoglobin.

(ii) White blood cells are bigger in size.

(iii) White blood cells are nucleated.

(iv) White blood cells are much less in number.

(v) White blood cells are amoeboid in shape.

(vi) The functions of W.B.C.'s are absolutely different from those of red cells.

(vii) There are several varieties of leucocytes, whereas red cells are only of one variety.

(viii) Their life span is shorter.

One of the most important functions of leucocytes is the body defence against infection. This is achieved by three processes: (1) phagocytosis, (2) production of antibodies, and (3) destruction and removal of toxins of protein origin.

Leucocytes are manufactured in spleen, lymph nodules, tonsils, Peyer's patches etc. According to *Osgood* and *Sabin* the life span of the different varieties of leucocytes differs as shown in the following lines:

(i)	Granulocytes	1-2 days (Sabin)	
(ii)	Neutrophils	2-4 days	Osgood
(iii)	Eosinophils	8-12 days	
(iv)	Basophils	12-15 days	
(v)	Lymphocytes	1-2 or 3 days	

White blood cells are sub-divided into two categories, granular and non-granular leucocytes, based on the presence or absence of cytoplasmic granules:

Various Types of Leucocytes in Different Animals

Animals	*Neutrophils*	*Eosinophils*	*Basophils*	*Lymphocytes*	*Monocytes*
Human	67	3	<1	23	7
Horse	54	4	<1	38	4
Cow	21	5	<1	64	10
Sheep	42	4	<1	48	6
Goat	45	2	<1	48	5
Pig	42	3	<1	47	8
Dog	57	10	<1	25	8
Cat	58	5	<1	27	10

Granular Leucocytes

The leucocytes contain cytoplasmic granules and lobulated nuclei are the *granulocytes.* The granulocytes arise in red bone marrow from precursor cells called *myeloblasts.* The nuclei of granulocytes appear in many shapes that is why also called *polymorphonuclear leucocytes.* The granules can be stained with Wright's stain, eosin or methylene blue. They are classified as neutrophils, eosinophils, or basophils on the basis of the shapes of their nuclei or the staining reaction of their granules.

Neutrophils: Neutrophils comprise about 67 per cent (or 3000-6000 per cubic mm.) of all white blood cells in peripheral circulation. They are about 10 to 12 microns in diameter and contain nuclei that have from three to five lobes. The cytoplasm of the mature neutrophil is filled with fine lysosomal granules containing phosphatase, nucleotidase, protease, amylase, lipase etc. They show amoeboid movement, and can move upon 40 microns per minute. Neutrophils are the chief phagocytic cells of the body. They are not confined to blood vessels, but, throughout the entire body where they function as *scavengers.* Neutrophils survive more than a few days after leaving the blood stream. If the infection is massive or the bacteria are very virulent, many neutrophils die; an accumulation of dead neutrophils and bacteria is known as pus. A localised accumulation of pus is called an abcess.

Some physioligists have described certain sex differences in the nuclei of neutrophils. About 3-5% of neutrophils from a female show the sex chromatin attached to one of the nuclear lobes by a thin stalk forming the so called "drumstick bodies."

Eosinophils: Also known as *acidophils* and comprise only 1 to 3 per cent of all white blood cells, 100-400 per cubic mm. They are about 10 to 15 microns in diameter. They have bilobed nuclei and contain large lysosomal granules that stain red with Wright's stain. Eosinophils in the peripheral blood increase in allergic diseases, such as asthma or hay fever, and in parasitic infections, such as trichinosis. Some people believe that the eosinophils contain much of the *histamine* that is present in the blood. Histamine causes the symptoms of allergic reactions.

Basophils: Basophils are also known as *cyanophils.* They are even rarer and make up only about 0.5 per cent of all white blood cells or 25 to 200 per cubic mm. They are about 8 to 10 microns in diameter (smallest among W.B.C) having bilobed or kidney shaped nuclei and contain large granules that stain dark blue with Wright's blood stain. These granules contain *histamine* and *heparin,* which are released into the blood stream under conditions of stress or allergy. Basophils are non-phagocytic: they are similar to the most cells in loose connective tissue. They possibly have some role in local anticoagulation and formation of ground substance. They are believed to belong to cells of the reticulo-endothelial system. The number of basophils increases in chicken pox.

The increase of granulocytes in the blood is called as *granulocytosis.* Diminution of granulocytes in the blood is known as *granulocytopenia.* Complete disappearance of granulocytes is known as *agranulocytosis.*

Agranular Leucocytes

These are non-granular white blood cells that contain simple spherical non-lobulated nuclei. These cells comprise about 25-30 per cent of all leucocytes. These cells include monocytes, which are formed in lymph nodes and the spleen and lymphocytes, which are formed in all types of lymphoid tissue, including lymph nodes, spleen, tonsils and possibly the thymus.

Monocytes. These are the largest among all white cells ranging from 16-22 microns in diameter. Monocytes make up about 5 per cent of all white cells. The number of monocytes varies from 100-400 per cubic mm. of blood. The number increases in tuberculosis. Their nuclei are indented to horse shoe shape and stain purple. The nucleus is eccentric with a large amount of clear non-granular cytoplasm, may be, with vacuoles in it. They arise in the red bone marrow from precursor cells called *monoblasts.* The monocytes are motile and have the power of engulfing bacteria. These are most active in acid environment (pH ranges below seven). In general, they are found around walled off abscesses and infections which have been brought under control. They are also found in tissues, and in these locations the cells are differentiated into *macrophages* or scavenger cells. Monocytes live as macrophages for several months in the tissues and are commonly found at sites of chronic infection or inflammation. They play a vital role in removing damaged tissue and thus preparing the way for regeneration processes of the body.

	Monocytes		*Lymphocytes*
1.	Largest measuring about 16-22μ in diameter.	1.	Small 7.5 to 12μ in diameter
2.	Nucleus is indented to horseshoe shape and sometimes rounded.	2.	Nucleus is round or oval shaped.
3.	Nucleus is eccentric.	3.	Nucleus is centrally placed.
4.	Cytoplasm resembles the frosted glass	4.	It has clear glass appearance.
5.	Motile & phagocytic	5.	Non-motile and non-phagocytic.

Lymphocytes: They make up about 25 per cent of all white blood cells. The number varies from 1500-2700 per cubic mm. of blood. The number increases in tuberculosis. Two types of lymphocytes have been reported. *Small lymphocytes* are most common in blood. They have a diameter of 8 microns. They have relatively large, somewhat spherical, nuclei. Large lymphocytes have a diameter of 12 microns. They are primitive, proliferative cells, residing in the lymph nodules that give rise to the active, small, lymphocytes. Both small and large lymphocytes have spherical nucleus surrounded by a thin rim of cytoplasm. Lymphocytes arise from *lymphoblasts*. Mature lymphocytes are released into the lymphatic system and ultimately enter the cardiovascular system, which they leave very rapidly to enter the tissues. Once in the tissues, lymphocytes live only for a few days; they may survive for years in the lymphatic system.

Lymphocytes are non phagocytic and neutralize the toxicity produced in the body. The important function of these cells is to produce antibodies. They also contribute to scar formation after injury and thus facilitate wound healing.

The Blood Platelets

The platelets (thrombocytes) are the smallest of the formed elements of the blood, measuring 2 to 3 μm in diameter. They are formed by division of the cytoplasms of *megakaryocytes,* large cells 40-150 μm in diameter found in bone marrow, lungs and to a less extent in other tissues.

The megakaryocytes are polyploid cells containing, on average, four times the diploid number of chromosomes in a large, usually lobulated nucleus. The separation of individual platelets is an orderly process involving the formation and fusion of small cytoplasmic vesicles to form the platelet membranes. The rate of platelet production is partly controlled by the number of circulating platelets (normally 100000 to 500000 per mm^3) and it now seems likely that a humoral substance *thrombopoietin* mediates this influence in much the same way as does erythropoietin in haemopoiesis. Since megakaryocyte has a volume 3000 to 4000 times that a single thrombocyte it seems likely that each may produce more than a thousand platelets

The mature platelet is a biconvex disc with a complex structure, a living cell which, like the erythrocyte, consumes oxygen in spite of the absence of a nucleus. It shows the following elements. and exterior coat rich in glycoprotein and acid mucopolysaccharide; a unit membrane (cell membrane) with the usual trilaminar structure; a system of microfilaments (probably of actin-like protein) dispersed through the cytoplasm; an equatorial ring of 8 to 24 *microtubules* close to the cell membrane, each tubule consisting of 12 to 15 helical subfilaments; granules containing lysosome-like enzymes; glycogen particles; *electron dense granules* (probably serotonin storing bodies); a few mitochondria; a Golgi apparatus; a *dense tubular system* of membranes.

In man platelets have a life span of 7 to 14 days. Some 10 to 15 per cent are lost by consumption in haemostatis and the maintenance of vascular integrity. The remainder are destroyed by the reticulo-endothelial (macrophage) system, especially in the spleen, thus the platelet count rises, sometimes permanently, if the spleen is removed. Information about platelet life span has come from experiments using diisopropyl-phosphofluoridate (DFP) labelled with either 3P or ^{3}H. When injected DFP labels the platelets and enables their rate of destruction to be followed. Similar information has been obtained by labelling the platelets *in vitro* with ^{32}P or ^{51}Cr and transfusing them. The main functions of platelets seem to be in haemostatis but it has now been shown that labelled platelets can contribute part of their cytoplasm to endothelial cells and may therefore have a role in supporting the metabolism of injured intima. Platelets also contain, and can release, a protein able to increase vascular permeability and thus contribute to the humoral control of inflammatory raactions.

There are differences in the distribution of macrophages between species and also, within one species, in the behaviour of its macrophages towards different kinds of particulate substance. These differences demand great caution in arguing from circumstances in the experimental animal to those in man and from one type of substance or particle to another.

Tissue histiocytes. Cells of macrophage type occur in most connective tissues. Many of the cells appear to be long-term residents and are sometimes referred to as "fixed" tissue histiocytes or macrophages. In most sites they are scanty but they are relatively abundant in the omentum of the fetus and new-born where cells beneath the peritoneum appear as pale milky aggregates against the yellowish adipose tissue and have thus acquired the name of 'taches laiteuses'. When the need arises for histiocytes in greater number; as in certain forms of inflammation, those of 'fixed' origin are rapidly supplemented by others, the 'wandering' histiocytes, that appear to be constantly on patrol in most tissues. These in turn are supplemented by yet others, formerly circulating blood monocytes but now, in response to the stimulus, extravascular. It may be that most if not all 'wandering' histiocytes are in fact of intravascular origin.

Microglia. Within the central nervous system, especially around small arteries and arterioles, metallic-impregnation methods reveal cells that are neither astrocytes nor oligodendrocytes. Such cells, in areas of brain damage, change their appearance and become clearly recognizable as macrophages. They are known collectively as the microglia or central nervous system histiocytes; another commonly used name derived from the frequent foamy appearance of their cytoplasm is compound granular corpuscclel. It has long been believed that these cells are of mesenchymal origin, derived from the tissues of the perivascular sheaths, and that they enter the brain along with the blood vessels during its early development. More recently the use of labelled blood monocytes has shown that in areas of injury cells of apparently microglial type rapidly bacome supplemented by macrophages that were at one time certainly blood monocytes. The extent and frequency of this process is uncertain. The pericyte has also been regarded as possibly capable of becoming a macrophage in these circumstances. The exact histogenesis of the cells presently designated as the microglia is thus still debatable. It should be noted that leucocytes do not enter the substance of the brain from the blood stream during health, and also that even the microglial cells fail to engulf material from dyestuffs or colloidal suspensions injected intravenously into a healthy animal. These observations emphasize the existence of a so-called blood-brain barrier to which reference will be made later in connection with transfer between blood and cerebro-spinal fluid of various drugs or other substances.

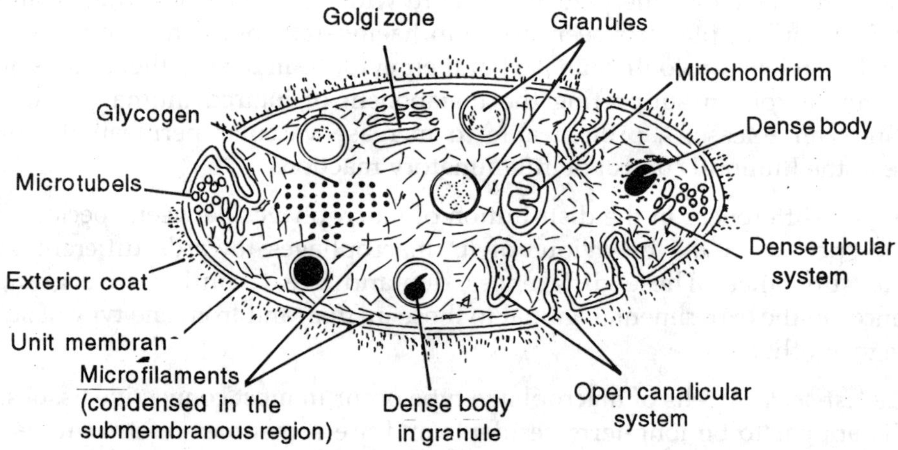

Fig. 1.7A A schematic cross section of a platelet showing the fine structure. Platelet morphology. In *The Circulating Platelet.*

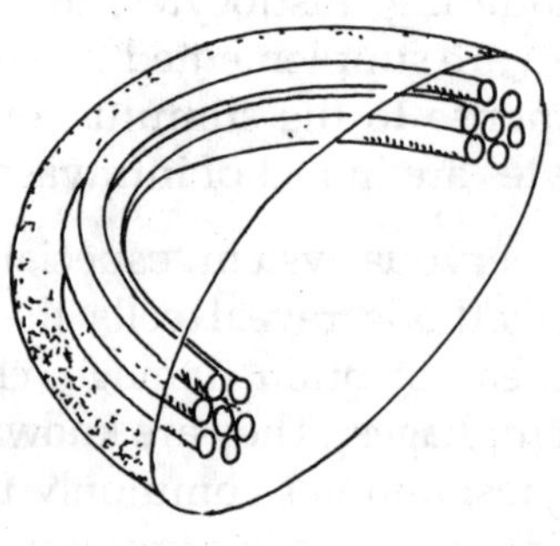

Fig. 1.8. Scheme of half-platelet showing the equatorial arrangement of tubules.

Cells lining sinusoids. Sinusoids are relatively wide channels, both haemic and lymphatic, through which the flow of blood and lymph is correspondingly slow. This type of structure is present in liver, spleen, bone marrow, adrenal and pituitary; and lymph nodes. A further feature of the liver, spleen bone marrow and nodes is that many of their endothelial cells are markedly phagocytic, the sinusoidal cells of the adrenal and pituitary by comprison show only minimal activity.

Liver. The origin of these cells is still in debate as is their relation to the sinusoidal endothelial cells that do not contain carbon. On the whole at present it seems likely (a) that all the endothelial cells have a highly phagocytic ability, and are therefore potentially 'Kupffer' cells but that some react more promptly or more avidly than others, perhaps due to their age or metabolic status at the time, (b) that some such cells, when laden with particles, become detached and pass in the hepatic veins or the lymphatics to the lungs and regional lymph nodes, (c) that replacement is achieved mainly by division of adjacent sinusoidal endothelial cells but also by lymphocytes that pass from the spleen and become transformed and incorported into the sinusoidal lining. It seems likely also that the different forms of endothelial phagocytic cell claimed to exist are but morphological variants of the one endothelial cell type with occasional transforming immigrant lymphocytes.

Spleen. The structure of the spleen is remarked that there is probably a double form of circulation of blood, one rapid and one slow. The slow type of circulation leads in effect to a sequestration of blood cells and affords ample opportunity for phagocytosis whether of aged erythrocytes or abnormal materials and substances of the kinds mentioned earlier. The exact mode of final disappearance of an erythrocyte is principally fragmentation and ingestion of the particles by the phagocytic endothelial cell; it is unlikely to be engulfed whole by these cells or to disappear by relatively sudden rupture.

Bone marrow. The experimental intravenous infection of appropriate suspension has shown that the distortion of phagocytes in the bone marrow is similar to that in the spleen. The endothelium of the marrow is discontinuous, and so particulate material (and ageing erythrocytes) has ready access to the extravascular of patene hymatous compartment of the marrow. Experimental observations of this kind have also shown that phagocytic cells are present not only in the endothelium but also in the non-endothelial parenchyma.

Lymph nodes. For present purposes the lymph node may be considered as having three types of cell (a) lymphoblasts/lymphocytes, (b) reticulum cells; that is, the cells, which, with their reticulin fibres, comprise the permanent population and skeleton of the node, and (c) the endothelial cells of the peripheral and penetrating sinuses. Of these, the lymphocytes series possesses virtually no phagocytic ability; the reticulum cells possess some but of low degree only. Lymph nodes are major sites of phagocytosis due almost wholly to the activity of the endothelial cells (endothelium of the immediately related afferent and efferent lymphatics has no such activity, a sharp, interesting and ill-understood functional difference). In some states of inflammation, macrophages containing lipid material may accumulate in large number in the substance of lymph node as well as in the endothellium of the sinuses. These cells might be reticulum cells, stimulated to greater-than-normal phagocytosis by unusally great demand, but seem more likely to be endothelial cells that have passed, fully laden, from the wall of the sinus into the pulp of the node until such time as they can digest and dispose of the engulfed susbtance.

Other functions. A few endothelial cells in the sinusoids of the adrenals and pituitary show phagocytic activity; they have little if any physiological significance. In the lung, phagocytes are abundant. They do not comprise a formal 'system' as do the Kupffer cells in the liver but are present as a relatively large and widespread patrol of wandering histiocytes. If no particulate material or micro-organisms ever entered the lungs, the macrophages might never be seeen. As it is, macrophages with engulfed carbon or other material are virtually always present in the alveoli and airways and can be easily seen in bronchial secretion or expectoration. The origin of these cells is still uncertain: it is till unsure whether and to what extent they are derived from circulating blood monocytes (which become wandering tissues histiocytes) or alveolar epithelial cells or the fibroblastic mesenchymal cells that support the alveolar epithelium. Most inhaled particulate material is trapped directly in the mucus of the respiratory tract and then expectorated or swallowed; much is engulfed by the macrophages which are likewise removed in the mucus; some is carried by the macrophages into lymphatics from which it eventually becomes deposited in the small foci of lymphoid tissue in the lung or in the regional (mediastinal) lymph nodes. In persons heavily exposed to dusty conditions, the material may travel even further; thus, in miners, carbon is commonly found in the lymphatics and lymph nodes of the diaphragm, posterior abdominal wall and neck.

The extent to which one form of mesenchymal cell may change or 'transform' into another is an interesting problem. At one time or another, each of the lymphocyte, monocyte, endothelial cell, fibroblast and macrophage has been regarded as capable of transforming into any of others; and this may be true. However, since most of the evidence so far has been mainly morphological, by which 'transitional' forms are easy to find but almost impossible to identify in a definitive way, some doubt remain. Continuing studies of the use of isotope-labelled cells, in the manner described earlier, give some hope that the uncertainty will gradually be dispelled.

Functions of the macrophage system. The earliest recognizable precursor of the macrophage is the primitive mesenchymal cell already mentioned as part of the population of lymph node, a *reticulum cell.* This type of cell occurs also in the bone marrow and is the precursor of the haemocytoblasts. It is thus, in turn, the precursor of all the formed elements of the blood and lymphoid tissue including the lymphocyte and its derivative, the plasma cell. Because of this common ancestry, it has been usual hitherto to regard these cells as all comprising one 'system', the reticulo-endothelial system, whose function was thus a combination of phagocytosis (macrophages and polymorphonuclear leucocytes, formerly microphages), antibody manufacture and transport with maintenance of immunity (lymphocytes and plasma cells), and haemopoiesis (the haemocytoblast). With increasing knowledge of these three processes, this association of functions has become increasingly artifical, hence the desirability, mentioned in the opening paragraph, of considering as a separate macrophage system those cells of which a major function is the phagocytosis of particulate matter.

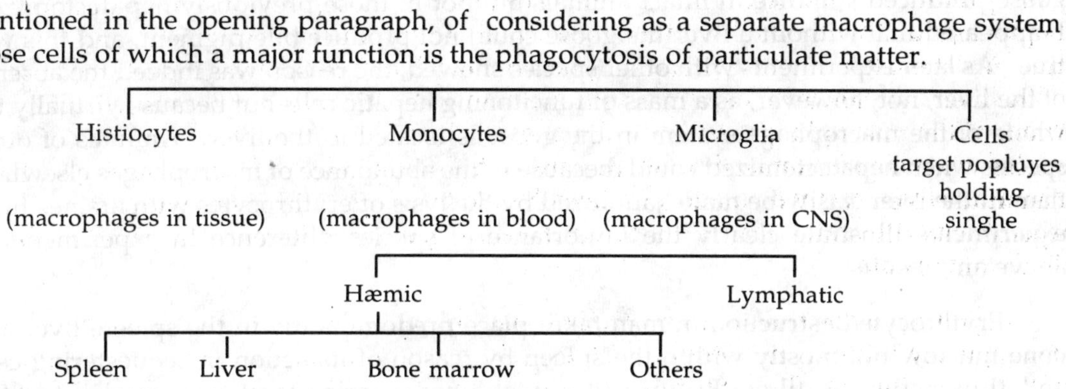

Fig. 1.9 The macrophage 'system'

Phagocytosis. Macrophages differ from polymorphonuclear leucocytes in their much greater avidity for or ability to engulf inorganic particulate material such as carbon and dust particles in general. Examination of bronchial secretion shows dust in abundance within macrophages but not in other leucocytes. Macrophages have also the unusual capacity, when confronted by particularly insoluble or foreign material, to fuse together with the formation of multinucleated giant cells. The presence within a tissue of some foreign material such as a surgical suture or a thorn is not, of course, a physiological situation; but neither also, perhaps, is the presence of dust in the bronchial tree. Macrophages can destroy many types of micro-organisms, mostly types that cannot be adequately or efficiently destroyed by the polymorphonuclears. Most forms of organic foreign material such as a spicule of fish-bone or the surgeon's catgut can be gradually destroyed by enzyme action and lysis. Most forms of inorganic material, whether exogenous or, like sterol crystals, endogenous, cannot be destroyed by lysis: these, therefore, remain undisturbed either throughout life or (possibly because of some tissue reaction) until surgical removal, or they may be transported to lymph nodes via the lymphatics by the macrophages Bile pigment, haemosiderin, melanin, lipid susbtances and carbon are all materials that may be seen in different circumstances within macrophages; so also, in association with tissue damage, are dead and dying micro-organisms and polymorphonuclears, tissue debris and fibrin. Besides phagocytosis, cells of the macrophage system are intimately concerned with the catabolism of haemoglobin, that is the further breakdown of the erythrocyte and its main constituent after phagocytosis has occurred.

Formation of bile pigment (bilirubin, haematoidin). Bile pigment is formed by and within the cells of the macrophage system, especially those of liver, spleen and bone marrow as a result of enzyme action upon the haemoglobin derived from effete or otherwise imperfect or damaged erythrocytes. Iron derived from the haemoglobin is retained within the macrophage as haemosiderin and ferritin the bile pigment is released into the plasma. It was at one time believed that bile pigment was formed only by the cells of the liver and this, belief appeared to derive sound support from an experiment showing that haemolytic anaemia produced by the administration of arsine (As I_3) to a goose produced jaundice in intact animals but not in those previously hepatectomized. It appeared that without a liver the goose could not produce bile pigment, and this was true. As later experiments with other species showed, the reason was indeed the absence of the liver, not, however, as a mass of funcitoning hepatic cells but because virtually the whole of the macrophage system in the goose is located in the liver. Animals of other species when hepatectomized could, because of the abundance of macrophages elsewhere than in the liver, easily be made jaundiced by the lysis of erythrocytes with arsine. Such experiments illustrate clearly the importance of species difference in experiments of above and results.

Erythrocyte destruction in man takes place predominantly in the spleen, liver and bone marrow but mostly within the spleen by reason of its action in sequestering cells and thus acting as filter. Erythrocyte breakdwon continues at a normal rate after splenectomy but a peripheral blood film will then usually show a greater than usual number of erythrocytes with minor morphological abnormalities such as undue thinness or retention of nuclear remnants; such cells are presumably filtered out by the spleen in the intact individual.

When blood is extravasated or escapes into the tissues from within the vascular compartment, as in bruising, the released haemoglobin is disposed of in essentially the same way as when it is released inside the vascular compartment, as in bruising, the released haemoglobin is disposed of in essentially the same way as when it is released inside the vascular compartment; that is, by absorption into macrophages and conversion to bile pigment and iron. In these circumstances bile pigment may accumulate locally in crystalline form both within macrophages and (presumably after extrusion from the cell) without. This form of the pigment has long been known to pathologists as haematoidin. The range of colours in the familiar 'black eye', from purple through dark and light green to brownish, is produced by the extravasated blood, its progressive conversion to bile pigment and gradual absorption. A massive escape of blood into the tissues or one of the body cavities may result in jaundice of varying intensity depending in the amount of bile pigment formed and transported in the blood.

Relation to antigens and antibodies. Almost as soon as the macrophage system was discovered and defined by the ability of its cells to take up and concentrate inert particulate matter and various dyestuffs, attempts were made to find out whether it behaved towards other substances in the same way. In many instances it does, and amongst the materials ingested and stored are certain types of lipid and foreign protein. We thus know that macrophages can ingest and store antigens, and from this the question immediately arises whether they also manufacture antibodies. In short, the answer is almost certainly they cannot; recognition of antigen and manufacture of antibody remain the prime responsibility of the lymphocyte/plasma cell system. It is possible, however, that the macrophage may in some way 'process' antigenic protein and by either excreting the modified protein or altering its own surface RNA facilitate in some way the immunogenetic activity of the lymphocytes. The matter is one of intensive current research.

PHYSIOLOGICAL CHANGES IN BLOOD IN INFANCY AND CHILDHOOD

The haemoglobin content of the blood at birth is about 21 g per 100 ml, but it declines from this high value during the first two or three months of infancy to about 12 g, rising again to about 13 g in the succeeding three months. The iron released by breakdown of the haemoglobin of the destroyed red cells remains within the body and is re-utilized for the synthesis of haemoglobin, but the initial fall in the red cell count is not prevented by the administration of iron even in large amounts. A proportion of the haemoglobin of the foetus differs both chemically and spectroscopically from the haemoglobin of adults, the difference lying in the globin fraction; this fetal haemoglobin (HbF) forms 55 to 98 per cent of the total circulating haemoglobin in the normal full-term infant. Small amounts (1 to 2 per cent) of a similar material are found in the blood of many adults. HbF can be detected in larger quantities in the blood of patients with certain blood disorders. Fetal haemoglobin takes up oxygen more readily and gives up carbon dioxide more easily than does adult haemoglobin.

A few nucleated red cells are found in the peripheral circulation for a short time after birth. About 5 to 10 per cent of reticulocytes occur in the blood of the new born but adult numbers (1 per cent or less) are reached in a few days. The red cells at birth contain only one quarter of the adult amount of carbonic anhydrase; premature infants have even less. The infant starts off with 300 to 500 mg of iron provided, of course, by the mother; after birth the iron requirements must be provided in the food.

At birth there is a polymorphonuclear leucocytosis lasting only several days; this is followed by a lymphocytosis which preside for a year or so. The former is probably the result of deficient supply of oxygen before birth and its disappearaence follows improved oxygen supply after birth.

The platelets, unlike the other cellular elements, are present at birth in reduced numbers, normal adult values being attained within the first 10 days of life.

The haemotological changes to premature infants are of particular importance. At birth many such infants have a very high haemoglobin level, often of the order of 20 or 21 g/100 ml. This appears to be due to fetal anoxia, particularly in the so-called dysmature infant suffering from placental failure. The tiny premature infant is born with poor iron stores and if his mother has not received prophylactic or therapeutic folic acid he often develops megaloblastic anaemia. Tocopherol may be important in protecting the erythrocyte of the premature infant from haemolysis. Soluble vitamin K analogues may cause haemolysis, and are thus of potential danger to the central nervous system from damage to the basal nuclei by unconjugated bilirubin.

COAGULATION OF BLOOD

One of the outstanding characteristics of blood is its ability to clot and within a short time after exposure to air, form an impervious cover for damaged tissue to prevent blood loss and keep out foreign matter.

Blood coagulation is the major chemical defence against blood loss. When a sample of human blood is taken, it turns into a jelly like mass within 3 to 10 minutes (average 6 minutes). This phenomenon is called *coagulation* or *clotting* of blood. Microscopically clot consists of blood corpuscles in a network of thread like fibrins. Inside blood vessels, the blood does not clot due to the presence of an anticoagulin substance - the heparin, secreted by mast cells which are found around capillaries. The blood coagulation is a very complicated process. Various theories have been proposed to explain the phenomenon of coagulation Some of the important theories are given below:

Best & Taylor's theory

According to the proposers of this theory, four chemical substances are required for coagulation. These are (a) *prothrombin* which is synthesized in liver and is found in small amount in blood plasma; (b) *thromboplastin* or *thrombokinase* is a fatty compound, found in the tissues; (c) *calcium ions* are the inorganic constituents found in plasma in their optimum concentration which is about 5 mg. per 100 ml. of blood; and (d) *fibrinogen* which is soluble plasma protein found in a dissolved form.

When the body is injured, the thromboplastin is liberated from the disintegrated blood platelets and the damaged tissues. It checks the activity of *antiprothrombin*, a substance that is found in blood to neutralize the activity of thrombin and then after, it converts inactive prothrombin into active *thrombin* in the presence of calcium. Now thrombin changes the soluble fibrinogen into insoluble fibrins in the presence of vitamin K. The fibrins constitute the *thrombus* or blood clot to trap the blood corpuscles to block the injured part of blood vessels.

Howell's Theory

Howell studied coagulation first in *Limulus* and then after in mammals. According to this theory, thrombokinase does not play any role in the conversion of prothrombin into thrombin. This conversion is done in the presence of calcium alone. It was suggested that an enzyme *tryptase* is released by the injured tissues. The tryptase inactivates *antiprothrombin* and thus initiates the conversion of prothrombin into thrombin in the presence of calcium ions.

Fuld and Spiro Theory

According to this theory, the injured platelets liberated *thrombokinase* or *thromboplastin* that converts prothrombin into thrombin in the presence of calcium ions. Then after thrombin converts soluble fibrinogen into insoluble fibrins to produce clot.

Mechanism of Blood Coagulation

When a blood vessel is injured, two reactions occur to stop the bleeding. One reaction closes the vessel. The damaged platelets release serotonin that brings about vasoconstriction to reduce or to stop the loss of blood. The second reaction involves clot formation to plug the rupture by means of various chemicals known as *coagulation* factors. In plasma, these factors are called *plasma coagulation* factors.

Clotting is a complex process and can be described as a sequence of three stages. Stage I is concerned with the formation of substance called *thromboplastin*. Stage 2 involves the conversion of *prothrombin*, a plasma protein into *thrombin*, an enzyme. This stage requires the presence of thromboplastin and several other plasma coagulation factors. In stge 3 thrombin catalyzes the conversion of *fibrinogen* into fibrin. Fibrin forms the threads of the clot.

Depending on whether thromboplastin is released by damaged tissues or formed by ruptured platelets, blood coagulation may proceed along one of the two routes: the extrinsic pathway or the intrinsic pathway.

Extrinsic pathway. The extrinsic pathway make use of a tissue factor which has been found in a variety of tissues and of plasma factors. The pathway begins when a blood vessel is ruptured. The damaged tissues surrounding the blood vessels and the ruptured area of blood vessel itself release a lipoprotein called tissue-*thromboplastin*. Tissue thromboplastin forms *extrinsic thromboplastin* along with plasma coagulation factors IV, V, VII and X. This process is stage I of the extrinsic pathway. In stage 2 prothrombin becomes active and called thrombin. This activation requires extrinsic thromboplastin and several plasma factors such as IV, V, VII an X. In stage 3, fibrinogen is converted to fibrin in the presence of factors IV and XIII.

Intrinsic pathway. The intrinsic pathway uses only blood plasma factors without the need of tissues clotting factors. This type of clotting is triggered when blood comes in contact with the rough surface. Under normal conditions, the *negatively* charged endothelium of blood vessel repels the *negatively* charged membrane of platelets. Thus platelets do not adhere to the endothelium of blood vessels. In the damaged blood vessels, the rough surface loses the negatively charged endothelium. Thus, the platelets adhere to the ruptured area. The clumped platelets release *platelet coagulation* factors in the plasma.

In intrinsic pathway, the *intrinsic thromboplastin* is formed when four platelet coagulation factors (Pf_1, Pf_2, Pf_3, Pf_4) react with seven plasma coagulation factors (IV, V, VIII, IX, X, XI, XII). It happens in stage I. In stage 2, prothrombin is converted to thrombin in the presence of intrinsic thromboplastin and plasma factors IV, V, VII & X. The stage 3 involves the conversion of fibrinogen into fibrin in the presence of thrombin and *plasma coagulation* factors IV and XII.

COAGULATION FACTORS

Factor I (Fibrinogen)

Fibrinogen is a glycoprotein of molecular weight 340,000. It consists of three pairs of non-identical polypeptide chains. It is synthesized in liver and remains soluble in plasma. During coagulation it is converted into fibrin.

Factor II (Prothrombin)

Prothrombin is a glycoprotein of molecular weight 70,000. It is produced by liver and its synthesis required vitamin K. Human prothrombin has nine per cent carbohydrates including hexos, hexosamin and neuraminic acid. In the presence of thromboplastin, it is converted into enzymatic thrombin which is having a molecular weight of about 34,000 daltons.

Factor III (Tissue Factor or Tissue Thromboplastin)

It is a lipoprotein complex. It is obtained from tissues. Purified preparations contain two fractions of M.W.330,000 and 220,000. Phospholipids greatly increase activity. It converts prothrombin into thrombin in the presence of calcium ions.

Factor IV (Calcium Ions)

This factor acts as a co-factor in coagulation. It is essential for the formation of both extrinsic and intrinsic thromboplastin and also in the conversion of prothrombin into thrombin. It is apparently involved in all three stages of clotting. Removal of calcium or its binding in plasma prevents coagulation.

Factor V (Pro-accelerin or Labile Factor)

It is a plasma glycoprotein of molecular weight 290,000 (bovine). It is a heat labile protein synthesized in liver. This factor is necessary for the complete conversion of prothrombin into thrombin by the intrinsic or extrinsic thromboplastin.

Factor VI (Accelerin)

It is no longer used in coagulation theory and its number has not been reassigned. This factor is a hypothetical activation product of pro-accelerin.

Factor VII Proconvertin or Stable Factor or Serum Prothrombin Accelerator (SPCA)

It is a plasma protein having molecular weight 63,000. It requires vitamin K for its synthesis. It is synthesized in liver and is required in stage I of extrinsic pathway. It is associated with prothrombin. It accelerates the formation of tissue thromboplastin from damaged tissues.

Factor VIII (Antihaemophilic Factor (AHF) or Antihaemophilic Globin (AHG) or Platelet Co-factor I)

It is a glycoprotein with a molecular weight of about 1.1 million. It is synthesized in liver and is required for stage 1 of intrinsic pathway. Its deficiency causes *haemophilia A*. It is closely associated with fibrinogen that is why it disappears when the blood clots.

Factor IX (Christmas Factor, or Plasma Thromboplastin Component (PTC) or Platelet Co-factor II)

It is a glycoprotein of molecular weight 55,400 (bovine). It is synthesized in liver and contains a single polypeptide chain. Its formation requires vitamin K. This factor is required for stage I of intrinsic factor. Deficiency causes disorder called *haemophilia B*, a disease similar to haemophilia A. The disease was first seen in a patient named Christmas hence named as *Christmas disease.*

Factor X (Stuart Factor or Stuart Power Factor)

Factor X is a glycoprotein with a molecular weight of 55,000. It is synthesized in liver in the presence of vitamin K. It is required for stage 1 and 2 of extrinsic and intrinsic pathways. Deficiency results in nose bleeding, bleeding into a joint, or bleeding into soft tissues.

Factor XI (Plasma Thromboplastin Antecedent (PTA)

It is a glycoprotein of molecular weight 160,000. It is synthesized by liver. It consists of two similar polypeptide chains. It is required for stage 1 of intrinsic pathway. Deficiency results in haemophilia C, a mild haemophilia of both males and females.

Factor XII (Hageman Factor or Surface Factor)

It is a glycoprotein of uncertain molecular weight (about 90,000). It is activated on the surface of contact or by contact with glass and may assume role in initiating coagulation outside body. It is required for stage I of intrinsic pathway.

Factor XIII (Fibrin Stabilizing Factor (FSF) or Fibrinase of Laki-Lovand Factor (LLF)

It is a glycoprotein of molecular weight 320,000. Also isolated from platelets as a protein of molecular weight 150,000. It is required for stage 3 of clotting.

Platelet coagulation Factors

There are four platelets coagulation factors as given below:

(i) *Platelet factor I (Pf_1) or platelet accelerator*. Essentially same as plasma coagulation factor V.

(ii) *Platelet factor 2 (Pf_2) or thrombin accelerator.* Accelerates formation of thrombin in stage I of intrinsic pathway and conversion of fibrinogen to fibrin.

(iii) *Platelet factor 3 (Pf_3) or platelet thromboplastin factor.*

(iv) *Platelet factor 4 (Pf_4).* Birds heparin, an anticoagulin, during clotting.

Anticoagulants

These are the substances preventing the coagulation of blood. Some of them are synthesized in the body of organisms, such as *heparin, hirudin, lamphredin* and *coumarin.* Among these, coumarin is of plant origin. It is also known as *dicumarol* and acts as a Vitamin K. It inhibits the release of factor VII.

Heparin is an acid (sulphated) mucopolysaccharide having molecular weight 16,000. It was first obtained from liver (hence the name), now prepared from beef lung or intestinal mucosa. It interferes with the formation of thrombokinase and also with the thrombin-fibrinogen reaction. The action of heparin in the circulation may be neutralized by administration of *protamine*—a low molecular weight basic protein from fish sperm heads. The salivary glands of leech contain *hirudin* which is a powerful anticoagulant (anti thrombin). In hospitals *Hirudinari medicinalis* is used for the study and use of this anticoagulant.

An extract from the venom of the Malayan pit viper has also been used to produce a different kind of anticoagulant effect, *defibrination*.

The citrates (sodium) and oxalates (sodium and ammonium) and EDTA, etc., are used by laboratories and blood banks to prevent blood samples from clotting. These substances react with calcium to form insoluble compounds. In this way, the blood calcium is tide up and is no longer free to catalyze the conversion of prothrombin to thrombin. Citrated blood can be used for transfusions. The liver metabolizes the citrate, freeing the calcium ions. Oxalated blood cannot be used for transfusions. There are some other synthetic coagulants such as *dicumarol, pelentan*, etc., which block the synthesis of prothrombin formation in liver and thus prevent blood coagulation.

Fibrinolysis

Clot formation is a vital mechanism that prevents excessive loss of blood from the body. Once the injured blood vessel is repaired, the clot dissolves. In many cases fibrin formed within the blood vessels is rapidly dissolved to restore the fluidity of the blood, in others the fibrin becomes hyalinized as is removed by phagocytes and replaced by connective tissue. The process of liquefaction of fibrin is known as *fibrinolysis*. At the beginning of the coagulation pathway, certain enzymes are released by damaged tissues. These enzymes activate an inactive plasma enzyme called *plasminogen* into an active form called *plasmin*. Plasmin is a trypsin like enzyme that dissolves the fibrin clot.

Thrombosis

Unwanted clotting may be brought on by the formation of cholesterol-containing masses called *plagues* in the walls of the blood vessels. They result in a rough surface that is perfect for the adhesion of platelets and is often the site of clotting. Clotting in an unbroken blood vessel is called *thrombosis*.

Coagulation Time. If normal blood is shed directly from a blood-vessel on to a clean watch-glass and the glass moved gently from side to side, the drop of blood ceases to move in three to ten minutes. Many mechanical devices have been invented to obtain a more accurate measurement but the practised observer usually prefers the simple method.

Bleeding Time. The time taken for a pricked ear, dried off with blotting-paper every quarter of a minute, to stop bleeding is known as the bleeding time, which is from two to four minutes. It depends not only on coagulability but on the power of the injured capillary to contract.

Prothrombase Time. Fullerton's method aims at the determination of the power of the prothrombase. It may also be used as a test for liver function as prothrombase is made there. The blood is kept at 37ºC., first decalcified by adding standard solution oxalate and made ready for clotting by the addition of brain extract. "The time between the addition of calcium and clotting is the *prothrombase time,* which is about twelve seconds."

Capillary Resistance Time appears also to be a valuable indication of the amount of cortisone circulating. A small cup is applied to the skin of the arm and a negative pressure produced in it (Robson and Duthie, 1950). The cup has interior illumination and a glass roof through which the skin can be seen. In the normal, about 300 mm. Hg. is necessary to produce ten petechiae (minute haemorrhages).

Fibrinolysis

In the living animal fibrin formation is an intermediate step in a variety of physiological and pathological processes; such as in haemostasis during menstruation and a parturition; in the inflammatory response to infection and trauma; and in reactions to cancer cells in the circulation and tissues. In many cases fibrin formed within blood vessels is rapidly dissolved to restore the fluidity of the blood, in others the fibrin becomes hyalinized or is removed by phagocytes and replaced by connective tissue. The process of liquefaction of fibrin is known as fibrinolysis; it may occur as rapidly as blood coagulation itself. Fibrinolysis also resembles blood clotting in being the end result of a chain of enzyme reactions involving components from both plasma and tissues.

The main plasma component of the fibrinolytic system is *plasminogen* (profibrinolysin), inactive precursor of the proteolytic enzyme *plasmin* (fibrinolysis). Plasmin also splits protein other than fibrin and fibrinogen such as gamma globulin, casein, gelatin, blood clotting factor V, VIII and IX, kinnogens (to produce vasoactive kinins) and chondromucoproteins. Plasmin is rapidly destroyed by *antiplasmins,* from the α_1 and α_2-globulin fractions of plasma. α_2-Antiplasmin acts by the rapid formation of a complex with plasmin. The complex is readily dissociated by attachment of the plasmin to insoluble protein substrates, especially fibrin. α_2 Antiplasmin acts more slowly to form a more stable, non-reversible complex with plasmin. There is sufficient of these two inhibitors in the plasma to neutralize the plasmin resulting from the total transformation of all of the blood plasminogen. For this reason plasmin is not detectable in blood unless fibrin is added to dissociate the α_2-globulins-plasmin complex. These unique inhibitory arrangements render the action of this non-specific proteins highly selective for fibrin. Many drugs have been used as inhibitors of fibrinolysis, the most effective are ε-aminocaproic acid (IACA) *tranexumic* acid (p-aminomethyl-cyclohexane carboxylic acid AMCHA) and trasysol (a polypeptide extract from bovine salivary glands, which also inhibits trypsin and kallikrein).

The transformation of the enzyme precursor, plasminogen, to the active form, plasmin, requires the presence of an activator simply referred to as *plasminogen activator.* Substances having an activating effect on plasminogen are found in small amounts in

PLASMINOGEN (A globulin)

↓ **ACTIVATORS** of plasminogen

(a) In blood

(b) In tissues

(c) In urine (urokinase)

(d) From micro-organisms (strep to leuine)

EACA blocks ------------------→

Two inhibitors in blood -------→

ANTIPLASMIN ---------------→ **PLASMIN** (a proteolytic enzyme)
(a_1 and a_2 globulins)

↓

EACA blocks ------------------→ **FIBRIN** (a protein)

↓

SOLUBLE PRODUCTS (polypeptides)

Fig. 1.10.— The fibrinolytic system of plasma. EACA is ε-amino-n-caproic acid which interferes with the system at two points. Its action in blocking the activation of plasminogen is an example of competitive inhibition, that is it competes with plasminogen for activation. It inhibits the action of plasmin on fibrin in a non-competitive way. Two inhibitors oppose plasminogen activator or the process of activation; one, stable at 37ºC appears in calculating plasma and a second labile at 37ºC is formed during coagulation or thrombus formation in the presence of calcium.

the blood and in high concentration in the tissues, especially in the endothelium of blood vessels. Urine contains an activator, urokinase; the activity of urine is more than that of blood but less than that of endothelial cells. Small amounts of proteolytic enzymes, such as trypsin and leucocyte protease, are also able to activate plasminogen, as can the lysosomal enzymes of many types of cell. The activating effect of these substances is, however, weaker and less specific than that of the plasminogen activators found in blood, urine and endothelium. In addition to endogenous agents,. activators of plasminogen have been obtained from various bacteria, moulds and plants. Of these the most important is *streptokinase,* a protein from cultures of haemolytic streptococci. In purified form this material is widely used to promote fibrinolytic activity in the circulating blood of patients with thrombosis. The mechanism of action of streptokinase on human plasminogen is still debated but appears to be more complex than that of endogenous activators and may involve an auto-catalytic mechanism.

Fibrinolysis has been studied by innumerable techniques. Fibrinolytic activity in whole blood is commonly measured by the *dilute whole blood clot lysis time technique.* Blood is diluted to diminish the effect of inhibitors clotted by thrombin and then incubated. The time taken for the clots to dissolve is a measure of spontaneous fibrinolytic activity. The other widely used method is the *euglobulin lysis time technique*. The plasma under test is diluted and acidified to precipitate the euglobulin fraction containing fibrinogen, plasminogen and plasminogen activator; much of the inhibitory activity remains in the supernatant. The precipitate is redissolved, clotted by the addition of thrombin, and the time taken for the clot to dissolve at 37°C is measured.

For testing the fibrinolytic activity of fluids other than plasma, such as urine and extracts of tissue the *fibrin plate* method is used. The substrate is fibrin prepared as a uniform layer in petri dish. The material to be tested is placed on the fibrin and the dish is incubated at 37°C to allow digestion of the fibrin substrate to take place. The diameter of the zone of digestion in the fibrin layer gives a measure of the fibrinolytic activity. A modification of this technique has been used to reveal the distribution of plasminogen activator in tissues. A thin section of fresh tissue is incubated on a thin layer of fibrin. Wherever there is fibrinolytic activity in the section the fibrin is digested. The areas of digestion show as clear spots when the preparation is stained and can be related to structures in the overlying section.

Fibrinolytic activity is detectable in the blood of normal subjects; is increased after exercise, after injection of adrenaline and in emotional stress; it shows a circadian rhythm being increased by day and diminished at night. Arterial blood contains less activator than venous and the activator content of the endothelium in arteries is generally less than that in the venous intima. The endothelium of arteries supplying the retina, myocardium and kidneys is an exception to this rule and has a high content of activator.

Some fibrinolysis seems to go on continuously in the circulating blood since fibrin degradation products (FDP) can be detected in the blood of healthy subjects. In cases of thrombosis and of excessive fibrinolysis the level of FDP may be greatly increased from the normal level of 2 to 10 μg/ml of plasma to as much as 760 μg/ml. At these high levels FDP have a heparin-like action on the thrombin-fibrinogen reaction and impair the stabilization of fibrin by factor XIII.

The physiological effects of fibrinolysis are still uncertain. There is no doubt about the existence of a thrombolytic effect but the influence of fibrinolysis on kinin systems and on the control of blood viscosity and flow have yet to be fully assessed.

2

The Lymph & Tissue Fluids

During its passage through the capillaries of the vascular system, the blood normally loses a certain quantity of water and protein as well as salts and other plasma constituents to the interstitial spaces, thereby forming the *interstitial fluid*, and as noted earlier, this fluid is the internal environment within which the cells and tissues of the body live and by which they are nourished.

The *lymph* essentially is interstitial fluid which enters the lymphatic vessels. Hence the composition of lymph is far more variable than that of the blood for a number of reasons. For example, the specific region of the body in which it originates, the nutritional state of the individual, and the degree of bodily activity all influence not only the composition but also the rates of formation and flow of this important body fluid. Following a discussion of the morphologic aspects of the human lymphatic system, the several factors affecting lymph composition and flow will be discussed.

General Functions of the Lymphatic System

Fundamentally, the lymphatic system provides an alternative and indirect route whereby interstitial fluid and its various constituents can be returned to the blood. Unlike the closed circulatory system, in which blood passes in a cyclic fashion throughout a complete circuit, the lymphatics provide a one-way system of drainage channels from the cells and tissues that lead back to the blood vascular system. Thereby fluids and substances which cannot be removed from the interstitial regions via direct reabsorption into the blood capillaries are removed continually from the interstitial compartment and at rates which are commensurate with their formation.

All of the tissues of the body have a lymphatic drainage system. Exceptions to this general statement are the superficial regions of the skin, the central nervous system, the deeper-lying regions of the peripheral nerves, the bones, and the endomysium of the skeletal muscles. Actually, however, even these tissues possess microscopic interstitial spaces through which fluid can percolate; therefore eventually the fluid from these regions also reaches a plexus of lymphatic vessels.

Approximately 90 per cent of the water which is filtered from the arterial end of a vascular capillary is reabsorbed by the time the blood reaches the venous end of the vessels as discussed. The remaining 10 per cent of the filtered water, now called interstitial

Table 2.1
Composition of Lymph Compared with that of Plasma[a,b]

Substance (Species[c])	*Lymph[d]*	*Plasma*
Na (M)	127.0 mEq/liter (T)	127.0 mEq/liter
K (M)	4.7 mEq/liter (T)	5.0 mEq/liter
Ca (M)	4.2 mEq/liter (T)	5.0 mEq/liter
Cl (M)	98 mEq/liter (T)	96.0 mEq/liter
Glucose (M)	124 mg % (T)	123.0 mg %
Urea (D)	23.5 mg % (C)	21.7 mg %
Creatinine (D)	140.0 mg % (C)	137.0 mg %
Amino acids (D)	4.8 mg % (C)	4.9 mg %
Phosphorus (D)		
Total	11.8 mg % (C)	22.0 mg %
Inorganic	5.9 mg % (C)	5.6 mg %
Protein (D)		
Total	4.89 gm % (T)	7.04 gm %
Albumin	2.34 gm % (T)	3.15 gm %
Globulin	2.36 gm % (T)	3.33 gm %

a. Data from Best and Taylor (eds). The physiological Basis of Medical Practice, 8th ed, 1996, Williams & Wilkins; Ruch, Patton (eds). Physiology and Biophysics, 19th ed, 1966, Saunders.

b. The data included in this table are approximate only, as the composition of the lymph can vary considerably depending upon many factors including the tissue and its state of metabolic activity. Thus lymph contains many enzymes, hormones, and metabolic by-products of the cells in addition to the substances listed. On passage through the lymph nodes, lymph also acquires a large cellular population, principally lymphocytes. Thus thoracic duct lymph may contain between 8×10^4 and 12×10^4 of these elements per mm^3, whereas peripheral lymph normally contains only a few hundred cells per mm^3.

c. M = man; D = dog.

d. T = thoracic duct lymph; C = cervical (peripheral) lymph.

fluid, enters the terminal lymphatic capillaries and as lymph is returned ultimately to the blood.

The fine structure of a single blind-ending terminal lymphatic capillary is shown in Figure 2.1. Note that the individual endothelial cells which form the walls of these

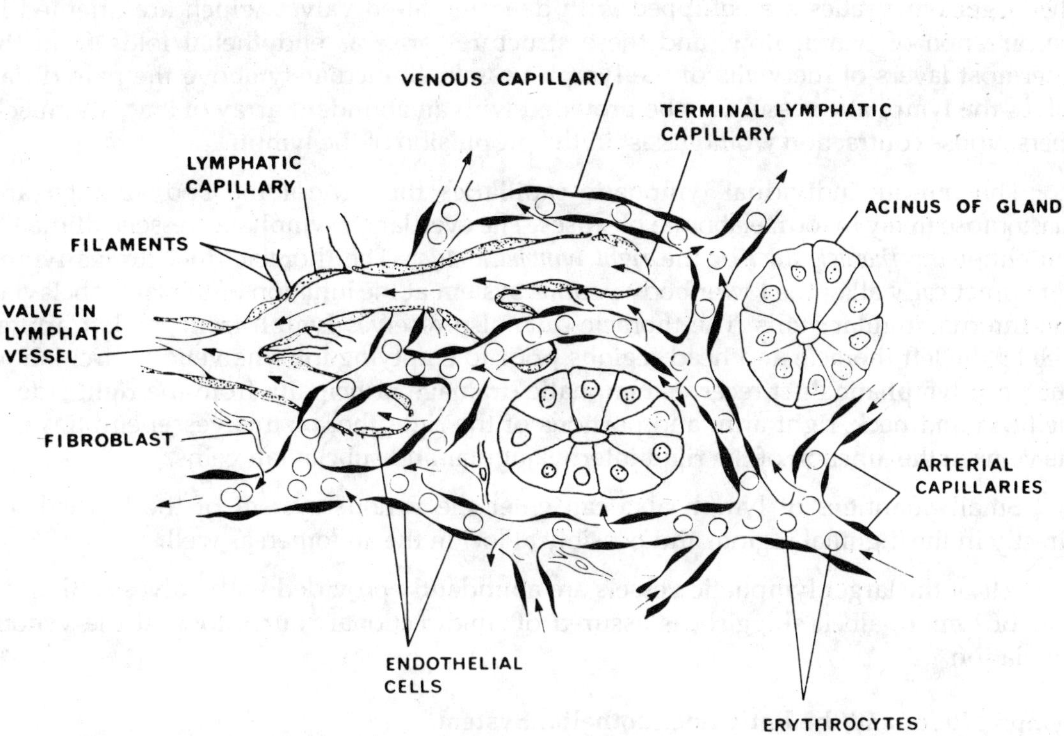

Fig. 2.1 The histologic relationships between a capillary network and the terminal lymphatics in an exocrine gland. The arrows signify the direction of flow of blood and lymph into and out of the interstitial fluid space.

vessels are contiguous but not continuous, as is the case with the endothelium of the vascular capillaries. The endothelial cells of the lymphatics merely overlap somewhat at their edges, thereby lending a high degree of permeability to the lymphatic capillaries. In fact, actual gaps may be present between the cells, and the basement membrane is imperfect or absent completely. Substances of high molecular weight, such as proteins, can pass almost unimpeded from the interstitial fluid into the lumen of the lymphatic vessels through the pores, a situation which is quite unlike that found in blood capillaries.

The inward-facing "flap-valve" disposition of the endothelial cells which permits only a one-way flow of interstitial fluid. The *anchor filaments* attached to the exceedingly delicate endothelial cells also tend to lend structural support to the vessels. As a consequence of this overlapping cellular arrangement, inteistitial fluid, once it has entered a terminal lymphatic capillary, cannot escape readily. This is true because an increased pressure within the vessel closes the pores in the vessel wall by causing mechanical apposition of the edges of adjacent endothelial cells. In addition, the lymphatic channels having a diamete larger than 100 to 200μ are invested with progressively heavier layers of elastic and collagenous connective tissue fibres, as well as smooth muscle bundles.

The larger lymphatics are equipped with delicate paired valves which are oriented in the direction of lymph flow, and these structures arise as endothelial folds from the innermost layers of the walls of the lymph vessels. Immediately above the paired flap valves the lymphatic vessel may be provided with an abundant array of smooth muscle fibers whose contraction would assist in the propulsion of the lymph.

The minute individual lymphatic capillaries throughout the body branch and anastomose freely to form elaborate plexuses. The ever-larger lymphatic vessels ultimately join either the *thoracic duct* or the *right lymphatic duct*. The thoracic duct drains lymph from practically all of the lower body venous system at the junction of the left subclavian and internal jugular veins. The thoracic duct also receives lymph from the left arm as well as the left thoracic and head regions prior to emptying into the venous circulation. The right lymphatic duct receives lymphatic drainage principally from the right side of the head and neck, right arm, and portions of the right thorax; this vessel empties into the veins at the junction of the right internal jugular and subclavian veins.

Small quantities of lymph also can enter the venous system of the lower body directly in the inguinal region, and possibly at loci in the abdomen as well.

All of the larger lymphatic vessels are abundantly provided with valves so that the flow of lymph, albeit sluggish, is assured of unidirectional course toward the venous circulation.

Lymph Nodes and the Reticuloendothelial System

Situated along the larger lymphatic vessels at intervals are found highly organized flattened and rounded structures known as the *lymph nodes*. These nodes range between 1 and 25 mm in diameter and are especially prominent during certain infections in the cervical, axillary, and inguinal regions. Lymph nodes essentially are filters composed of connective tissue penetrated by afferent and efferent lymphatic vessels.

As noted above, the lymphatic vessels, unlike the vascular capillaries, are freely permeable to large molecules, and even to foreign particulate matter such as microorganisms. Consequently all such foreign matter upon entry into the interstitial compartment of the body must traverse the lymphatic system prior to entering the general circulation.

The lymphatic tissue within the lymph nodes comprises an essential portion of the so-called *reticuloendothelial system* (RES) of the body. The reticuloendothelial system itself is composed of various cells lining many vascular channels in addition to the lymph nodes, and these cells are capable of actively phagocytizing foreign bodies such as bacteria and viruses in addition to forming antibodies against these infectious agents as discussed earlier. Phagocytic cells of the reticuloendothelial system are found in the bone marrow, spleen, liver (Kupffer cells), and lymph nodes among many other tissues. All of these phagocytic cells are closely related and described by the general term *reticulum* (or *mesenchymal*) cells.

The stem or reticulum cell is a primitive element regardless of where it is found;hence it retains the latent potentiality of undergoing differentiation into many quite specialized

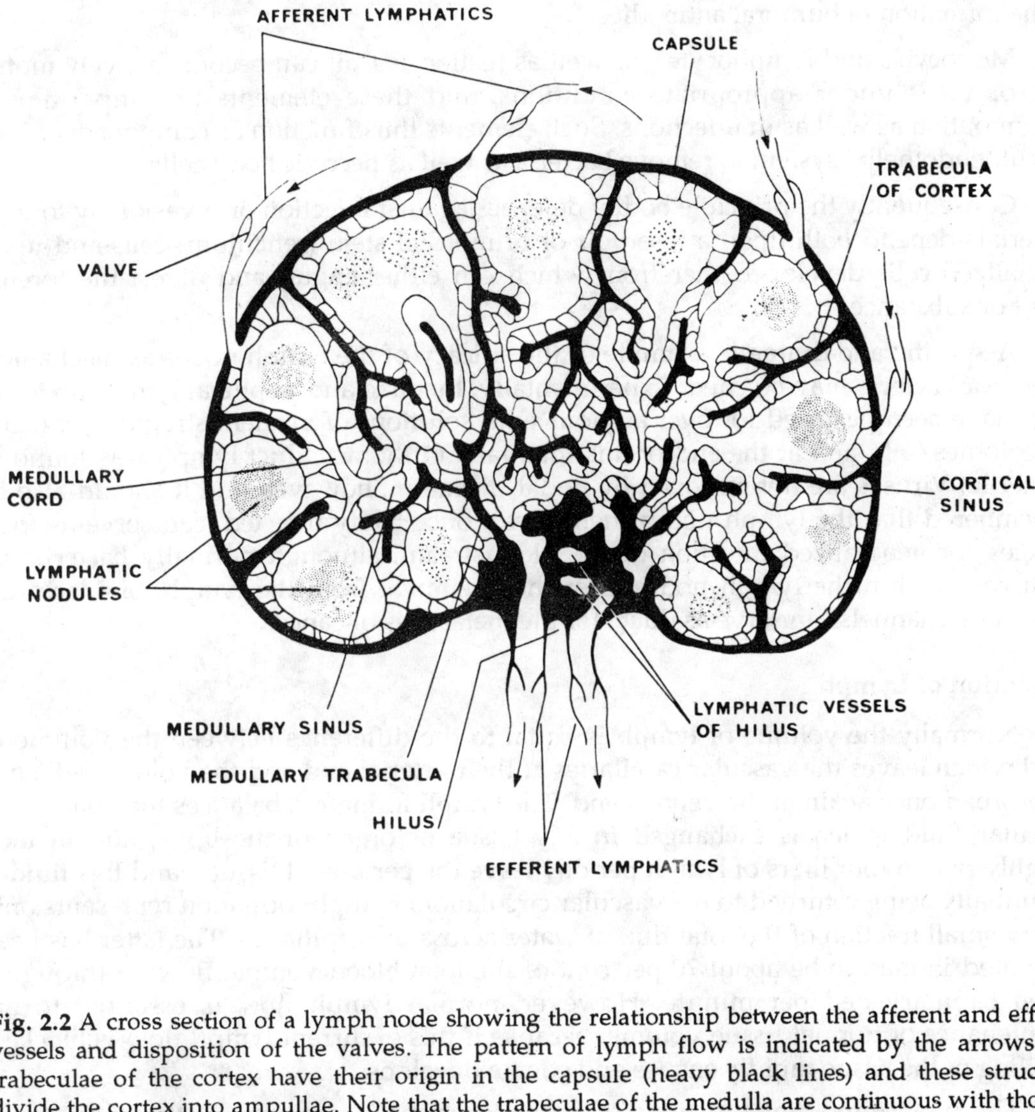

Fig. 2.2 A cross section of a lymph node showing the relationship between the afferent and efferent vessels and disposition of the valves. The pattern of lymph flow is indicated by the arrows. The trabeculae of the cortex have their origin in the capsule (heavy black lines) and these structures divide the cortex into ampullae. Note that the trabeculae of the medulla are continuous with those of the cortex. Blood vessels are not indicated.

cell types. Thus, reticulum cells in bone marrow (stem cells) can form either hemocytoblasts, which in turn form erythrocytes, or else may evolve into myeloblasts for the production of leukocytes. The reticulum cells also can form lymphocytes in the lymph nodes. The actively ameboid tissue *histiocytes* (or *clasmatocytes*) which wander constantly through the tissues as macrophages are related closely to the reticulum cells. These macrophages ingest and digest foreign particulate matter, microorganisms, and dead or necrotic body cells themselves. Histiocytes in traumatized tissues also can turn into fibroblasts and thereafter form collagen fibers to assist in wound healing. Primitive reticulum (or stem) cells also can develop into specialized *plasma cells*, which are essential to the formation of humoral antibodies.

Monocytes and lymphocytes, as well as histiocytes, all can become actively motile macrophages under appropriate conditions, and these elements are important in inflammation as well as in infections. Such elements thus function as components of the reticuloendothelial system to remove bacteria as well as necrotic body cells.

Consequently the principle bodily defenses against infection or invasion by foreign materials depend both upon a reservoir of primordial stem (reticulum) cells and upon specialized cells developed therefrom which can either engulf and digest the foreign agent or substance.

A specific and dramatic example of the efficacy of the lymph nodes as mechanical filters for bacteria may be cited. Experimentally, the iliac and popliteal lymph nodes of dogs have been perfused for over an hour with solutions of virulent streptococci (2.5×10^7 colonies/ml), and at the end of this interval and thoracic duct lymph was found to be sterile! Viruses are not removed by nodal filtration, however, and it should also be remembered that the lymph nodes themselves, once badly infected, can serve as focal sources for generalized infection of the bloodstream, although normally bacteria are destroyed within the lymph nodes after their removal from the lymph. Similarly the lymphatic channels can serve as ducts for the metastasis of cancer.

Formation of Lymph

Normally the volume of lymph is equal to the difference between the volume of fluid which leaves the vascular capillaries at their arterial end and the volume which is reabsorbed once again at the venous end. The lymph formation balances the quantity of vascular fluid which is exchanged in any tissue or organ of the body, and in man roughly two to four liters of lymph per day leave the peripheral tissues, and this fluid is continually being returned to the vascular circulation. Lymph formation represents only a very small fraction of the total flux of water across the capillaries. The latter has been estimated in man to be about 70 per cent of the total blood volume flowing through a given capillary bed per minute. However, normal lymph flow is essential to the maintenance of normal tissue volume, because if this excurrent lymph flow is blocked, swelling of the tissue rapidly ensues and edema develops.

The most important functions of normal lymphatic drainage of the body are to remove excess proteins and fluid from the interstitial spaces. There is no other channel than the lymphatics whereby proteins can be returned to the circulatory system, so that the continual removal of the protein from the interstitial space is critical to the life of the individual; and if this process is interfered with in any major way, normal capillary dynamics become so deranged that continued survival is impossible.

As stated earlier in this section, lymph is interstitial fluid which has entered the lymphatic vessels; the composition of this fluid reflects in nearly identical fashion that of the interstitial fluid in that part of the body whence it was derived.

The interstitial fluid protein concentration is low, on the average being about 1.8 gm/100 ml; this value also is the average protein concentration in the lymph which is derived from most of the peripheral tissues. Lymph produced in the liver, however, may have a protein concentration as high as 6 per cent, and intestinal lymph may contain 3 to 4 gm per cent protien. Since about one-half of the total lymph formed in the body is derived from the liver and intestines, the thoracic duct lymph contains roughly between 3 and 5 gm per cent protein in contrast to about 7 gm per cent in plasma.

The important role of the lymphatics in the absorption of nutrients, especially fats, from the gastrointestinal tract. It should be mentioned in passing, however, that after a fatty meal the thoracic dict lymph may contain a concentration of fat that can be as high as 1 or 2 per cent.

The fluid that is filtered out through the arterial end of the peripheral capillaries under the driving force of a hydrostatic pressure head developed by the heart normally contains around 0.15 per cent protein, although the interstitial fluid itself usually contains about 10 times more protein than this. The final concentration of about 1.5 per cent protein in the lymph results largely from the reabsorption of water at the venous end of the capillary, a process which concentrates the protien, whereas the concomitant reabsorption of protein back into the vascular capillary is negligible. The net result of the operation of these factors is that a marked concentration of the interstitial fluid (hence lymph) proteins develops.

Capillary Dynamics and Interstitial Fluid

Certain functional aspects of capillary dynamics now must be considered in relation to the formation of interstitial fluid, hence the lymph.

The vascular capillaries are the actual functional portion of the cardiovascular system, as it is here that the actual exchange of materials between the blood and the interstitial fluid takes place and vice versa. The true capillaries are the smallest vessels found in the blood vascular system, and these vessels have a diameter that ranges between 7 and 9 M. The capillaries are composed of a single layer of endothelial cells covered by a thin basement membrane so that the entire capillary wall is about 0.5 M. The ultrastructure of the capillary wall is such that minute pores between adjacent endothelial cells are present which have a diameter between 80 and 90 A. Although these submicroscopic pores represent only 0.001 per cent of the total surface area of the capillaries, they are of considerable functional importance as through these regions water and dissolved substances pass from the blood to the interstitial fluid and vice versa.

Diffusion is the major process whereby water and other substances traverse the capillary membrane, and this process can be exceedingly rapid. For example, the rate of diffusion for water across the capillary wall is about 40 times greater than the linear flow rate of plasma through the capillary.

The volume transfer of water between the capillaries and interstitial fluid across the endothelial interface is regulated by four major factors, and these factors in turn

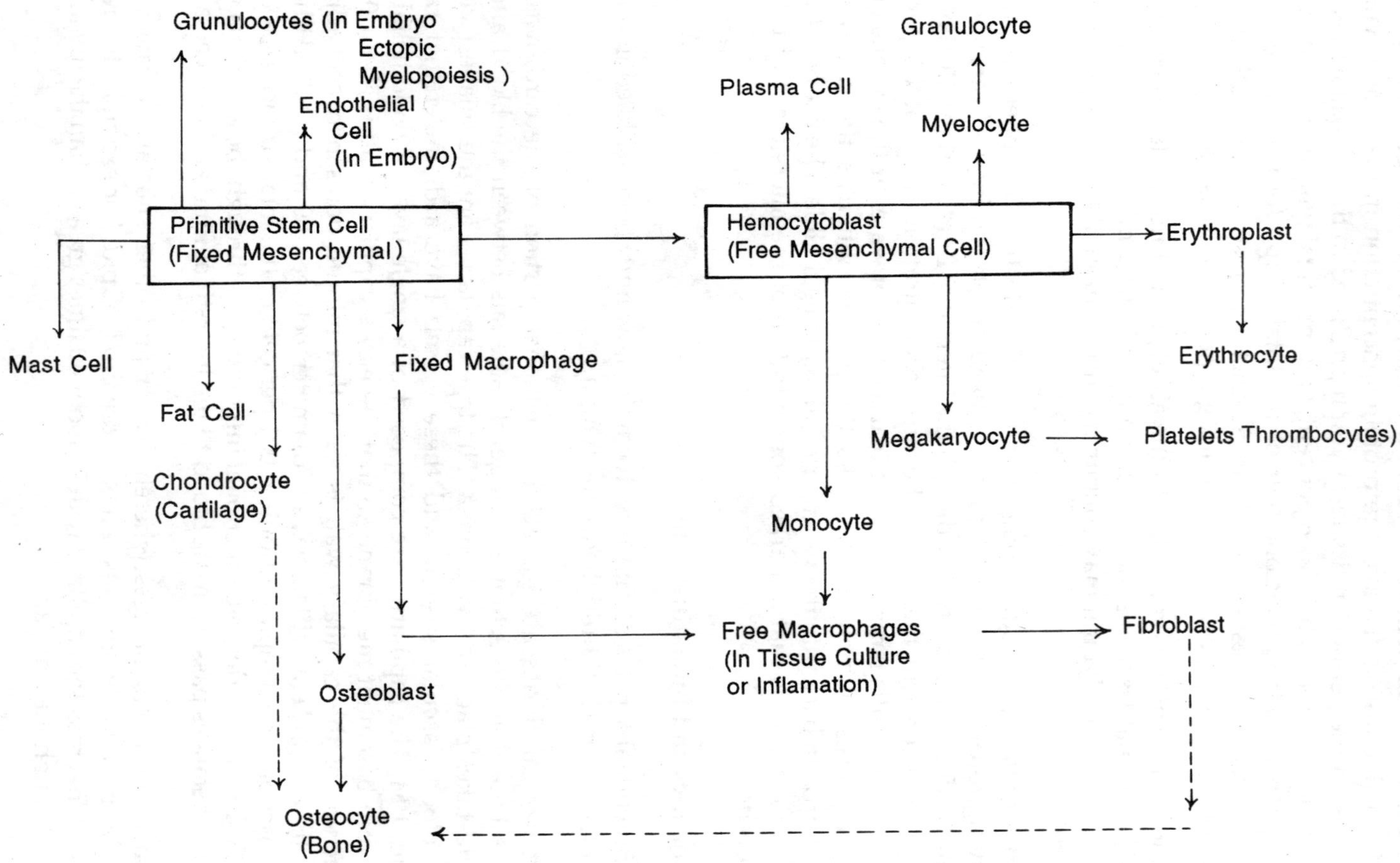

Fig. 2.3 The overall relationships among the primitive fixed stem (or reticular or mesenchymal) cell and the various cells of the blood and connective tissues. The dashed lines indicate potential transformations which can occur under special circumstances only (eg, neoplastic growth). Not all steps in the development of each cell type are indicated.

determine whether fluid moves out of, or into, the plasma. These important parameters involved in capillary dynamics may be considered individually (refer to Fig. 2.5).

First, the functional mean intracapillary pressure, which has been measured experimentally both directly and indirectly, appears to be approximately 17 mm Hg. Although the intracapillary pressure fluctuates widely under various physiologic conditions, it is generally conceded that at the arterial end of the capillary the average hydrostatic pressure tends to force fluid out of the capillaries.

Second, the interstitial fluid colloid osmotic pressure also tends to cause movement of fluid out of the capillaries, and this osmotic flow of water results from the movement of a normally small quantity of plasma proteins through the larger pores in the capillary membrane, thereby increasing the net osmotic pressure of the interstitial fluid (average 4.5 mm Hg; range 0-10 mm Hg). The plasma proteins found in the interstitial fluid are chiefly albumin and globulin, which are able to penetrate the capillary wall far more readily than the much larger fibrinogen molecules. Parenthetically, however, it should be noted that lymph clots when withdrawn from the body, and presumably the mechanism involved in this process is similar to that which is present in plasma. Therefore some fibrinogen must be able to escape from the lumen of the vascular capillaries into the extracellular fluid.

As the total volume of interstitial fluid in the human body is around 12 liters, the total quantity of protein in the interstitial fluid compartment is almost equal to that present in the plasma, despite the lower net concentration of protein that is found in the interstitial fluid.

Third, the interstitial fluid (or tissue) pressure tends to move fluid inward across the vascular capillary membrane. This pressure, like the capillary pressure, has been found extremely difficult to measure directly because of the tiny spaces involved (on the order of 1μ). However, indirect measurement of this factor by several techniques has indicated that this pressure normally is around - 7 mm Hg; that is, the interstitial fluid pressure actually is 7 mm Hg below atmospheric (ambient) pressure. Most investigators, however, consider the hydrostatic pressure of the tissues to range from 0 to +10 mm Hg. Hence this positive tissue pressure would, on the other hand, tend to steepen the outward hydrostatic pressure gradient between the capillary lumen and the interstitial fluid. This process must be subjected to further experimental evaluation before a definitive statement can be made insofar as any physiologic role can be ascribed to the negative interstitial fluid pressure in capillary dynamics.

Fourth, the plasma colloid osmotic pressure (or oncotic pressure) also tends to move fluid into the capillaries. This osmotic force is developed by the plasma proteins which are found in solution in the plasma at a total concentration of about 7 gm per cent, compared to around 1.8 gm per cent in the interstitial fluid. Most of the osmotic pressure developed in the plasma is due to the presence of these proteins which behave as a colloidal suspension even though they are in true solution within the plasma.

Furthermore, since the capillary membrane is impermeable to the vast majority of the plasma protein molecules that are present, these molecules increase the total colloid

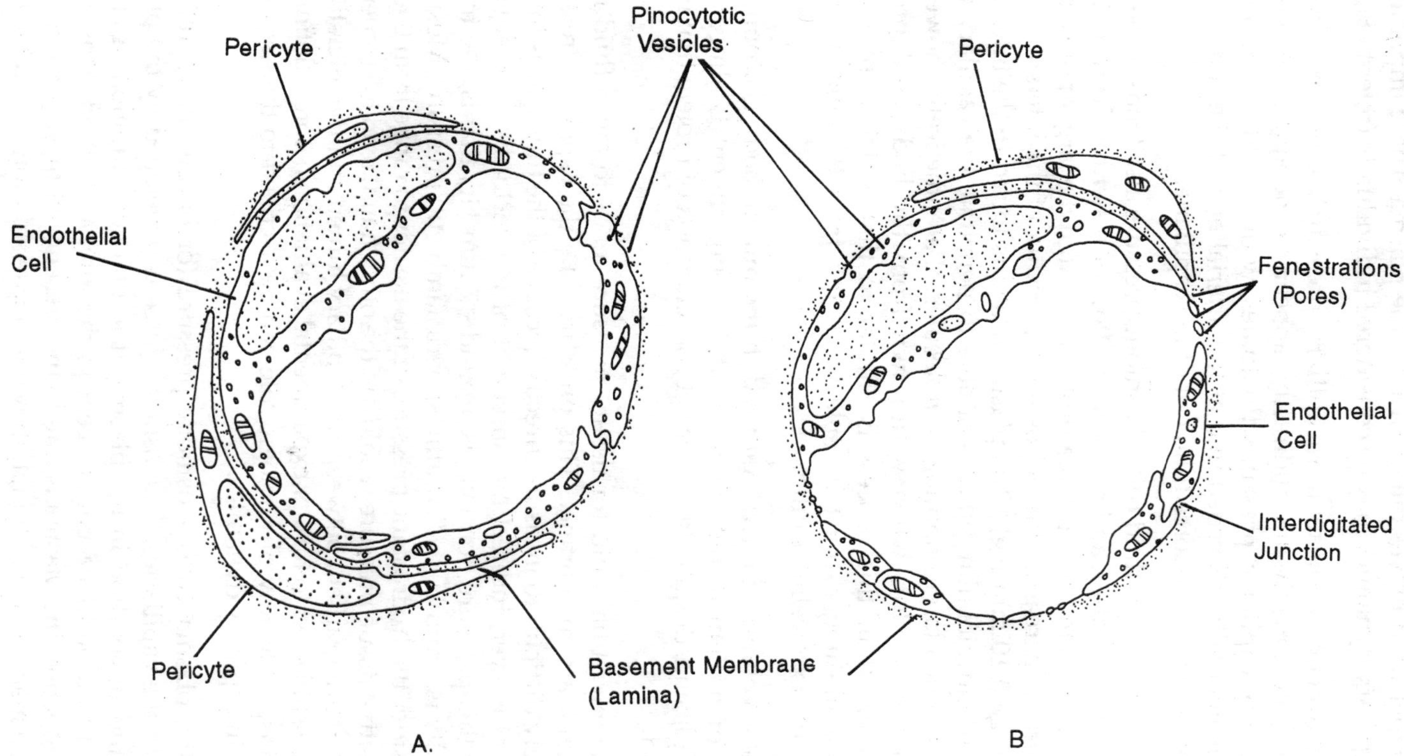

Fig. 2.4 The ultramicroscopic relationships among the principal elements that comprise a continuous (or "muscular") capillary having an uninterrupted endothelium (A), and a fenestrated capillary in which the endothelium varies in thickness, the thinnest areas having pores that are closed by extremely thin diaphragmatic membranes (B). The average wall thickness of both of these commonly-encountered types of capillary measured through the cytoplasmic portion of their component endothelial cells is about 0.5μ.

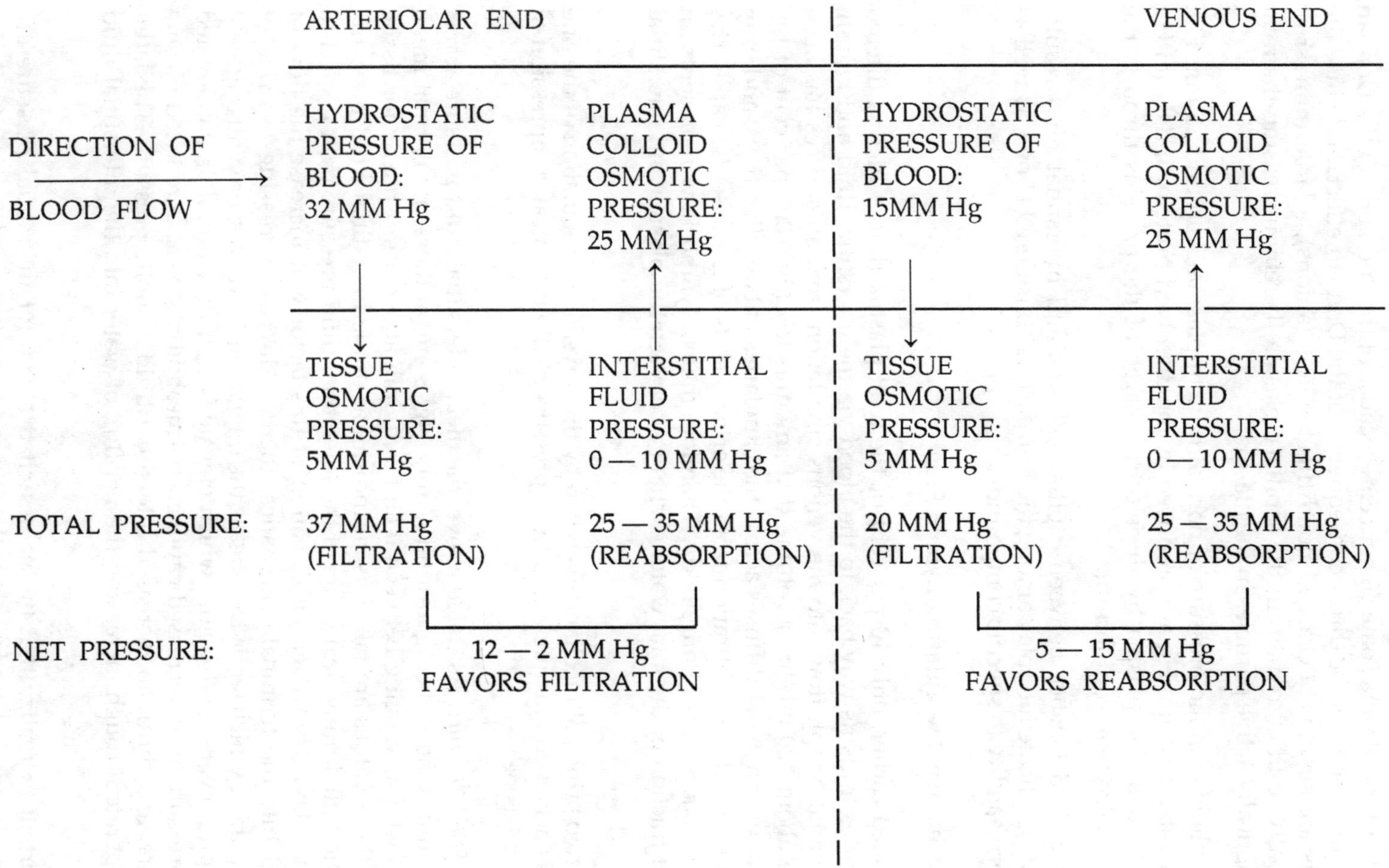

Fig. 2.5 Normal capillary dynamics in man according to the Starling hypothesis. The integrated mean capillary hydrostatic pressure is 17 mm Hg (Note: this mean pressure is not the arithmetic mean pressure. It is important to realize that there is a smooth and gradual transition in the magnitude of the hydrostatic pressures of the blood between the arteriolar and venous ends of the capillary and not a sudden and abrupt change as indicated between the left and right halves of the figure (vertical dashed line).

osmotic pressure of the plasma some 50 per cent, because of the operation of the Donnan equilibrium as discussed. As the direct consequence of the Donnan effect, and since the plasma proteins are negatively charged nondiffusible ions (anions), a large number of cations, principally sodium, remain in the capillary plasma thereby increasing the total number of osmotically active particles in the plasma.

The total colloid osmotic pressure of normal human plasma is around 25 mm Hg; and of this total, about 17 mm Hg are produced by the dissolved protein, and 8 mm Hg by the cations held in the plasma by the electric charge of the proteins through the participation of the Donnan equilibrium.

The relative fluid balance between capillary plasma and interstitial fluid results from an extremely delicate interplay among the four factors considered above, as well as the capillary permeability to specific compounds.

Physiologic Mechanisms Regulating Lymph Flow

As mentioned earlier, only 10 per cent of the total plasma fluid which is filtered from the capillaries finds its way back to the blood via the interstitial fluid and lymph. In humans, the total lymph flow into the venous circulation from all sources has been estimated to be about 120 ml/hr, a volume that amounts to only 0.001 per cent of the calculated rate at which water diffuses across the capillaries in both directions, and only 10 per cent of the rate of water filtration from the arterial ends of the vascular capillaries to the interstitial spaces in the entire body. Therefore the net lymph flow represents an extremely small fraction of the total water exchange between the plasma and interstitial fluid.

There are two principal mechanisms whereby the physiologic regulation of the rate of lymph flow is achieved, the interstitial fluid pressure and mechanical compression of the lymphatic vessels per se.

Interstitial Fluid Pressure. As stated above, the mean interstitial fluid pressure at rest normally is subatmospheric, being around -7 mm Hg. Some authors cite normal mean values for this factor as ranging between 0 and + 10 mm above atmospheric for tissue pressures, and these values are taken as an indication of the interstitial fluid pressure. Regardless of the actual numerical value of the interstitial fluid pressure with respect to the outside of the body, however, an elevation of this factor will increase the flow of interstitial fluid into the terminal lymphatics, thereby directly increasing the rate of lymph flow. Anything which tends to increase the interstitial fluid pressure will augment the rate of lymph flow. Several factors which elevate lymph flow are, first, an elevated intracapillary pressure or an increased capillary permeability; second, a reduced plasma osmotic pressure; and third, an increased interstitial fluid osmotic pressure. The latter factor would operate through increasing the net flux of water into the interstitial fluid compartment.

It is important to realize that the values cited above for interstitial pressure are mean levels only, and that under physiologic conditions these values can (and do) fluctuate markedly and rapidly both above and below the average values which are recorded under experimental conditions in anesthetized animals.

The "LYMPHATIC PUMP". Since not only the larger lymphatic capillaries but also the entire system of lymphatic vessels are supplied liberally with valves, then any mechanical pressure or massage, regardless of its cause, exerted upon a tissue or lymphatic vessel will cause movement of lymph in one direction only. This "lymphatic pump" ensures the slow but steady one-way progression of the lymph back into the blood vascular system. The rate of lymph flow thus may be augmented between 3 and 14 times above the resting level during exercise, because of the active muscular contractions, as well as by passive movements of the body, arterial pulsations, or external manipulation (compression) of the tissues.

Contraction of the smooth muscle fibers in the lymphatic vessels per se also would assist in the propulsion of lymph, although man lacks rhythmically pulsatile lymph hearts such as are found in the frog, bat, rat, and guinea pig.

Any process which impedes normal lymph flow or which increases the rate of interstitial fluid formation without a concomitant increase in the rate of lymph flow leads to a net accumulation of interstitial fluid of *edema*.

Miscellaneous Body Fluids

In this section a number of specialized extracellular body fluids will be discussed. These transcellular fluids, although present in the human body in rather small total individual volumes (Fig. 2.1), all serve a number of important and specific physiologic roles. The reader should note the intimate relationship that exists among the various transcellular fluids, the capillary blood, the interstitial fluid, and the lymphatic drainage. Although the individual transcellular fluids may have a composition that differs considerably from that of plasma, nevertheless water provides the continuum among these various fluids, and ultimately all are derived from blood constituents.

Cerebrospinal Fluid

The total volume occupied by the brain and spinal cord is approximately 1,650 ml; approximately 140 ml of this total volume is occupied by the cerebrospinal fluid (CSF). A principal function of this fluid is to act as a cushion for the brain, and as both brain and cerebrospinal fluid have essentially the same specific gravity, the brain literally floats within the skull.

Cerebrospinal fluid is found within the ventricles of the brain and in the subarachnoid space (between the arachnoid membrane and pia mater) which surrounds both the brain and spinal cord as well as in the cisterns, which are merely dilatations of the subarachnoid space in certain regions. The most important of these dilatations are the *cisterna magna*, which is located beneath and behind the cerebellum, the *cisterna pontis*, found on the ventral aspect of the pons, and the *cisterna basalis*, which also contains the arterial loop known as the circle of Willis.

Formation and circulation of cerebrospinal fluid. The principal site of formation of the cerebrospinal fluid is in the *choroid plexuses* which are located within the ventricles of the brain. These choroid plexuses are found in the temporal horns of the lateral ventricles, in the posterior region of the third ventricle, and in the roof of the fourth ventricle. These highly vascular tufted structures are composed of many small pouches which project into the ventricles of the brain, and are composed of pia mater, capillaries, and the ependymal cells which line the ventricles. The choroid plexus has an afferent arterial and efferent venous blood supply. The pia and ependymal cells form a richly vascular double-layered membrane termed the *tela choroidea.* The cerebrospinal fluid probably is formed by the ependymal cells lining the ventricles and spinal cord, although the total volume of CSF derived from this source probably is quite low.

The cerebrospinal fluid is being formed continually and reabsorbed at a rate of approximately 750 ml per day, and the net pressure of the CSF is regulated by a balance between these two factors. An average value for the cerebrospinal fluid pressure in a normal supine individual is 130 mm water (about 10 mm Hg), although considerable variations above and below this value may be encountered in practice.

The circulation of the cerebrospinal fluid takes the following pathway. From the lateral ventricles, the fluid passes through the foramina of Monro into the third ventricle; together with the additional fluid formed in the latter chamber, the cerebrospinal fluid then traverses the aqueduct of Sylvius into the fourth ventricle where more fluid is produced. The combined CSF fluid volumes thence pass through the two lateral foramina of Luschka as well as the antral medial foramen of Magendie into the cisterna magna. Thence the cerebrospinal fluid passes upward to the arachnoid villi of the cerebrum through the subarachnoid spaces and the small tentorial opening of the mesencephalon, whence it is reabsorbed.

Absorption of cerebrospinal fluid. The main route of absorption of the excess cerebrospinal fluid produced each day is through the arachnoid villi. These structures project from the subarachnoid spaces into the venous sinuses of the brain, and the trabeculae of the arachnoid membrane bulge through the venous walls, and thus provide highly permeable regions which allow free passage of cerebrospinal fluid, including protein molecules and particulate matter smaller than 1μ in diameter, into the blood. The interstitial fluid which is formed in the brain is absorbed partly by the arachnoid villi; hence together with the perivascular spaces these velli perform an important lymphatic function in the central nervous system as this structure lacks any true lymphatic drainage as mentioned earlier.

The perivascular spaces themselves are formed as the superficial vessels of the brain penetrate inward, thereby carrying a layer of pia mater with them as they course away from the subarachnoid space. The open space which is located between the pia and the vessel is termed the *perivascular space*, and these regions persist along the course of the vessels down to the level of the arterioles and venules. There is no pia mater present about the capillaries of the brain. The perivascular spaces thus provide the main channels for the transport of interstitial fluid formed by the brain to the arachnoid villi, and the subarachnoid space capillaries from which this fluid is absorbed.

Composition of cerebrospinal fluid. Certain major constituents of the cerebrospinal fluid were listed in Table 2.4 compared with plasma. Note that the composition of cerebrospinal fluid differs in certain important features from that of plasma. For example, the sodium content is about 7 per cent higher, whereas glucose is 30 per cent lower and the potassium content also is lower, being around 40 per cent less than that found in plasma. Note also the considerably lower concentrations of protein and glucose in cerebrospinal fluid compared to plasma. Obviously the cerebrospinal fluid is not a simple plasma filtrate; rather it is a secretion which is produced actively by the choroid plexus. Furthermore, judging from the quantitative differences between CSF and plasma for specific solutes, the choroid also is quite selective in its functions.

It is believed that the cuboidal choroid epithelial cells secrete sodium ions into the cerebrospinal fluid by an active transport mechanism. This active process in turn builds up a net positive charge; hence chloride and other anions move passively together with the sodium into the cerebrospinal fluid. This ionic surplus increases the osmotic pressure of the fluid to about 160 mm H_2O within the ventricles of the brain; therefore large volumes of water, containing other permeable solutes, move across the choroid membrane and into the ventricles. The glucose concentration remains low, as this substance is not as freely diffusable as water. Potassium ions, presumably, are transported actively out of the cerebrospinal fluid; hence their concentration is maintained at low levels.

Interestingly, the total concentration of osmotically active constituents within cerebrospinal fluid is 9 milliosmols above the plasma, and this value corresponds to an osmotic pressure of 160 mm H_2O as noted above, a fact which provides the basis for the osmotic theory of cerebrospinal fluid formation presented above.

Cerebrospinal fluid pressure. The pressure of cerebrospinal fluid within the central nervous system depends upon two reciprocal factors: the relative rates of secretion and absorption of the CSF. Normally these factors are in an exceedingly delicate balance so that the total volume, hence the pressure, remains essentially constant when measured under identical conditions in any particular individual. Any imbalance between these two factors can lead to severe defects.

Blood-Brain and Blood-Cerebrospinal Fluid Barriers. The membranes between the blood and cerebrospinal fluid as well as the blood and the brain per se are not freely permeable to all substances. These so-called *blood-brain* and *blood-cerebrospinal fluid barriers* are present in the choroid plexus and in the vascular tree of all other regions of the brain parenchyma, save the hypothalamic region, which is particularly sensitive to variations in the concentrations of extracellular fluid components. Functionally, both of these barriers are freely permeable to water, oxygen, and carbon dioxide; however, they are only slightly permeable to electrolytes (eg., sodium, potassium, and chloride ions), and practically impermeable to certain drugs that are used therapeutically.

The blood-cerebrospinal fluid barrier is caused by the high functional impermeability of the choroid epithelial cells to certain substances, as the passage of such materials into the cerebrospinal fluid requires that the substance first must pass through both the capillary endothelium and subsequently the epithelial cells of the choroid plexus.

Perilymph and Endolymph

Periotic Fluid Or Perilymph. The perilymph fills the periotic labyrinth of the inner ear, which consists of the vestibule, semicircular canals, scala vestibuli, and scala tympani. The perilymph also is in direct communication with the cerebrospinal fluid in the subarachnoid spaces which surround the brain via the *perilymphatic duct.*

The perilymphatic fluid is considered to be an ultrafiltrate of blood. The capillaries of the spiral ligament have been implicated both in the formation as well as in the reabsorption of perilymph.

Otic Fluid Or Endolymph. The endolymphatic fluid is found within the otic labyrinth, i.e., in the cochlear duct (scala media), utricle, saccule, and within the three semicircular canals. The endolymph probably is secreted by cells of the stria vascularis, as well as by secretory cells which are associated with the neuroepithelial structures of the vestibule. The endolymphatic sac, which lies between the dura and periosteum of the interior surface of the petrous bone, has been implicated in the reasbsorption of endolymph.

Despite the minute volume of endolymph which is available for sampling and analysis, it has been established definitely that the ionic composition of this fluid is quite different from either perilymph or cerebrospinal fluid as indicated. Endolymph contains very high concentrations of potassium ions, and thus resembles intracellular fluids in this regard. Perilymph, on the other hand, is similar to other interstitial fluids insofar as its ionic composition is concerned.

The fluid within the organ of Corti(tentatively named *cortilymph*) must have a composition at least resembling perilymph, as the high potassium ion concentration of the endolymph would completely preclude impulse conduction within the unmyelinated fibers of the hair cells. Possibly the ionic constitution of the endolymph plays a role in the genesis of the endocochlear potential, although this statement is conjecture which at present is unsubstantiated by any direct experimental evidence.

Intraocular Fluids: Aqueous Humor and Vitreous Humor

The intraocular fluids of the eye perform the important function of distending the eyeball mechanically; hence the intraocular fluids maintain the retina and cornea in an exceedingly precise alignment with respect to the lens and other elements of the eye.

The Aqueous Humor. This clear, freely flowing liquid portion of the intraocular fluid is found to the front, as well as at the sides, of the lens.

Formation, Composition, and Properties of Aqueous Humor. In the human eye, aqueous humor is formed at an average rate of about 0.1 ml^3 per minute, and nearly all of this fluid is secreted by the ciliary processes. These structures are folds having a total area of about 6 cm^2 in each eye, and they extend from the ciliary body into the posterior chamber. This latter region is circumferentially located around the eyeball, behind the iris, and just behind the ligaments of the lens.

The exceedingly transparent aqueous humor has a composition resembling that of an ultrafiltrate of plasma; hence the protein concentration is quite low, ranging between 10 and 20 mg per 100 ml in humans. Other significant differences between the plasma and the aqueous humor are that the latter fluid has a lower glucose and higher lactic acid content. Furthermore, the ascorbic acid (vitamin C) concentration in aqueous humor is between 15 and 20 times higher than that of plasma. The pH of the aqueous fluid is between 7.1 and 7.3, the specific gravity is 1.002 to 1.004, and the refractive index is 1.33.

The aqueous humor presumably is derived from the blood within the capillaries of the ciliary processes by a mechanism similar to that already described for the formation of the cerbrospinal fluid. That is, active intraocular transport of sodium results, in the osmotic movement of water and additional solutes into the eyeball. In partial support of this concept for the formation of aqueous humor, it has been determined that the osmolar activity of his fluid is 3 to 6 milliosmols higher than that of the plasma. This difference is far more than sufficient to produce water movement across the membrane which is quantitatively adequate for the normal production of aqueous humor. Furthermore, studies conducted directly upon the epithelial membrane of the ciliary processes have revealed that sodium is transported actively by this tissue in quantities which again are quantitavely adequate to account for the intraocular osmotic activity that is essential to the operation of an osmotic mechanism for the production of aqueous humor. Other substances, including amino acids, also are transported actively thereby secreted into the aqueous humor of the eye.

The capillaries of the choroid and the retina function primarily to maintain the integrity of the latter structure; however, minute quantities of fluid from these vessels also can pass into the aqueous humor of the vitreous body.

The capillaries within the iris are concerned primarily with the nutrition of this structure. However, because of its strategic position in the middle of the aqueous humor, approximately 40 per cent of certain ions in the aqueous humor can diffuse rapidly both into and out of the iris. Phagocytic properties are well developed in the surface epithelial cells of the iris; consequently particulate matter is eliminated readily from the aqueous humor by this mechanism, and this in turn helps to maintain the crystal clarity of this fluid.

Circulation and Absorption of Aqueous Humor. Following its secretion by the ciliary processes, the aqueous humor flows between the ligaments supporting the lens, through the pupil, and into the anterior chamber of the eye. Thence the aqueous humor passes into the angle between the lens and the iris, the so-called iridocorneal angle, through the trabeculae, and into the canal of Schlemm. The latter structure actually is a thin-walled vein running circumferentially around the eye. This vessel is unusual in its extremly high degree of permeability (even small particulate material and proteins can pass readily through its wall), and also for the fact that it is usually filled with aqueous humor instead of blood, despite its being a true vein in the anatomic sense. In addition, the small veins which drain the canal of Schlemm also are usually filled with aqueous humor; hence these vessels are called *aqueous veins*. As one consequence of this unusual venous arrangement, a lymphatic drainage system for the eye is unnecessary because of the direct removal of proteins together with water and other susbtances by their direct passage into a vein (the canal of Schlemm). This situation is unique, as only in the eye do proteins pass directly into the venous circulation.

Vitreous Humor. Sometimes also called the *vitreous body* (or *corpus vitreum*) because of its gel-like consistency, this portion of the introcular fluid owes its viscosity to a dense fibrillar network of transparent proteinaceous fibers. The aqueous humor which fills the eyeball behind the lens is freely, but vey slowly, interchangeable within this matrix. Thus very leisurely diffusion is the process whereby the vitreous humor and the substances contained therein are exchanged, a fact that is in marked contrast to the active flow of liquid within the aqueous humor proper which fills the anterior part of the eyeball.

Intraocular Pressure. Normally the average intraocular pressure when measured directly with a manometer connected to a needle inserted within the anterior chamber ranges from 10 to 22 mm Hg (average about 16 mm Hg). Indirectly, the intraocular pressure can be measured by means of a tonometer, a device which is placed directly upon the surface of the anesthetized cornea. A pressure sufficient to deform the cornea is applied by a piston within this instrument, which is calibrated in such a way that the applied force can be related directly to the intraocular pressure.

Although not entirely understood in detail, the mechanism for regulating the introcular pressure at a constant level throughout the lifetime of individual is remarkably precise. It is believed that the principal regulatory mechanism for the intraocular pressure resides in the outflow resistance against the flow of aqueous humor into the canal of Schlemm. Thus an augmented intraocular pressure presumably lowers the outflow resistance by distending the trabeculae leading to the canal of Schlemm, thereby increasing the outflow of aqueous humor until the pressure becomes stabilized at normal levels once again.

Obviously alterations in the rate of secretion of the aqueous humor at a constant outflow resistance, as well as variations in the resistance to outflow of the aqueous veins themselves, also could effect the intraocular pressure markedly.

Fluids Within the "Potential" Body Spaces

The transcellular fluids included within this broad classification are in the *pleural, pericardial, peritoneal,* and *synovial cavities* (or both the joints and the bursae) as well as the *tunica vaginalis* surrounding the testes. Normally, these regions of the body are "dry" (actually, moist), and contain at most only a few milliliters of fluid which serves to lubricate the surfaces of the various organs and structures which move in contact with each other. In certain pathologic circumstances, however, these regions can swell to contain enormous volumes of fluid, hence the term "potential" spaces is applied to such regions of the body.

Since the membranes surrounding each of the several potential spaces listed above are freely permeable to water as well as to most solutes, they offer little resistance to the passage of fluid and electrolytes in either direction between the space and the surrounding interstitial fluid.

Protein collects in the various potential spaces, as it does in the interstitial fluids, by leakage out of the capillaries. However, each of these spaces is related either directly or indirectly to terminal lymphatic vessels as discussed below, so that normally only very small quantities of free liquid are present.

The lymphatic pump as discussed earlier, operates almost continuously to move fluid into or toward lymphatic drainage vessels from the potential spaces. Therefore various movements of the body are associated in general with maintenance of the potential spaces, as each of these movements, may exert a mechanical compression which forces (or "milks") the fluid into or toward lymphatic vessels. Protein and other osmotically active substances thus are removed continuously, and the spaces normally remian "dry" save for a thin film of liquid on the surface of the various structures which are present in any particular space.

Any pathologic changes in capillary dynamics and which cause extracellular edema, also can produce a greatly increased fluid volume and higher pressures wihin the potential spaces. Consequently, a decreased plasma colloid osmotic pressure, an increased colloid osmotic pressure of the fluid wihin the space, an increased capillary pressure or permeability, or an obstruction of the lymphatics which drain a potential space all can produce an increased fluid volume within that space. The fluid which collects following the operation of any one of these mechanisms is known as a *transudate* if it is characterized by a low content of cells and/or by a low concentration of materials derived from cells, e.g., protein. Thus transudates in general are characterized by a low viscosity, i.e., a high fluidity. An *exudate*, on the other hand, typically contains high concentrations, of protein, cells and the solid material derived from cells such as is seen following the operation of an inflammatory process. Consequently the viscosity of an exudate is much higher than that of a transudate. Furthermore a transudate usually (but not invariably!) is sterile, whereas exudates usually are not, since they frequently are produced by the action of microorganisms such as bacteria. Excessive fluid in the peritoneal cavity is referred to specifically as *ascites*, whereas a generalized edema or interstitial fluid accumulation is known as *anasarca*.

The several potential spaces and certain unique features which are related to each of them now may be considered.

The Pleural Cavity. The mechanism whereby diffusion of fluid into and out of this space takes place is exactly the same as that which obtains in the tissues, save that a very permiable serous membrane, called the parietal and visceral pleura (depending upon its location) is situated between the capillaries of the thoracic structures and viscera of the pleural cavity itself. The mediastinal and lateral surfaces of the parietal pleura contain numerous lymphatics; therefore during expiration the intrapleural pressure rises thereby forcing fluid into, as well as along, the lymphtics.

Within the pulmonary capillaries, the blood pressure is relatively low, about 5 to 10 mm Hg. The plasma proteins and electrolytes, however, exert a net colloid osmotic pressure of some 25 mm Hg; thus a continuous pressure exists at the surface of the visceral pleura of some 20 mm Hg, and this pressure tends to withdraw fluid from the pleural cavities into the pulmonary capillaries. As a consequence, the net pressure of the film of fluid within the intrapleural space averagee - 10 to - 12 mm Hg with respect to atmospheric. Since this continuous negative pressure is greater than the elastic (or "collapse") force of the lungs (-4 mm Hg), these structures remain permanently expanded. The thin film of fluid that lines the pleural cavity is essential, however, to the lubrication of the lungs during normal respiratory excursions.

The Pericardial Cavity. This potential space surrounding the heart has similar fluid dynamics to those found within the pleural cavity. The intrapericardial hydrostatic pressure also is negative, and like that of the pleural cavity, the pressure within the pericardial cavity also fluctuates rhythmically due to contractions of the heart as well as the respiratory motions. The small quantiy of pericardial fluid functions like that present in the pleural cavity.

The Peritoneal Cavity. The fluid dynamics of the peritoneal cavity are similar to those found in other potential spaces of the body. Hence fluid is filtered through both parietal and visceral peritoneal membranes, and this serous fluid also is reabsorbed through them. However, the pepritoneal cavity is more subject to the development of a fluid excess than are the other potential spaces for two reasons. First, whenever the pressure within the hepatic sinusoids increases above 5 to 10 mm Hg large quantities of fluid containing a high concentration of protein exude through the surface of the liver directly into the peritoneal cavity. The result is increased osmotic pressure within the peritoneal fluid that results in an osmotic movement of water into the peritoneal cavity; thus the volume of fluid increases until equilibrium is attained. Second, the capillary pressure within the visceral peritoneum is much higher than in other regions of the body because of the vascular resistance to blood flow to the liver that is present within the portal veins. Any increase in the intrahepatic resistance is reflected in a retrograde increase in the vascular pressure within the visceral capillaries, and this pressure increase can lead directly to an increased filtration of fluids from the visceral peritoneal capillaries directly into the abdominal cavity.

Infection is a very common cause of increased fluid volume (or *ascites*) in the peritoneal cavity; the exuded cells and debris may obstruct the lymphatics, thereby leading to an increased protein concentration and resultant increased osmotic pressure in the ascites fluid with an attendant failure of fluid reabsorption. Elevated central venous pressures which may be inducted by portal vein occlusion, hepatic cirrhosis, carcinoma, or cardiac failure all can lead to ascites fluid accumulation within the abdominal cavity.

Lymphatic drainage from this potential space is effected principally through large vessels located throughout the peritoneal cavity and especially on the inferior surface of the diaphragm. The latter structure, of course, moves rhythmically during respiration thereby pumping large quantities of lymph into the thoracic duct with each movement.

The Synovial Cavities. The synovial cavities include the bursae of the skeletal muscles as well as the joint cavities and the tendon sheaths. These tissue spaces contain large quantities of mucopolysaccharides of unknown origin which add viscosity to the synovial fluid (or synovia), thus augmenting its lubricant function. In fact, the viscosity of the synovia resembles that of raw egg white.

The synovial fluid is a typical interstitial fluid, save for the polysaccharides referred to above, and the fibrous tissue membranes lining the several synovial cavities normally offer only slight resistance to reabsorption, hence drainage, of this fluid from these spaces.

Intracellular Fluids

Because of their special significance to the bioelectric aspects of excitation, conduction, and contraction, the intracellular ionic and other constituents of muscle and nerve have received more research attention than the intracellular components of many other cell types. The intracellular composition of erythrocytes also has been investigated in some detail because it is a simple matter to prepare large quantities of these elements for analysis.

It is, of course, impossible to make any accurate generalizations about the intracellular fluids of different cell types because extremely wide qualitative as well as quantitative differences are found normally in the cell populations that make up the various body tissues. Furthermore, even the same cell type may exhibit marked differences in its compositions depending upon such factors as age, state of functional activity, and so forth. In addition to the tables referred to above, specific data concerning the intracellular components and biochemical structure of particular cell types will be cited in context throughout the remainder of the is book.

Abnormalities of Cerebrospinal Fluid Pressure

As noted earlier, the normal pressure of the cerebrospinal fluid is maintained by an exceedingly delicate balance between the rate of formation and the rate of absorption of this fluid. Any factor or agent which alters this balance likewise can change the pressure of the CSF greatly. For example, a brain tumor which blocks the normal reabsorptive pathway for cerebrospinal fluid (e.g., in the tentorial opening), can produe tremendous increases in CSF pressure which may range up to 500 mm of water (37 mm Hg). Infection and intracranial hemorrhage also can induce marked elevations in the cerebrospinal fluid pressure. Normally, free cells are almost completely absent from this fluid, and the large quantities of these elements which appear during infection and in conjunction with an inflammatory swelling can block reabsorption of CSF by the arachnoid villi almost totally, thereby inducing massive increases in cerebrospinal fluid pressure.

Hydrocephalus, or excessive water within the cranium, also can augment the cerebrospinal fluid pressure greatly, and this condition may assume one of two clinical forms. Noncommunicating hydrocephalus, such as is caused by a block in the aqueduct of Sylvius, causes massive dilatation of the two lateral ventricles as well as the third ventricle of the brain, with a concomitant increase of cerebrospinal fluid pressure and a flattening of the brain against the skull. In newbron infants the entire head may swell to enormous dimensions because of such a defect. Permanent psychomotor damage may be extensive. Communicating hydrocephalus generally is caused by excessive development of the choroid plexus in newborn infants. Therefore in this condition the rate of formation of cerebrospinal fluid, consequently its pressure, are increased greatly, although the functional reabsorptive capacity as well as the anatomic channels for reabsorption are normal. Here, too, severe brain damage may result from the mechanical deformation of the neural tissue together with marked enlargement of the head.

Blockage of the central canal of the spinal cord (as by a blood clot or tumor) results in a marked fall in the pressure of the cerebrospinal fluid below the obstruction, as the cerebrospinal fluid normally must pass upward to the brain in order to be reasbsorbed.

Anatomically, the dura mater of the brain follows the optic nerve to the eye as a connective tissue sheath which terminates at the sclera. If the pressure of the cerebrospinal fluid is elevated markedly, this pressure is transmitted directly to the sheath of the optic nerve, thence to the retinal artery and vein which enter this sheath just behind the eyeball to pass into the retina of the eyeball together with the optic nerve. Therefore an elevated pressure in the optic sheath hinders the outflow of the blood in the retinal veins, thereby inducing increase capillary pressure throughout the eyeball with an attendant retinal edema. The tissues of the optic disc are especially sensitive to an increase capillary pressure; the edema developed within this region of the eye is much greater than elsewhere in the retina, and thus the degree of papilledema of the optic disc can be observed directly by an ophthalmoscope. This observation in turn is indicative of the alteration in cerebrospinal fluid pressure.

Edema

The rate of formation of interstitial fluid by the filtration of water and solutes from the plasma must be balanced precisely by the rates of lymph formation and lymph flow in order that a net accumulation of interstitial fluid, or *edema* not develop. Therefore under normal circumstances the fluid which is filtered from the capillaries in excess of that reabsorbed by the same vessels is prevented from accumulating in the interstitial spaces by lymph formation at a rate which balances that of production of interstitial fluid. If, however, there is a disturbance in any one (or more) of the physiologic regulatory mechanisms so that excess interstitial fluid accumulates within the tissues, then the condition of edema develops as the consequence of the derangement of the normal interchange and distribution of fluid. Edema per se is not a particular disease; rather this condition is a sign of an underlying disorder.

Edema may be generalized throughout the body or else localized in certain regions, depending upon the mechanism involved in its production. The four specific types of edema and some of their potential causes are given here, as they illustrate clearly the effects produced by a derangement of the normal mechanisms of fluid balance among blood, interstitial fluid, and lymph. The distinction among these mechanisms is important clinically as therapy is directed toward ameliorating the causative factor.

A.

(A) Mean Hydrostatic Pressure : 40 MM Hg
Colloid Osmotic Pressure : 25 MM Hg — 15 MM Hg ↓

Interstitial Fluid Pressure : 8 MM Hg
Tissue Colloid Osmotic Pressure : 1 MM Hg — 7 MM Hg ↑

B.

Mean Hydrostatic Pressure : 17 MM Hg
Colloid Osmotic Pressure : 14 MM Hg — 3 MM Hg ↓

(A)

Interstitial Fluid Pressure : 5 MM Hg
Tissue Colloid Osmotic Pressure : 10 MM Hg — 5 MM Hg ↓

C. Mean Hydrostatic Pressure : 17 MM Hg
(A) Colloid Osmotic Pressure : 5 MM Hg — 12 MM Hg ↓

Interstitial Fluid Pressure : 5 MM Hg
Tissue Colloid Osmotic Pressure : 1 MM Hg — 4 MM Hg ↑

D. Mean Hydrostatic Pressure : 17 MM Hg
Colloid Osmotic Pressure : 25 MM Hg — 8 MM Hg ↑

Interstitial Fluid Pressure : 17 MM Hg
(A) Tissue Colloid Osmotic Pressure : 25 MM Hg — 8 MM Hg ↓

Fig. 2.6. The four possible mechanisms for the genesis of edema. In all instances, blood flow is from left to right in the capillary (horizontal parallel lines). In each example, the principal abnormality (A) is indicated. The vertical arrows to the right signify the direction of the net pressures for filtration (downward) or reabsorption of fluid (upward). **A.** An elevated mean hydrostatic pressure results in an abnormally high outward (filtration) pressure of 8 mm Hg at the venous end of the capillary, hence an elevated rate of interstitial fluid formation and edema. **B.** An elevated capillary permeability (dashed lines) results in an excessive loss of plasma protein from the capillary to the interstitial fluid. Hence a concomitant decrease in the plasma colloid osmotic pressure as well as a neat increase in the tissue colloid osmotic pressure develps so that a greater-than-normal loss of fluid from capillary to interstitial fluid occurs (net outward pressure = 8 mm Hg) and edema develops. **C.** Hypoproteinemia results in a marked decrease in the colloid osmotic pressure of the plasma; hence an excessive net loss of fluid to the interstitial space occurs along an 8 mm Hg gradient, resulting in edema formation. **D.** Blockage of the lymphatic drainage channels results in a net accumulation of protein in the interstitial fluid and a concomitant increase in the tissue colloid osmotic pressure. Although the filtration and reabsorption pressures are about equal, edema develops nevertheless, because any excess fluid filtered out of the capillaries above that reabsorbed cannot be removed by the lymphatics; hence a massive edema ensues. Furthermore, any increase in the concentration of protein in the interstitial fluid would result in an osmotic removal of still more water from the plasma, thereby worsening the edema. The numerical values presented in this figure are indicative, but not necessarily absolute. For the normal interrelationships among the four dynamic factors which normally are responsible for regulating the volume of interstitial fluid (thus preventing edema).

First, an elevated capillary pressure induces edema as more fluid is filtered out of than is returned to the capillary. Hence excess fluid collects in the interstitial spaces until the interstitial fluid pressure increases sufficiently to balance the abnormally high intracapillary pressure.

Pathologic factors which increase the venous pressure produce this type of edema. For example, cardiac failure (principally of the right side of the heart), tends to produce an increased systemic venous pressure, and this results in a serious and generalized "cardiac edema" because the increased venous pressure is transmitted in retrograde fashion to the capillaries. venous thrombosis, on the other hand, causes a localized edema peripheral to the obstruction due to the increased intracapillary pressure in the vessels that normally are drained by the occluded vein.

Second, an increased capillary permeability causes excessive loss of plasma proteins to the interstitial fluid with an attendant rise in the colloid osmotic pressure of this extravascular compartment, whereas the osmotic pressure of the plasma concomitantly decreases as the plasma proteins are lost. The resulting osmotic imbalance causes the interstitial fluid pressure as well as volume to tend to increase, thereby producing edema.

Burns, insect bites, drugs, and bacterial toxins which interfere with the normal capillary permeability all may cause this type of edema.

Third, a decreased net plasma protein concentration, if of sufficient magnitude, can reduce the normal colloid osmotic pressure of the plasma to such an extent that edema develops. In this situation, more fluid leaves the capillary than can be reasbsorbed and progressive edema develops as the excess fluid accumulates in the interstitial space. Not only are severe burns attended by a loss of protein at the site of the injury due to an increased capillary permeability which causes edema as described above, but also this localized protein loss is complicated by an overall reduction in the circulating plasma protein concentration. If this net protein loss from the plasma is severe enough, then a generalized edema develops. Severe malnutrition with an attendant decrease in the total plasma protein concentration also can produce this type of edema.

Fourth, lymphatic obstruction produces edema directly because the protein normally drained from the tissue spaces via these channels is retained in the interstitial space, increasing the interstitial fluid colloid osmotic pressure markedly. As a consequence, excess fluid tends to collect in the tissues producing lymphatic occlusion to such an extent that a liimb or the scrotum may become enormous; the resulting severe edema is referred to specifically as *elephantiasis*. Lymphatic obstruction and edema also may occur following radical surgery for cancer in which malignant lymph nodes are deliberately extirpated and their vessels tied off in order to prevent spread (*metastasis)* of the tumor.

3

Blood-Forming Tissues

In body tissues generally, most cellular differentiation takes place in embryonic stages once and for all, proliferation and differentiation of blood cells continue throughout life. The life of an individual blood cell is short; mammalian erythrocytes, for example, appear to live, at the most, only a few months, and the life of some leukocytes appears to be measured in days or even hours. In consequence, an animal must retain throughout its existence **hemopoietic tissues** in which blood cells are constantly formed and must, in addition, provide for the removal of worn-out cells.

Students of the blood have devoted much study to blood cell formation; and some features of the process are still in doubt. Most other differentiated cells are parts of

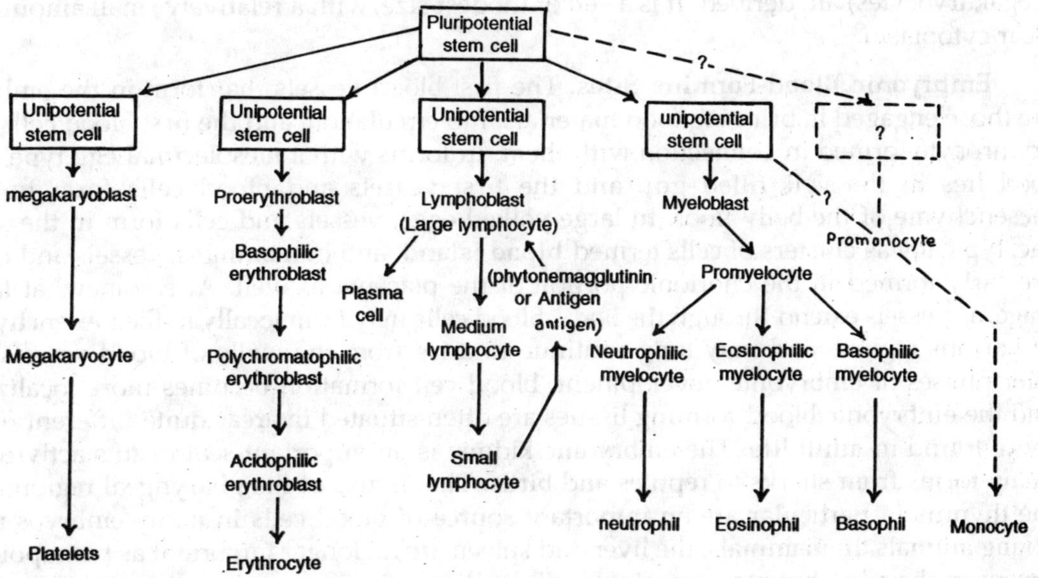

Fig. 3.1. Development of the various types of blood cells from pluripotential stem cells. This, representing the stages found in mammalian bone marrow, is still not completely worked out (note the quesiton marks along the possible paths to monocytes). We shall not attempt to describe or define the many types of cells that are involved.

tissues that are fixed in positions; their development takes place on the spot. But blood cells are free agents, and it is immaterial where they are formed, as long as the area is in communication with the blood vessels. Thus, blood-forming tissues are found in the most varied places in various vertebrates. Unlike most organ systems, little or none of the circulatory system is derived from any of the epithelial sheets laid down in the early embryo. Instead it is derived from mesenchyme cells—vessels and blood corpuscles alike—and thus from the same elements that give rise to the connective tissues.

Except for certain sites used in early embryonic stages, areas in which blood cells arise or are stored have, in general, common structural features. All are spaces that are enlargements of circulatory vessels or lie adjacent to such vessels. A network of fibers forms the "skeleton" of the tissue. Along the course of the fibers lie **reticular cells,** which are responsible for the formation of the fiber network. They are part of the **macrophage** system of the body—cells of phagocytic nature, having the power of engulfing waste or foreign materials, such as bacteria or damaged blood cells. Macrophages are not restricted to blood-forming tissues but may be found along the course of blood vessels, notably in the liver and spleen, or occur as free, ameboid, scavenging elements in the connective tissues.

Enmeshed within the reticular framework of a hemopoietic tissue are found masses of blood cells in process of multiplication and differentiation. The **pluripotential stem cell** or **hemocytoblast**—derived from the embryonic mesenchyme—is the primary unspecialized cell type, from which blood corpuscles of all sorts (erythrocytes, leukocytes, megakaryocytes) are derived. It is a cell of modest size, with a relatively small amount of clear cytoplasm.

Embryonic Blood-Forming Sites. The first blood vessels that form in the embryo are those engaged in bringing food materials into circulation, and the first blood cells are erythrocyte formed in connection with them. In forms with a mesolecithal egg type, the food lies in the yolk-filled gut, and the first vessels and blood cells form in the mesenchyme of the belly floor. In large-yolked eggs, vessels and cells form in the yolk sac, typically as clusters of cells termed **blood island**, and in mammals, vessels and cells are early formed in the chorionic portion of the placenta as well. At a somewhat later stage, as vessels extend through the body, blood cells may form locally in the mesenchyme of various regions and may long continue to arise from the walls of blood vessels. In later phases of embryonic development, blood cell formation becomes more localized, and the embryonic blood-forming tissues are often situated in areas quite different from those found in adult life. The embryonic kidney is an important seat of this activity in many forms from sharks to reptiles and birds. The tissues of the pharyngeal region and the thymus in particular are an important source of blood cells in many embryos and young animals. In mammals, the liver and spleen are no longer important as hemopoietic organs in the adult but play prominent roles in the embryo.

Thymus Gland. Almost universally present and highly important in early life is the thymus gland. This consists of clusters of soft glandlike material found in variable arrangement in the bronchial or throat region. When well developed, the thymus tissue is arranged in lobules, each containing a cortex and medulla. Characteristic are **reticular**

cells that form a network throughout the gland and constitute most of the bulk of the medulla. The cortex mainly consists of lymphocytes. In addition, there may be other histologic features—elongate muscle-like cells, spherical corpuscles that perhaps are masses of degenerating cells in the medulla, and so on. A thymus has not been definitely identified in hagfishes, although cells in some of the pharyngeal muscles show certain thymic characteristics. A thymus is however, found in all higher fishes (including lampreys), usually as a paired series of soft, irregular masses of tissue situated deep to the surface above most or all of the gill slits. In amphibians, the thymus is found deep within the lateral surface of the neck behind the pharynx. In frogs, it consists of a single pair of compact oval bodies; in addition, a pair of **jugular bodies** are thymus-like lymphoid structures that are derivatives of branchial pouches. In the other two amphibian orders, the thymus is generally a rather diffuse, lobulated mass of tissue. In young reptiles, it is frequently in the form of a strand of tissue running the length of the neck on either side. It retains this form in adult crocodilians but usually in reptiles forms more compact bodies—two pairs of them in *Sphenodon*, lizards, and snakes; a single pair in most turtles. In birds, as in their crocodilian relatives, the thymus is generally a long strand of tissue extending the length of the neck; it is somewhat irregularly and variably lobate. Among mammals, the most common condition of the thymus is that of a pair of structures that have migrated from the throat back to a position in the anteroventral part of the thorax, deep to the sternum and near the point at which the major vessels leave the heart. However, the thymus is sometimes cervical in position, and, in some mammals, both cervical and thoracic bodies may be present.

The reticular portion of the thymus is derived from the endodermal lining of the embryonic gill pouches, generally from epithelial thickenings formed at the dorsal side of such pouches. There is, however, much variation in the specific pouches concerned. In fishes, every typical gill pouch may produce a thymic bud, and even the spiracle is implicated in many sharks. Among the amphibians, the Gymnophiona produce thymic material from every embryonic pouch; but, in salamanders, the number concerned is usually reduced, and, in frogs and toads, only the first posthyoid cleft contributes. Reptiles also show a variable condition, but usually only two pairs of pouches contribute to the adult thymus. In birds, the thymus usually comes from the second and third posthyoid pouches. In mammals, the second postspiracular cleft is the usual seat of thymic origin. The mammalian thymic buds are, in contrast to the usual situation, derived from the ventral rather than the dorsal parts of the branchial pouches. Another odd feature in mammals is that the cervical part of the thymus, which we have mentioned as present in various forms, does not come from the endoderm at all, but from an inpouching of skin in the neck of the embryo; it is, seemingly, a new development, comparable in structure to a true thymus, but not homologous with it. The lymphoid cells of the thymus develop (as do other blood cells) from mesenchyme, which migrates into the thymus from other blood-forming organs.

The thymus grows rapidly during embryonic life and is frequently a massive structure of the throat region of young or larval vertebrates (the calf thymus forms a good proportion of commercial sweetbreads). By the time the adult stage is reached, however, the thymus has ceased to grow and often shrinks; it thus becomes relatively, and often absolutely, smaller than in earlier stages. Its tissues tend to degenerate, and, in many adult mammals, the thymus has disappeared entirely. Its function includes the rapid production of lymphocytes during development and early life; in older animals, lymphocytes may proliferate in the spleen, bone marrow, and (in mammals) lymph nodes. The thymus is always essential in the establishment of immunity reactions in the developing vertebrate; these reactions are, as we have noted, associated with the lymphocytes.

Adult Blood-Forming Tissues. A great variety of organs may give rise to blood cells in adult vertebrates of one group or another. In fishes, much of the maturation of erythrocytes takes place in the blood vessels. Except in birds and mammals, the spleen is an important area of blood-cell formation. In lampreys, elasobranchs, many teleosts, and amphibians, the kidney continues throughout life as a great source of blood cells. In cartilaginous fishes, the gonads are areas in which white blood corpuscles are formed. In teleosts, amphibians, and turtles, hemopoietic tissue is associated with the liver, and, in urodeles, this is a large source of leukocytes. In the sturgeon and paddlefish, blood-forming tissue surrounds the heart. As a persistence of embryonic conditions, masses of lymphoid tissue are present in the intestinal walls, and many vertebrates show in adult life blood-cell formation in the throat region. Masses of lymphocytic tissue are present in the walls of the mouth and pharynx in amphibians and in many mammals as **tonsils,** palatine, lingual and pharyngeal. Peyer's patches in the wall of the intestine and, in some forms (like ourselves), in much of the wall of the appendix are further knots of lymphoid tissue. The esophagus of sharks shows a large mass of lymphocyte-forming tissue, and similar esophageal "tonsils," as well as the thymus, may be found in a number of amniotes.

The **bone marrow** is a great center of blood cell formation in higher vertebrates. The hollowing out of large bones appears to be primarily an adaptation for greater efficiency in the use of bony tissue and weight reduction. The resulting "waste" space is, however, available for other purposes; fat storage and blood cell formation are the uses to which the marrow cavities are put in. In frogs, some hemopoiesis takes place here, especially in the males at the breeding season, and, among reptiles, the lizards are notable for considerable utilization of bone marrow. In birds and mammals, this site is universally used and highly important as a source of blood cells. In reptiles and birds, the bone marrow produces blood cells of all sorts; in mammals, however, although some lymphoid cell formation occurs in bone marrow, the lymph nodes are the center for their proliferation, and production in marrow cavities is largely of erythrocytes, granular leukocytes and monocytes.

Bursa of Fabricius. Another lymphoid organ quite similar to the thymus in many ways, the **bursa of Fabricius,** is found in birds. This develops as a dorsal pouch off the cloaca. Its history—an early development from near the end of the gut, rapid growth, production of lymphocytes in the embryo, and reduction or loss with maturity—parallels that of the thymus closely. Histologically, the lymphoid tissue is like that of the thymus, but the bursa also retains fairly normal mucosal epithelium; this epithelium may be the source of the lymphocytes, but (as usual) their origin is open to dispute. In birds, the lymphocytes produced here differ in their function in the immune system from the thymic lymphocytes. Interestingly, mammals, which lack the bursa, still produce, from an unknown source, lymphocytes of the bursal type.

Spleen. It is only in the spleen and in the lymph nodes characteristic of mammals the adult hemopoietic tissues assume the condition of descrete organs. The spleen is the largest mass of reticular tissue in the vertebrate body and is an important organ in the formation, storage, and destruction of blood corpuscles; it is, further, of importance in defense against disease. In most vertebrates, it is a reddish body situated in the dorsal mesentery close to the stomach; it is surrounded by a connective tissue capsule. Inwardly

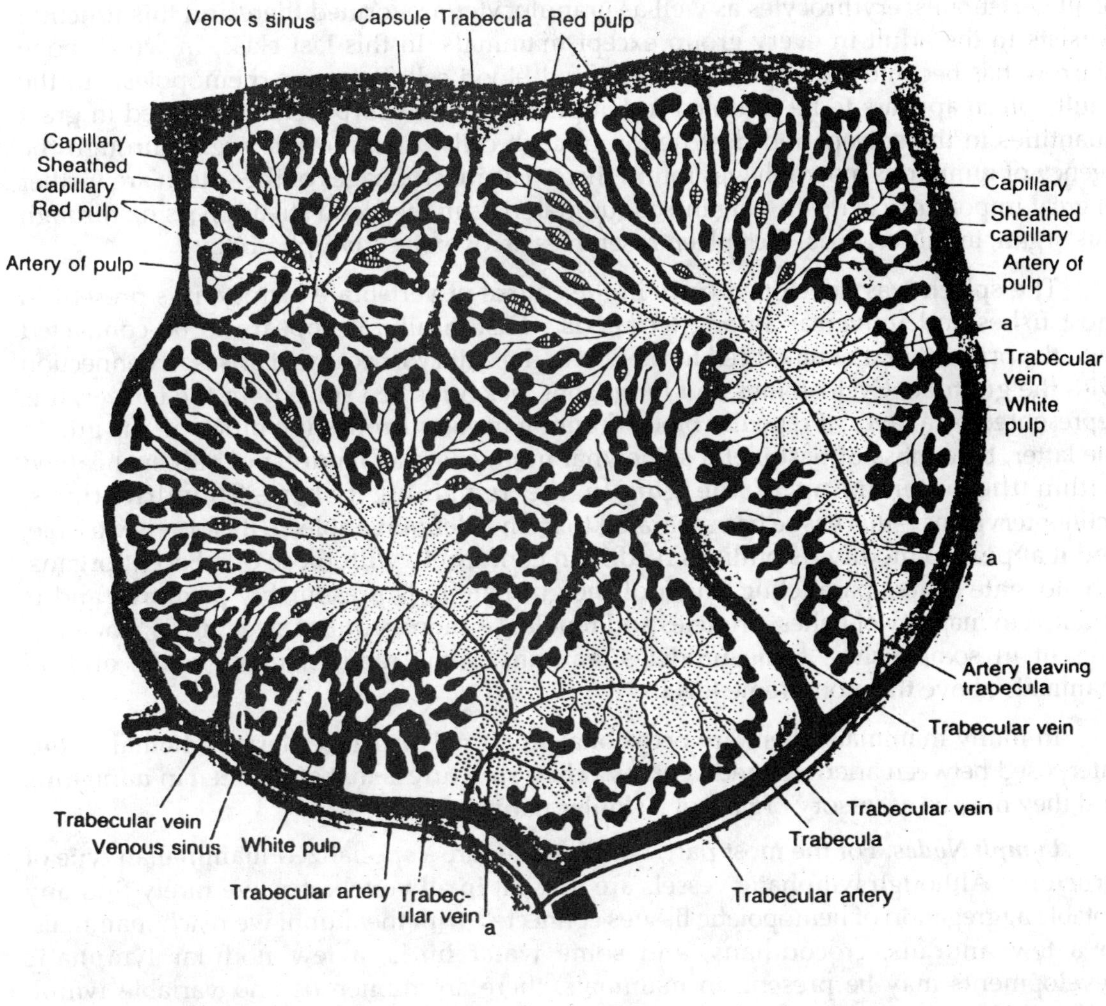

Fig. 3.2. Diagram of a part of the mammalian spleen. Venous spaces in black; white pulp, heavy stipple; connective tissue capsule and trabeculae, light stipple; red pulp, unstippled. "Sheathed arteries" are surrounded by white pulp, here shown as hatched areas.

extending connective tissue partitions form an extensive reticular network, in the spaces of which are contained tissues of two types, a **white pulp** and a **red pulp**. As may be inferred, the former contains clusters of white corpuscles; the red pulp consists of thick masses of all the elements of the blood, including, of course, a large percentage of erythrocytes. In fishes and some amphibians, the pulp is dominantly red; in higher tetrapods, white pulp is also quite common. The spleen is fed by an artery and is drained by a vein; lymphatic vessels are rarely well developed. The internal circulation of the spleen is obviously complicated, with much of the blood passing through an "open" circulatory system. The white pulp clusters about the terminal arterioles; the red pulp lies near the venous outlets.

The spleen is always an important center of blood cell production. In the embryos of all vertebrates, erythrocytes as well as granulocytes are formed there and this function persists in the adult in every group except mammals. In this last class, in which bone marrow has become the important seat of red blood cell formation, hemopoiesis in the adult spleen appears to be confined to lymphocytes. Red corpuscles are stored in great quantities in the spleen, and destruction of such cells occurs in this organ through the agency of numerous macrophages found there. The macrophages of the spleen are further of great importance in destroying infectious materials in the blood stream passing through this organ; in this regards, the spleen resembles an oversized lymph node.

The spleen was developed early in the course of vertebrate history, it is present in most fishes and universal among tetrapods. Historically, it appears to be connected with the primary seat of blood cell formation in the embryo, because it arises in connection with the gut tube. Cyclostomes and lungfishes lack a formed spleen. In the former, it is represented by a layer of reticular blood-forming tissue surrounding much of the gut: in the latter, by a mass of tissue of a somewhat more compact nature, but still ensheathed within the outer lining of the gut. In the remaining fishes—Chondrichthyes, actinopterygians—this tissue has separated to form a definitive spleen. Its form is variable, and it appeas to modify its outlines readily in conformity with those of adjacent organs. An elongate shape, paralleling much of the gut length, is presumably primitive and is retained in majority of fishes, urodeles and reptiles. A more compact structure is, however, present in some fishes, some urodeles, anurans, some reptiles, many birds, and all mammals above the monotreme level.

In many mammals, there are occasional small red structures termed **hemal nodes** interposed between arterioles and venules. Their structure is that of a spleen in miniature, and they may be accessory organs of a similar nature.

Lymph Nodes. For the most part, lymph nodes are a specialized mammalian type of structure. Although lymphatic vessels are present in all vertebrates, we rarely find any notable aggregation of hemopoietic tissues connected with them until we reach mammals. In a few anurans, crocodilians, and some water birds, a few nodular lymphatic developments may be present; in mammals, there are numerous and variable lymph nodes, both in the subcutaneous tissues and in the interior of the body.

These are small, rounded encapsulated masses of reticular tissue, comparable to a small spleen in general structure, but sharply distinguished from that organ by being

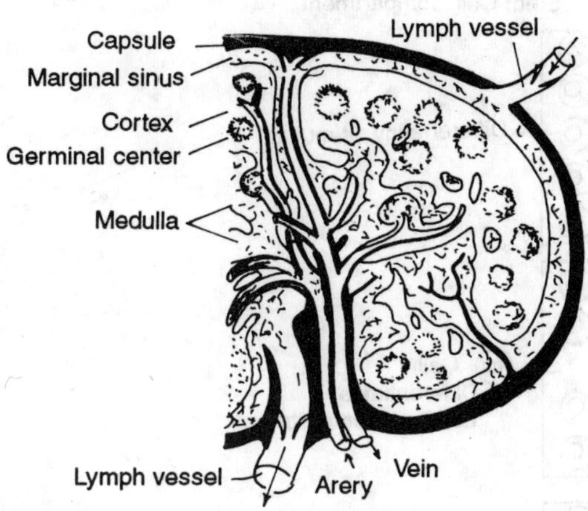

Fig. 3.3. Diagram of the structure of a lymph node. In addition to the lymph vessels, a node is supplied by a small artery and vein.

situated along the course of lymphatic rather than blood vessels. Their cellular contents consist almost entirely of lymphocytes of various sizes. These nodes are, in mammals, a special seat of lymphocyte proliferation; in adult lower vertebrates, the lymphocytes develop in the same organs as the other types of corpuscles.

Hematopoietic Stem Cells

In the normal steady state, all of the cellular systems of the blood-erythrocytes platelets, neutrophils, lymphocytes, monocytes, eosinophils, basophils—are in a balanced system of cell loss and cell renewal. In order for cell renewal to occur, there must be a stem cell for each of these systems. For purposes of this review, we shall define an hematopoietic stem cell as a cell that has two capabilities. (1) the ability to reproduce itself by mitosis, implying that the daughters of mitosis in the stem cell compartment have all the capabilities of the mother cell; and (2) the ability to differentiate into mature hematopoietic cells.

In a normal steady state, it must be assumed that the stem cell compartment remains constant in size. One reasonable mechanism for maintaining a stable stem cell compartment size is illustrated in Figure 3.4, which shows the stem cell compartment as containing five cells. If a differentiating stimulus hits one of the cells in the compartment, it thereby removes it from the stem cell compartment through the mechanism of differentiation. In order to return to the original compartment size, another stem cell undergoes mitosis, producing two daughter stem cells. Thus, by self-replication, the compartment is maintained in a balanced state.

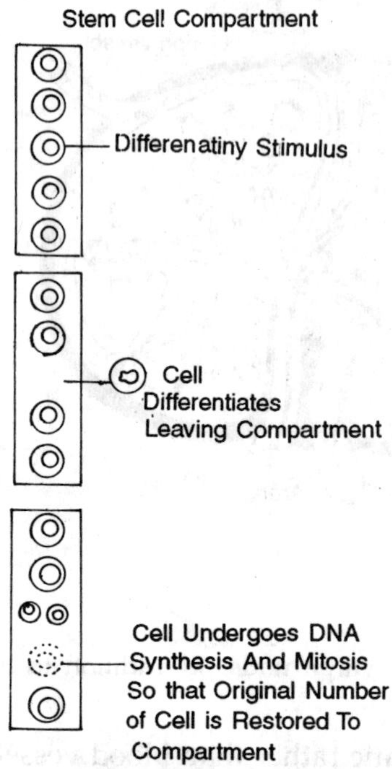

Fig. 3.4. A proposed model of differentiation and self-replication in a steady state stem cell compartment.

Until the last decade, the nature of hematopoietic stem cells was entirely speculative. It was suggested that there might be a single stem cell capable of differentiating into all of the recognized mature blood cells and, conversely, that each of the cellular systems might be entirely separate. There were many speculative variations between the two extremes of these monophyletic and polyphyletic schools of thought. For reasons discussed below, evidence now suggests that there are both differentiated unipotential stem cells as well as pluripotential hematopoietic stem cells.

Evidence for Pluripotential Hematopoietic Stem Cells in Man

Chronic myelocytic leukemia is a disease we often consider as primarily involving neutrophils. However, such patients usually have evidence for increased platelet, eosinophil, and basophil productions as well as evidence for increased neutrophil production. Thus it is not a disease of a single cellular system. Most patients with typical chronic myelocytic leukemia have a defect in chromosome 21. Whang and co-workers demonstrated that this chromosome defect was found not only in neutrophil precursors but also in the erythrocytic precursors in the bone marrow as well as megakaryocytes, and other investigators have demonstrated its presence in immature eosinophils. Since this defect is not present in lymphocytes, skin, or buccal mucosa, the most reasonable explanation for its presence in neutrophils, erythrocytes, megakaryocytes, and eosinophils is to suggest that this disease is a clonal disease that began by mutation in a single cell that then repopulated the entire bone marrow. Other evidence suggesting a clonal evolution of chronic myelocytic leukemia has been obtained by studies of phenotype distribution of 6-phosphogluconate dehydrogenase.

In yet another disease in man, there is evidence to suggest that neutrophils, platelets, and erythrocytes arise from a common precursor. Paroxysmal nocturnal hemoglobinuria has a membrane defect of red cells. This membrane defect has also been demonstrated in neutrophils and platelets but not in other cells of the body. Thus, in this disease as in chronic myelocytic leukemia, the most reasonable explanation is that the difficulty began in a single stem cell, which was pluripotential for these three cellular in systems, and that the single cell competed successfully with normal hematopoietic stem cells to repopulate the bone marrow.

HEMATOPOIETIC SPLEEN COLONIES

Although from the studies above we have evidence for pluripotential hematopoietic stem cells in man, it is only through studies of the spleen colonies of the irradiated mouse that we have obtained more definitive information and have been able to carry out studies of the behaviour of this cellular system. Brues and Stroud (1964) observed macroscopic nodules of cirumscribed hematopoietic tissue on the suface of the spleen following whole body irradiation in mice. Till and McCulloch (1961), following similar observations, delineated the character of these nodules and demonstrated that these were colonies of hematopoietic tissue arising from a single cell.

The methods used in the study of hematopoietic spleen colonies in irradiated mice. In the first and most simple method, the mouse is simply given sub- or midlethal irradiation and allowed to recover. Some eight to 10 days later, macroscopic nodules are visible on the spleen, the result of growth of surviving hematopoietic stem cells. The number of endogenous colonies declines exponentially with increasing irradiation dose. If the mouse is lethally irradiated so that no endogenous colonies appear prior to death, death can be averted by transplanting a sufficient number of bone marrow or spleen cells following irradiation. With a proper number of cells, spleen colonies are demonstrable following such transplanations. Till and Mcculloch (1961) demonstrated a linear relationship between the number of transplanted cells and the number of spleen colonies that developed. This observation suggested that the colonies might be clonal in nature. They and their co-workers then carried out a more definite demonstration of the clonal nature of hematopoietic nodules. Irradiation induces chromosome defects in cells in a random fashion so that it is exceedingly unlikely that two cells would have the same chromosome defect following recovery from irradiation. Donor animals sublethally irradiated were used for cellular transplantation into lethally irradiated recipients. If a chromosome defect was present in a colonly, it was present in virtually all of the cells. Conversely, if no defect was present in a colony, no cell in the colony had a defect, and the same chromosome defect was not observed in any two colonies. This indicates that colonies are clonal in nature and, since certain colonies contain a mixture of neutrophils, erythrocytes, megakaryocytes and eosinophils, strongly suggests that the colony-forming cell is a pluripotential cell capable of differentiating into the above elements.

In these studies, a common colony-lymphocyte chromosome defect was not detected. However, when similar studies were repeated using more heavily irradiated donors, the same defect was noted in certain colonies as well as in lymphoid tissues. These observations suggest that with a greater degree of destruction to the hematopoietic system, regeneration occurs from very primitive cell, which is pluripotent for all blood cells, and destruction is less severe, regeneration occurs from a more mature but still pluripotential stem cell that does not contain the lymphocyte among its progeny.

Concatenated stem cell compartments of differing degrees of differentiation and maturity were suggested on the basis of the shape of labeling curves for neutrophils following injection of diisopropylfluorophosphate. Recently, further evidence for concatenated granulocytic stem cell complements has been obtained by Bennett and co-workers. The W/W^v mouse has an hereditary defect in the colony-forming cell compartment. If this animal is used as a donor for lethally irradiated animals, no visible spleen colonies are formed in the normal recipient. However, if the spleen is examined microscopically, tiny colonies are observed. Thus, it would appear there is a qualitative defect in the ability of the colony-forming cell to proliferate. Bradley and Metcalf (1966) observed that if mouse marow was dispersed in soft agar and plated over a proper cell

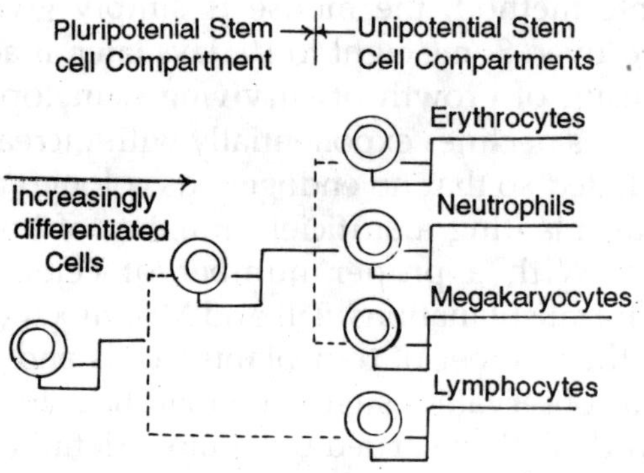

Fig. 3.5. A proposed model for concetenated stem cell compartments. Under ordinary circumstances cell systems are maintained by unipotential stem cell compartments and only under special circumstances do the pluripotent compartments enter a generative cycle.

feeder layer and incubated *in vitro*, colonies of neutrophilic and macrophagic cell arose from the bone marrow. Bennett and co-workers plated the marrow of the W/W^v mouse in this system and observed a normal concentration of neutrophilic colonies *in vitro*. Thus it would appear that the W/W^v mouse's defect in the pluripotential colony-forming cell is not propagated into more mature neutrophilic series. This suggests that there is a separate and more mature perhaps unipotential, stem cell for neutrophilic cells. There is similar evidence for a more mature differentiated stem cell in the erythrocytic series, which is distinct from the spleen colony forming cell. For example, following irradiation, or irradiation and transplantation, the rate of recovery of the colony-forming compartments differs from the rate of recovery of erythropoietic responsiveness. This suggests that the erythropoietin sensitive cell is a more mature stem cell than the spleen colony-forming cell.

There is evidence suggesting the spleen colony-forming cell compartment is at rest rather than in an active generative cycle under normal circumstances. Bruce and co-workers have done extensive studies concerning the effect of chemotherapeutic agents on the colony-forming cell compartment as studied by cell transplantation. If donor animal are injected with chemotherapeutic agents that act only in cells in a generative cycle, there is little or no effect on the colony-forming compartment. This suggests that this compartment is at rest and is entirely compatible with the thesis that there are concatenated stem cell compartments.

In Figure 3.5, a tentative working model summarizing the foregoing observations of the normal concatenated stem cell compartment is portrayed. Mature cell systems are considered to be renewed from differentiated unipotential stem cells in the normal steady state. The spleen colony-forming cell compartment is considered to be at rest in the normal steady state. If increasisng demands are made for mature cells or if the mature cell stem cell compartments are destroyed, they regenerate from the colony-forming cell compartment. If the destructive insult is extremely severe, regeneration may occur from the still more primitive compartment, which is also pluripotential for lymphocytes.

COLONY-FORMING CELL KINETICS

Methods of Study. Morphological identification of hematopoietic stem cells has not been accomplished. However, from studies of the changes in spleen colonies under various perturbed situations in the mouse, a great deal concerning the kinetics of this cellular compartment has been learned. The first method termed the "endogenous method" is in many senses the simplest and perhaps the least subject to experimental error. The primary difficulty with this method is that the clonal nature of the colonies has not been established. By analogy with the transplant method, it is assumed that these colonies are clonal. There is reasonably good evidence to support the concept that the number of endogenous colonies reflects the size of the total body colony forming cell pool. That the colonies observed on the spleen in this method reflect migration of cells to the spleen rather than growth of cells in the spleen at the time of irradiation was demonstrated. In this system, a lethal dose of irradiation was delivered to the spleen while the remainder of the mouse was shielded. Thus any colonies observed on the spleen must have migrated following the splenic irradiation. Since the number of colonies observed with Method #1 or Method #5 when a comparable dose of whole-body irradiation is given is virtually the same, it is apparent that most endogenous colonies are the result of migration.

Method #2, in which the mouse's own colony-forming cell compartment is destroyed by irradiation and colony-forming cells are supplied by transplantation, also has a number of advantages and disadvantages. It primary advantage is that the colonies have been demonstrated to be clonal. However, it is apparent from many studies that the number of transplantable colony—forming cells in marrow or spleen do not necessarily reflect the total size of the colony-forming cell compartment. Thus, the injection of foreign plasma that leads to a tenfold increase in endogenous colonies and that is accompanied by increased irradiation survival and an increased rate of hematopoietic regeneration almost certainly induces an increase in the total body colony-forming cell compartment. However, this increase is not demonstrable by transplantation of cells from the spleen or marrow of a plasma treated animal. Furthermore, although it is generally assumed that transplantation must at least reflect the number of colony-forming cells in the organ being transplanted, there are problems in this interpretation as well. For instance, the fraction of cells from the transplant that lodge and grow in the spleen can be influenced by treatment of the donor or treatment of the recipient. Furthermore, if the number of transplantable cells from an animal's marrow are compared to the number of cells that can migrate from a shielded marrow as shown in Method #3, discrepancies arise. In the third method in the mouse is lethally irradiated, but a portion of the marrow is shielded and regeneration of the entire system occurs from the shielded femur. A migration of colony-forming cells from this femur leads to visible colonies on the spleen some ten days later. If mice are subjected to 200 R irradiation and the curve of recovery of colony-forming cells in the marrow is followed by either transplanting marrow or shielding marrow, discrepant curves of recovery result. Thus, at the present time interpretation of quantitative changes utilizing transplantation studies are difficult.

Location of the Colony-Forming Cell Compartment. No exact quantitative data are available concerning the entire size and exact location of the colony-forming cell compartment within a normal animal. However, by transplantation studies it would appear that the marrow is the richest source of such cells, and considering the overall size of the marrow, it is probable that this is the primary location of the compartment in the normal animal. The spleen is also an efficient source of transplanted colony-forming cells and from transplantation studies the concentration of colony-forming cells in the spleen is approximately one tenth that of marrow. Colony-forming cells are also demonstrable in the buffy coat of the blood or in washings, from the normal peritoneal cavity. They are also present in fetal liver but not in adult liver, and attempts to demonstrate colony-forming cells in lymph nodes, thoracic duct drainage, or thymus have been negative. The mobility and migrating ability of this colony-forming cell compartment is indeed remarkable. This is perhaps best demonstrated by the method of study shown in #4 in which the mouse is lethally irradiated and an entire encapsulated spleen is placed free in the peritoneal cavity within four hours after irradiation

Table 3.1
Factors Influencing Hematopoietic Spleen Colonies

Pretreatment	Endogenous Colonies	Effect on Transplantable colony Forming Spleen (% of untreated control)	Cells in Marrow	Post-Irradiation Survival
Foreign plasma:				
(0.5 ml/day × 4 days)				
dog plasma	1,020	120	75	increase
human plasma	3,000			
rat plasma	550			
allogeneic mouse plasma	340			
isogeneic mouse plasma	90			
Bleeding (0.5 ml/day × days)	3,630	81	58	increase
Endotoxin injection				
(25 µg × 1 day)	3,600	998	86	increase
Sheep red cells (0.25 ml × 4 days)	210			
Mumps vaccine				
(0.1 ml/day × 4 days)	820			
Influenza vaccine				
(0.1 ml/day × 4 days)	600			
Phytohemagglutinin				
(0.5 ml/day × 4 days)	800			
Hypertransfusion	30			
Erypertransfusion				
(1 unit/day × 4 days)	200	165	86	none
Cobait for 4 days	100			
Testosterone for 4 days	220			
Cobalt and testosterone for 4 days	300	116	86	? increase

(Chervenick *et al* 1968a). From the peritoneal cavity, colony-forming cells can migrate from the viable transplanted spleen to the host's own spleen and form colonies.

Factors Influencing the Number of Hematopoietic Spleen Colony-Forming Cells. The age of the mouse is a significant factor in the number of endogenous colonies formed after a fixed dose cf irradiation in the strain of mouse used in our experiments. F_1 hybrid of a C57 black female and a DBA; Marsh *et al* 1767). After 600 R, 11-week-old mice had an average of eight colonies, 17-week-old mice had an average of 12 colonies, 23-week-old mice 15 colonies, and those 29 to 35 weeks of age had more than 30 colonies per spleen by the endogenous method. Female mice produce a significantly larger number of endogenous spleen colonies.

Preirradiation treatment of mice with a wide variety of substances significantly influences the number of endogenous spleen colonies. Foreign plasma, whether from a foreign mouse strain, rat, man, or dog, induces a very significant increase in spleen colonies. Other substances such as endotoxin, sheep red cells, mumps vaccine, influenza vaccine, and phytohemagglutinin also have a very significant effect, indicating that the foreign plasma effect has no particular specificity.

Hypertransfusion of mice prior to irradiation results in complete loss of erythroid colonies from the spleen. O'Grady and co-workers studied serial sections of the spleen from hypertransfused animals, and, while they could demonstrate no erythroid colonies in these spleens, there was no evident compensatory increase in other types of colonies. In the nonhypertransfused animal, the amount of radioactive iron taken up by the spleen is a relatively direct reflection of the number of erythroid colonies, and in hypertransfused animals the absence of erythroid colonies is reflected by virtually absent iron uptake. The absence of erythropoiesis in spleen colonies following hypertransfusion indicates that the progeny of the colony-forming cell are subject to standard hormonal control, and indeed if hypertransfused mice are injected with erythropoietin following irradiation, the erythroid colonies reappear. The observation that bled mice respond with an increased number of colonies, like those treated with erythropoietin, cobalt, and testosterone, suggest that the colony-forming cell compartment might be under the control of a regulating substance. However, preliminary attempts to demonstrate a colony-stimulating substance in isogeneic plasma from irradiated mice proved negative.

As noted in Table 3.1, the increase observed in endogenous colonies after the injection of foreign plasma or after bleeding often could not be demonstrated by transplanting marrow or spleen from animals treated in this fashion. In the case of foreign plasma injections, extensive experiments indicated that this did indeed reflect an increased number of colony-forming cells within the mouse's total compartment. The observation that bleeding and endotoxin injection lead to increased survival following irradiation suggest that these also reflect an increased total compartment size. The failure of transplantation studies to reflect this indicates that this technique cannot be used as a measure of total compartment size. Thus for the present, the only technique that would appear to hold any promise for measuring the total compartment size for colony-forming cells would be the endogenous technique. Whether all substances that change endogenous colonies when given before irradiation do so by changing total compartment size remains to be determined.

These studies do suggest, however, that the size of this compartment is very easily changed by a wide variety of stimuli and further indicate that the location of colony-forming cells within the mouse can shift rapidly and dramatically.

Kinetics of Recovery of the Colony-Forming Cell Compartment. Since increasing doses of irradiation induce an exponential loss of colony-forming cells, for the mouse to recover following irradiation, this compartment must undergo self-replication as well as differentiation for replacement of mature cells. Because of the difficulties inherent in

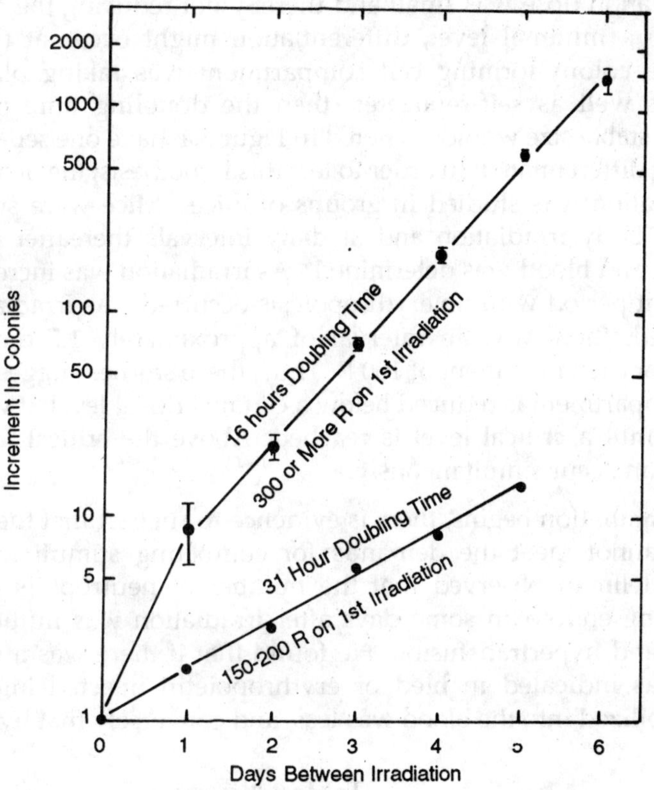

Fig. 3.6. Colony cell compartment regeneration after irradiation induced depletion. An exposure to whole body irradiation was given to all mice at time 0, and to different groups within minutes thereafter and then at daily intervals. Mice were killed ten days after the second irradiation and spleen colonies were counted. The upper curve is the mean and standard error derived from eleven separate such experiments and the lower is the mean of three experiments.

transplantation studies, we chose to study the rate of recovery of the colony-forming compartment in a strict endogenous system. Mice were subjected to sublethal whole body irradiation and at intervals thereafter a second exposure was given. Ten days after the second exposure, the number of colonies present on the spleen were determined. The change in the number of colonies as the space between the two iradiation is increased should reflect regrowth of the colony-forming cell compartment following the first irradiation. As noted in Figure 3.6, rapid regrowth of the colony-forming cell compartment occurred as measured by this technique. If the first irradiation exposure was 300 R or more, an exponential increase in colony-forming cells occurred with a doubling time averaging sixteen hours. However, if the first dose of irradiation was 200 R or less (lower curve in Fig. 3.9) a much slower doubling time for the colony-forming compartment was observed.

A possible explanation for this difference in doubling time would be to suggest that if the first irradiation dose was small and thereby not reducing the colony-forming cell compartment to a minimal level, differentiation might occur at the same time that regrowth of the colony-forming cell compartment was taking place. If a stem cell differentiates as well as self-replicates, then the doubling time must be slower. A compartment of stable size would, as noted in Figur 3.4, have one self-replicative division for each cell that differentiated. In order to test this hypothesis, the onset of differentiation following irradiation was studied in groups of mice. Mice were subjected to varying doses of whole body irradiation and at daily intervals thereafter iron uptake in the spleen, marrow, and blood was determined. As irradiation was increased from 200 R to 300 R, a transient period with no erythropoiesis occurred. As irradiation exposure was further increased, there was an interval of approximately 1.7 days before onset of erythropoiesis for each increment of 100 R. Thus, these studies suggest that if the colony-forming cell compartment is reduced below a certain critical level, it will regrow without differentiating until a critical level is reached. Above the critical level, regrowth and differentiation can occur simultaneously.

Once differentiation begins, there is evidence to suggest that the depleted stem cell compartment cannot meet the demands for competing stimuli for neutrophils and erythrocytes. Hellman observed that the number of neutrophils mobilized into the blood by injecting endotoxin some days after irradiation was influenced by bleeding, erythropoietin, and hypertransfusion. He found that if there was a strong stimulus for erythropoiesis as indicated in bled or erythropoietin injected mice, the number of neutrophils mobilized into the blood was less, and conversely that hypertransfused mice

Table 3.2
Effect of Altered Rates of Erythropoiesis on Marrow Granulocytes After 400 R Whole Body Irradiation

Procedure	*Absolute Number of Granulocytes Per Humerus* (% of control)*
Increased erythropoiesis	
bleeding + 400 R	52%
erythropoietin + 400 R	80%
Decreased erythropoiesis	
hypertransfusion + 400 R	170 %
hypoxia + 400 R	235 %

* Absolute number of granulocytes was determined 10 days after irradiation; control animals had an average of 3×10^6 cells/humerus.

could mobilize more. This suggested that there was competition for differentiated progeny from the depleted stem cell pool. We studied the question of such competition using a more direct measure of neutophils. The total number of neutrophils and neutrophil precursors was measured in the humerus of mice by a technique described in detail. These were measured at seven and 10 days following 400 R irradiation in mice subjected to changing demands for erythropoiesis. If an increased demand for erythropoiesis as indicated by bleeding or erythropoietin injection was introduced, the number of neutrophils observed in the marrow was decreased. Conversely, if mice were hypertransfused or made polycythemic by hypoxia, thus decreasing erythropoietic demands, an increased number of neutrophils was observed in the bone marrow. Thus, it would appear that the depleted stem cell pool cannot meet the demands for mature cell production and is responsive to competing levels of humoral stimulation for each cell type.

QUALITATIVE COLONY-FORMING CELL DEFECTS IN THE MOUSE

As noted in the introduction, there is suggestive evidence that chronic myelocytic leukemia and paroxysmal nocturnal hemoglobinuria are diseases of the pluripotential hematopoietic stem cell compartment in man. By analogy, it is reasonable to suggest that other diseases—such as acute myeloblastic leukemia, polycythemia rubra vera, and certain forms of aplastic anemia—may also represent defects in this cellular compartment. Two types of inherited anemia in the mouse suggest that the type of disease that may be anticipated in this cellular compartment may be quite variable. The W/W^v mouse has a qualitative defect in the colony-forming cell compartment and this mouse's cells, upon transplantation into a normal recipient, form microscopic rather than macroscopic colonies as previously noted. Conversely, if normal colony-forming cells are injected into an uniradiated W/W^v mouse the mouse's hematopoietic system is entirely repopulated by the transplanted cells. The W/W^v mouse is not only anemic but has decreased numbers of neutrophils and magakaryocytes in the marrow. Therefore, it would appear that this mouse has a qualitative defect in the colony-forming cell compartment in which this compartment cannot produce differentiated progeny at a normal rate so that this is a cellular defect leading to pancytopenia.

The SL/SL^d mouse also has an inherited form of anemia. However, if this mouse's marrow is used for transplantation into a lethally irradiated recipient, colonies of normal number, size, and cellular composition are produced. If normal marrow is injected into this anemic mouse after irradiation, colonies grow very poorly. Therefore, it would appear that in this animal the defect lies not within the cell itself, but the environment in which the cell must grow. These observations suggest that as methods become available for studying the stem cell compartments of man, a variety of defects may be found responsible for a number of disease processes.

IRON

Iron has been valued for its medicinal qualities since ancient times. Long before the

Christian era, it was known to the Egyptian, Greek and Indian physicians as a metal capable of imparting vigour and strength to patients suffering from many types of illness especially those accompanied by marked pallor. In early days, these patients were given drinking water in which old swords had been allowed to rust.

It was Sydenham, in the 17th century, who was the first to use iron, which was known as Mars, clinically in a manner that would be approved today. He prescribed for the treatment of chlorosis, iron or steel filings steeped in cold Rhenish wine, the dose being about 0.5-1.0 gms. of iron daily. In the 18th century, the presence of iron in blood was demonstrated and also that foods rich in iron could increase this amount in blood. Blaud, a French physician, formulated his famous pills in the early 19th century which provided 64 mg. of elemental iron per tablet and reported a cure for chlorosis. About the last decade of the 19th century, iron therapy was discredited probably as a result of clinical failure due to doses too small to show any effect. Soon, however, a host of investigators demonstrated its efficacy and dispelled all doubts about its value, though the major breakthrough in the understanding of the pathways of its absorption, turnover and excretion has occurred only in the last few decades, utilizing radioisotopes of iron.

Absorption

Iron absorption varies according to the body's needs and iron balance is maintained more by regulation of absorption rather than excretion of unwanted excess (Whitby and Britton, 1963). Absorption is enhanced when there is increased need and diminished when there is decreased need. Absorption of iron can occur along the length of the alimentary tract, but is greatest in the duodenum. Practically all the absorbed iron enters the body via the blood stream rather than the lymphatics (Drill, 1965). Absorption normally balances excretion thus maintaining fairly constant body levels.

The precise mechanism of iron uptake and transfer is controversial and various theories have been put forward without any one being universally accepted.

Probable Mechanisms of Iron Uptake

(1) Iron, in the ferrous state, passes directly through the mucosal cell into the bloodstream where it is attached to transferrin. The receptor cells of the intestinal mucosa contain a protein called apoferritin which is capable of combination with iron to form ferritin. When the cells are saturated, no more iron is absorbed till the saturation is reduced by transfer of iron to the plasma.

(2) Brown and Rother (1963) have suggested that there are two mechanisms involved. They found that during absorption, iron is *bound* to two factors—the *aminoacids,* glycine and serine and to a *protein.* They believe that the aminoacid-bound iron mediates principally when absorption is enhanced while the protein-bound form is a slowly mobilized storage form.

(3) Dowdle *et al* (1960) and Manis & Schachter (1962), believe that absorption of iron is an *active process* requiring energy and dependent on oxidative metabolism.

Regulation of Iron Absorption

The small intestine is both the absorptive and excretory organ for iron, and is also mainly connected with the control of body iron. This is now believed to depend on the iron content of the deciduous cells of the duodenal mucosa.

Hahn and Granick (1943) proposed a *"mucosal block"* to absorption of excess iron since they noticed that oral administration of a large dose of iron reduced absorption of a second dose given within six hours.

Iron is most easily absorbed in the ferrous state which passes through the mucosal cell directly into the blood stream and is attached to transferrin. An excess remaining in the villous epithelial cells is reconverted to the ferric state and combines with apoferritin to form ferritin. Granick (1954) also postulated that the *quantity* of ferritin was important, rejecting iron when it was high and accepting it when it was low. This excess iron is excreted in the faeces along with the exfoliated epithelical cells at the end of their life span of about 3 days, but it is believed that it acts only with small excesses of iron and is overwhelmed by large amounts. Increasing the size of the oral iron dose increases the amount absorbed but decreases the fraction of the administered dose that is absorbed.

Recently, studies by Luke *et al.* (1967), led them to postulate a gastric luminal mechanism operating in the regulation of iron absorption. They had previously (1966) suggested that normal gastric juice has, as one of its components, an iron binding potein gastroferrin, which is absent in the gastric juice of patients with haemochromatosis. In this study, they found that the gastroferrin content was low in iron deficient states. This led them to believe that gastroferrin production is concerned with the regulation of iron absorption in health, normal levels acting to inhibit the absoption of excessive amounts of iron in the diet and reduced level permitting enhanced absorption.

Koepke and Stewart (1964), proposed a different function for gastric juice after experimenting on dogs. They believe that the stomach secretes a substance which potentiates iron absorption and that this substance is produced in increasing amounts in iron deficiency anaemia and also in haemochromatosis.

Conditions when Absorption is Increased

(1) Ferrous form or haem iron.

(2) Presence of acid or reducing agents as they favour the reduction of ferric to ferrous iron.

(3) Iron deficiency anaemia.

(4) Last months of pregnancy.

(5) Phosphorus-poor diet.

(6) Pyridoxine deficiency.

(7) Chronic pancreatic or hepatic disease (as pancreatic secretion contains an inhibitor of iron absorption).

(8) After portocaval shunt.

Conditions when Absorption is Decreased

(1) Ferric state of the iron.
(2) Presence of phytates.
(3) Presence of phosphates.
(4) Administration of iron with food.
(5) Achlorhydria.
(6) Administration of antacids.
(7) After partial or total gastrectomy.
(8) Tissue iron overload.
(9) Malignant, inflammatory or infectious disease.

Transport

After absorption from the intestine in the ferrous state, iron is transported to the storage depots by glycoprotein β-globulin in the plasma called transferrin. The combination with globulin involves conversion of iron to the ferric state (Whitby & Britton, 1963). Normal adult transferrin value is 7-15 grams. Transferrin probably also carries iron from the storage sites to the bonemarrow, where iron is incorporated into haemoglobin. However, a saturated transferrin alone is not enough to furnish iron to the erythron. It appears to be essential to have proper functioning, iron-storing reticulum cells in the bone marrow.

Under normal conditions, the iron-binding capacity of the plasma is about one-third saturated. Normal plasma iron levels are 80-160 micrograms per 100 ml. Total iron binding capacity is 300 micrograms per 100 ml. plasma. The plasma iron concentration and total iron binding capacity of the plasma vary in different physiological conditions and disease states.

Plasma iron is Decreased in

(1) Iron deficiency anaemias }
(2) Late pregnancy } — total iron binding capacity is increased.
(3) Anaemias of infection — total iron binding capacity is decreased.

Plasma Iron is increased in

(1) Haemochromatosis.
(2) Acute hepatitis.
(3) Transfusion haemosiderosis.
(4) Pernicious anaemia in relapse.

Regulation of Plasma Iron

The primary factor regulating the rate of plasma iron turnover is haemoglobin synthesis. Plasma iron is normally in equilibrium with iron stores. Detailed studies of iron turnover have been possible because of radioactive tracer techniques. It is now believed that 35 mg. of iron are turned over per day. Pollycove and Mortimer (1961) account for about 32 mg. leaving the plasma to enter the 'erythropoietic labile pool', which is a poorly defined compartment in the bone-marrow. The major source of iron entering the plasma to achieve a balance is from senescent red blood cells (about 21 mg.). A fairly large amount (11 mg) re-enters from the 'erythropoietic labile pool' which is probably the fraction not used in haemoglobin production. Small amounts (about 1 mg. each) are destined for and return from storage depots and extracellular fluid.

Fate and Distribution

Total body iron of a normal adult male (70 kg.) is about 4 grams.

In the body, iron exists attached to protein (transferrin, ferritin) or in haem (haemoglobin, myoglobin, haem enzymes). About two-thirds is in haemoglobin and about one-quarter is in reserve stores as ferritin and haemosiderin. The remaining fraction is in myoglobin, parenchymal iron and various haem containing enzymes.

Two methods of iron transfer from transferrin to the immature erythrocytes have been postulated. It probably mainly occurs by an energy requiring process where the iron is released to specific receptor sites on the membrane of the red cell precursors. The other method is by 'ropheocytosis' where erythroblasts engulf the ferritin iron, which has been transferred from reticulum 'nurse' cells in the bone-marrow.

Mature red cells are not capable of taking up iron.

Stores

The stores of iron are mainly in the reticulo-endothelial cells and thus are found in organs rich in these cells, especially liver, spleen, bone-marrow. Storage iron is the reserve derived from the diet and from the continuous physiological destruction of the red blood corpuscles. It is presently mainly as ferritin and haemosiderin and is available for use by the bone marrow in contrast to enzyme to enzyme and parenchymal iron. About 10% constitutes a 'labile pool' which can be very rapidly mobilized. The rest is made available more slowly. A healthy adult in good nutritional condition can compensate, within a relatively short period, for the loss of 30% of his circulating red cells without recourse to iron therapy, provided the iron stores can be adequately mobilized. (Goodman & Gilman, 1967).

After oral administration, more iron is taken up by the bone-marrow and spleen. On intravenous administration it is deposited mainly in the liver.

Normal iron stores in the adult male range from 0.5 to 1.5 gms. (Drill, 3rd ed.).

Excretion

Iron is a precious metal and is tenaciously conserved. The capacity of the body to

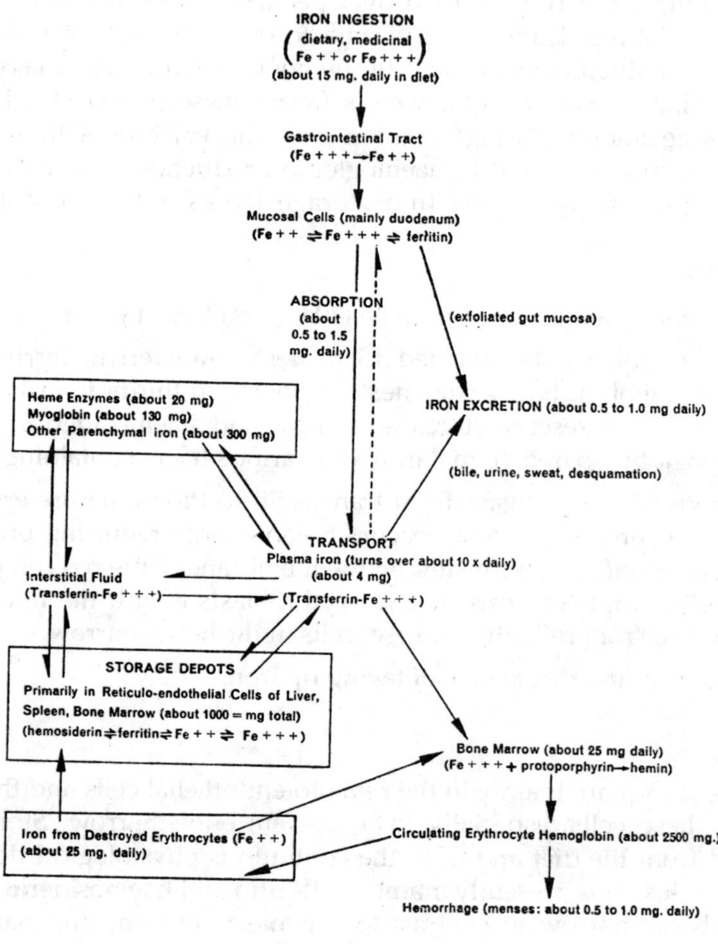

Normal absorption, metabolic pathways, and excretion of iron. (All amounts are for iron content.)

excrete iron is very limited as demonstrated by McCance and Widdowson (1943). Normally, excretion is about 0.5-1 mg. daily in an adult male. The greater part of the excretion is by sloughed off, mucosal epithelial cells of the bowel which contain ferritin. Excretion also takes place in sweat, nails, hair, faeces and urine mainly as enzyme iron of exfoliated cells. There are also trace losses in bile and cell-free sweat. Excretion of iron in sweat becomes of significance in geographical areas where excessive sweating occurs. Hussein *et al.*, (1960) believe that as much as 2-3 mg. per day may be lost in this way. In the female, there are added losses through menstruation, pregnancy and lactation.

Normal Values of Iron Excretion

Adult male or non-menstruating female—0.5-1 mg/day.

Loss in normal menstruation spread evenly over 28 days is about 0.5-1 mg/day.

Therefore, a female during her menstruating years loses about 1-2 mg/day. The iron 'cost' of a normal pregnancy may vary from 0-732 mg. The net loss is from 200-500 mg.

Table 3.3

Estimated Iron "Cost" of a Normal Pregnancy with and Without Lactation

	mg.
Iron taken be fetus	201-372
Iron in placenta and cord blood	34-170
Iron in blood lost at delivery	100-250
Iron lost in milk, lactation 6 months	100-180
Total Iron Loss	435-972
Iron conserved by 15 months' amenorrhea	480-240
Net Cost, Pregnancy Plus Lactation:	0-732
Iron Conserved by 10 months' amenorrhea	320-160
Net Cost, Pregnancy Without Lactation:	15-632

Requirement

Requirements for iron vary in different periods of life according to the demands of growth, menstruation and pregnancy.

Values of Iron Requirement to Balance Iron Excretion

(1) Men and post menopausal women 0.5-1 mg/day

(2) Menstruating women 1-2 mg/day

(3) Pregnant women 1.5-2.5 mg/day

(4) Children (average) 1 mg/day

(5) Girls (12-15 years) 1-2.5 mg/day

(Drill, 3rd ed.)

A well-balanced diet with an iron content of about 15 mg. will normally keep men and post-menopausal women in adequate iron balance. The margin for women and children, though, is very small, therefore, women during their childbearing years, girls during adolescence and babies from 6.24 months very readily become iron deficient. In countries where dietary iron intake is low, iron deficiency may be found in the whole population.

About 10% of food iron is taken to be normally absorbed. Therefore, the amount of iron ingested with the food must be ten times the daily requirement.

In iron-deficiency anaemia, dietary iron cannot be enough to compensate for the loss of iron. That can be easily understood if the following values are worked out.

> Total body iron is about 4 gms. in an adult of 70 kg. He has about 750 Gms. of circulating haemoglobin. As previously mentioned, about two-thirds of the body iron is in haemoglobin. Therefore, the 750 Gms. of circulating haemoglobin will contain 2.5 Gms. iron. 1 per cent of circulating haemoglobin requires 25 mg. of iron for its formation. Also, haemoglobin contains 0.335 iron; with every 100 ml. blood (containing 15 Gms. of haemoglobin) lost by haemorrhage, a total of 50 mg. iron is lost (Goodman & Gilman, 3rd ed.)

Dietary iron, even if fully absorbed, is not able to provide the 25 mg/day necessary to raise the haemoglobin level by 1 per cent per day. Therefore, it is essential to administer medicinal iron deficiency anaemia.

Preparations if Iron

Table 3.4 shows the average effective dose of the common preparations of iron, as well as the amount of iron administered, and the percentage used for haemoglobin formation.

Foods Rich in Iron

Of much greater importance than the total iron content of foodstuff, is the ionizable nature of the iron so that it is *available* for absorption and synthesis into haemoglobin (Whitby & Britton, 1963). The *most efficient iron containing foods* are liver, oatmeal, brown bread, dried fruits (especially figs and apricots) beans, lentils, peas, green vegetables, cocoa, chocolate, sardines.

Red meat, though rich in iron, has relatively little iron available.

Table 3.4

Preparation	*Daily dose in grams or ml.*	*Iron content in mg.*	*Utilization (per cent)*
Ferrous—			
Ferrous carbonate	0.31-0.62	150-300	10-12
Ferrous chloride	0.25-0.5	100-200	12.5-25
Ferrous sulphate exsic	0.6-1.2	180-360	14
Ferrous fumarate	0.6-1.2	195-390	-
Ferrous gluconate	0.9-1.8	104-208	11
succinate	0.45-0.9	111-222	15
Ferric —			
Ferric citrate	2.0	400	6
Colloidal ferric hydroxide	5.25-10.5	600-1,200	14
Complex ferric —			
Ferri et ammon. cit.	4.0-8.0	800-1,600	1.5-3.0
Iron Chelates —			
Iron aminoates	1.05-2.1	105-210	—
Iron choline citrate	0.96-1.92	120-240	5-25
Intravenous—			
Saccharated oxide iron	5.0-10.0	100-200	85+
Iron-dextran complex	5.0	250	85+
Intramuscular			
Iron-dextran complex	5.0	250	60+
Iron-sorbitol complex	2.0	100	60+

Foods with a poor or poorly available iron content are fish, chicken, milk, white bread, most fruits.

For haemoglobin synthesis however, the protein or globin part of the haemoglobin has also to be considered. Therefore, it is important that the diet contains a large amount of first class protein in addition to adequate iron.

LIVER AND LIVER EXTRACTS

The therapeutic value of liver feeding in pernicious anaemia was first discovered by Minot and Murphy in 1926. Before this, pernicious anaemia was invariably fatal. The efficacy of liver in this condition indicated that it was a deficiency state but how pernicious anaemia occurred in persons on a normal diet was not understood till 1929. In that year, Castle demonstrated that normal gastric juice contains an "intrinsic factor" which bind an "extrinsic factor" contained in animal protein and facilitates the intestinal absorption of this extrinsic antipernicious-anemia-factor (APAF) found in liver. The treatment involved ingesting half-a-pound a day of raw or lightly cooked liver. This was not palatable for long periods and investigations were started, lasting years into the extraction of the active substance from liver. Various processes were devised which led to the production of dried and fluid liver extracts for oral use, followed by parenteral preparations of greater and greater potency, and finally the isolation of vitamin B_{12}.

Other factors were then gradually discovered to have an effect on pernicious anaemia. These were:

(1) *Animal protein factor*—During the 2nd world war attempts to raise pigs and poulty on purely vegetable rations were not successful till fish animal waste was included in their diets. This fermentation product was named the Animal Protein Factor (APF). Some years earlier, liver extract had been shown to have APF. When the fermentation product was found successful in pernicious anaemia, it indicated that APF and APAF were identical or closely related. However, it is probable that the crude APF may contain other unidentified substances as well as Vitamin $_{12}$.

(2) *L.L.D. factor*—This factor was known to be present in yeast and liver extracts and was essential in the nutrition of Lactobacillus lactis Dorner. A relation was noticed between the activity of liver extract in supporting Lactobacillus Lactis Dorner and potency in pernicious anaemia, and it was suspected that this may be identical with APA factor.

(3) *Cobalt activated ruminant factor*—This was later identified as Vitamin B_{12}.

Wills Factor

Wills and associates described in India, a macrocytic anaemia usually associated with pregnancy which responded to "Marmite" and autolyzed yeast extract. They discovered that a similar anaemia, induced by keeping monkeys on the same type of diet as that of these patients, responded to crude liver extracts which were then said to contain a "Wills factor". This "Wills factor" was not present in the purer fraction which was effective in pernicious anaemia. It is now believed that the Wills factor was folic acid.

Haemopoietic Principle

"Liver itself and all liver preparations contain vitamin B_{12}. They also contain folic acid and a number of other factors. Highly concentrated and purified extracts for parenteral use depend for their activity upon the vitamin B_{12} content and are, indeed, assayed for potency in this way, but such preparations—like B_{12} itself—are ineffective when administered by mouth. It is evident, therefore, that liver itself, as well as the simple extracts which are effective by mouth, contain either some comprehensive haemopoietic principle which is effective upon simple absorption, or is not dependent upon intrinsic factor for potentiation or absorption.

The nature of this haemopoietic principle in liver has defied identification for more than a quarter of a century; in proper dose it is clinically as effective as Vitamin B_{12} itself, and, in contrast to folic acid, affords protection against neurotrophic complications. For these reasons various liver extracts, liver preparation and even liver itself still have a place in the therapeutics of anaemia."

The accepted theory is that liver contains all the anit-anaemic principles Vitamin B_{12}, Wills factor (related to or identical with folic acid), members of the B-complex group of vitamins in natural proportions, proteins, and accessory factors of Jacobson and Subbarow.

The following references show that liver and liver extracts play a continuingly important part in therapeutics.

"There is some suggestive evidence that crude liver extracts may contain haemopoietically active material other than Vitamin B_{12} and folic acid".

The superiority of the bound form of vitamin B_{12} in crude liver extracts over cyanocobalamin or hydroxycobalamin given separately in equal dosage becomes evident by a study of the effects of the three drugs. It has been reported "that urinary excretion of Vitamin B_{12} in the first 24 hours was least with the Vitamin B_{12} which was present in liver in natural form. This is probably due to better utilization and slower release".

Because of the protein content, whole liver may act in certain cases of resistant anaemias other than pernicious anemia.

Jacobson and Bishop, (1948) claim that the haemopoietic potency of whole liver extract is much higher than its vitamin B_{12} content.

Meacham and Heinle (1953) reported an antimacrocytosis factor in whole liver extract different from folic acid and Vitamin B_{12}.

Types of Preparations for use in Therapy

(1) Desiccated liver (desiccated liver substance)

Desiccated Liver is the dried, defatted or underfatted powder prepared from mammalian livers suitable for use as food by man. Each gram of Desiccated Liver contains the equivalent of not less than 2 mcg. of cyanocobalamin; it contains not less than 10 per cent of nitrogen.

Desiccated liver is prepared from sound, clean and entire glands that are free from external connective tissue and external fat, and dried in a vacuum at a temperature not exceeding 60 degrees. It is free from diluents or preservatives. One part of desiccated liver is obtained from approximately 4 parts, by weight, of fresh glands.

(2) Liver Concentrate

Liver concentrate is the dried, unfractionated product resulting from the water or acidified water extract derived from mammalian livers suitable for use as food by man. Each gram of liver concentrate is derived from not less than 15 grams of fresh liver and contains not less than the equivalent of 7.5 mcg. of cyanocobalamin, and not less than 9 per cent of nitrogen. Liver concentrate is prepared from finely minced fresh or frozen livers by extaction with water, with or without the addition of acid. The protein is coagulated by heat, the insoluble material removed, and the solution is concentrated and dried in vacuum or a spray dryer.

(3) Liver Fraction 1 (Soluble Liver Fraction)

Liver Fraction 1 is the product in paste form, containing that portion of liver concentrate soluble in 70 per cent alcohol, and free from diluents. Each gram of liver fraction 1 is derived from not less than 25 grams of fresh liver and contains the equivalent of not less than 6 mcg. of cyanocobalamin. It contains not less that 6 per cent of nitrogen. It may contain 0.1 per cent of benzoic acid or a sutibale concentration of another harmless preservative.

(4) Liver Fraction 2 (Insoluble Liver Fraction)

Liver fraction 2 is a product containing that portion of liver concentrate insoluble in 70 per cent alcohol. It does not contain added diluents or preservatives other than an amount not to exceed 5 per cent of a harmless substance to prevent caking. Each gram of liver fraction 2 is derived from not less than 25 grams of fresh liver; it contains no less than 6 per cent of nitrogen.

(5) Proteolysed Liver

Proteolysed liver is a mixture of the products of digestion of edible mammalian livers, and may be prepared by digesting mammalian liver with a proteolytic enzyme at a temperature of 50-60 degrees and a pH of 5 to 6. The product is heated at 100 degrees for 5 minutes to inactivate the enzyme, filtered concentrated under reduced pressure, and evaporated to dryness in vacuum or a spray dryer. It may contain up to 5 per cent of a harmless substance added to prevent caking.

Each gram of proteolysed liver is derived from not less than 6 grams of fresh liver and contains the equivalent of not less than 2 mcg. of cyanocobalamin; it contains not less that 11 per cent of nitrogen.

Effects of Parenteral Liver Therapy

When the bone marrow has been stimulated by parenteral liver containing the haemopoietic principle, the first noticeable response is the increase of reticulocytes in the circulating blood. The normal number of reticulocytes in the blood is about 1% (i.e. one reticulocyte to every 100 red blood cells.) However, when active blood regeneration takes place, as happens when a potent liver extract has been administered, they may increase up to 40%. This increase is known as the *Reticulocyte Response* and when it reaches its maximum level it is known as the *Reticulocyte Crisis.* This crisis usually occurs between the 4th and 12th day. After the crisis, the reticulocytes rapidly mature into erythrocytes and the reticulocyte level drops to the original 1%. It naturally follows that after good reticulocyte crisis, the red cell count increases. Thus after injections of Liver extract, an increase of red cells will be noticed after about ten days. The usual crisis day after injection is the 7th day. The average increase in red cells from a quarter to a half million red cells per ten days, but this varies according to the initial erythrocyte deficiency.

Two schemes are recommended; the first being useful in hospitals and nursing homes; the second in general practice. In hospitals, and with the patient in bed, large infrequent injections may be given. By this means, the number of liver injections are cut down, leaving time and space for any other injecitons, and a more concentrated stimulus is given to the bone marrow. Initially, 5 ml. of liver extract may be injected daily for the first two days. This is followed by 2 ml. on alternate days until a satisfactory reticulocyte response occurs. Later 2 ml. are given biweekly until a normal blood picture is obtained. This will meet the need of most cases.

In private practice where cases are naturally not so severe, more frequent and less bulky injections are advised. 2ml. daily up to a total of 10 ml. and/or a good reticulocyte response should be adequate. Thereafter 2ml. weekly may be sufficient to bring the blood picture up to normal. There are, however, no hard and fast rules and the dose should be adjusted to the severity of the aneamia and the degree of haematological response.

The strength of a liver extract is usually denoted as an extract from so many grams of fresh liver.

In general, the more refined a liver extract, the more potent it is in the treatment of Addisonian Pernicious Anaemia and the less effective it becomes in the treatment of Tropical Macrocytic Anaemia. This suggests that there are several parts to the haemopoietic substance in liver. Thus when one refines it down to merely a bone marrow stimulant, several substances also needed in blood formation, (such as Vitamin B-Complex) are excluded. Therefore, it is usually advisable and also economical to use a crude liver extract in the tropics.

It can easily be seen that whatever the type of anaemia, an extıact of the storage depot, namely the liver, will give a good response, provided there is no aplastic tendency of the bone marrow.

A well extracted whole liver (or crude liver) extract contains a high percentage of Vitamin B-Complex. These are what may be termed in the "natural" form.

Parenteral whole liver extracts are now standardised according to the Indian Pharmacopoeia. These standards are as follows:

(1) Liver Injection Crude is a sterile solution in water for injecion of that soluble thermostable fraction of mammalian livers which increases the red blood corpuscles in the blood of persons suffering from pernicious and other types of macrocytic anaemias. It is obtained by stopping the processes of extraction at such a stage that the final product is derived from an alcohol solution of a concentration not higher than 70 per cent by volume of ethyl alcohol.

Each ml. of liver Injection Crude has Vitamin B_{12} activity equivalent to either 1 microgram or 2 micrograms of cyanocobalamin. The preparation shall contain not more than 0.5 per cent of cresol or of phenol as a bacteriostatic agent.

(2) *Proper Name*: The proper name of the preparation shall be Liver Injection Crude.

(3) *Description*: A brownish Liquid which at times may show a slight turbidity.

(4) *Tests*:

(a) Reaction; pH 5 to 7.

(b) *Total Solids*: The total solids shall not be less than 15 per cent w/v in the case of a preparation containing 2 micrograms of cyanocobalamin per ml. and 7.5 per cent w/v in the case of a preparation containing 1 microgram of cyanocobalamin per ml. respectively.

(c) *Limits for proteins*: The protein nitrogen shall not exceed 0.08 per cent w/v.

(d) *Absence of undue toxicity*: On white mice.

(e) *Sterility and Pyrogen Test*: Liver Injection Crude shall comply with the sterility and pyrogen tests laid down for "Injection" in the Indian Pharmacopoeia.

(f) *Potency*: The B_{12} activity per ml. should either be 1 microgram or 2 micrograms.

(5) *Container*: The container used for Liver Injection Crude shall comply with the requirements laid down in the Indian Pharmacopoeia for container of Injection.

(6) *Storage*: Liver Injection Crude shall be stored in a cool place preferably at a temperature not exceeding 20^{0} C and protected from light.

(7) *Label*: The label on the container shall state the following details in addition to any other particulars prescribed in these Rules:

1. The amount of vitamin B_{12} activity (Cyanocobalamin) per ml.

2. The average amount of raw liver processed to produce 1 ml of extract.
3. The date of expiration of potency which should not be later than 24 months from the date of manufacture. (No F.I. 45/58-D)
4. The name and quantity of the bacteriostatic agent added

FOLIC ACID

Folic acid is a yellow crystalline substance consisting of three structural units (1) a pteridine, (2) p-aminobenzoic acid and (3) glutamic acid. It is also known as pteroylglutamic acid and was originally isolated from spinach, but is now known to be widely distributed in nature in conjugated forms which are biologically inert but are capable of liberating the free acid under the action of enzymes called conjugases. The reduced derivatives of folic acid are unstable and difficult to preserve except N^5 — formyl FH_4 also called the citrovorum factor or folinic acid or leucovorin.

Neither folic acid nor its conjugates are identical with extrinsic factor, intrinsic factor or the haemopoietic principle.

Folic acid has the character of a vitamin and is probably concerned with enzyme systems essential for metabolism.

Sources

Folic acid is found in leafy vegetables, mushrooms, liver, kidneys, yeast, nuts, grain, fruits, eggs and milk. The highest folate content per unit is in yeast, liver and fresh green vegetables. It should be noted that a large fraction (50-95%) of the folic acid from foods is removed or destroyed by excessive cooking or canning. The average diet contains 0.6 mg. daily before cooking, and 0.15 mg. after cooking. The daily intake is not likely to be more than 1 mg.

Absorption, Fate and Excretion

The major site of absorption of folic acid is the jejunum. Therefore, even though this substance is synthesized by intestinal bacteria, little is absorbed since most of this synthesis occurs in the colon (Drill, 3rd ed.). That this microorganism-synthesized folate is not available to the host can be also proved by the fact that dietary folate deficiency can be produced in man.

The percentage absorption of total folate from rich sources such as liver, yeast and egg yolk is high but only 10% of the forms of folate in most foods, is absorbed. However, the absorption of pteroylglutamic acid itself is almost total.

The exact mechanism of folic acid absorption is not completely definite but is probably an energy requiring mechanism for physiological amounts but by diffusion for greater quantitities.

Absorption is rapid since the vitamin appears in the plasma half hour after ingestion.

The total body content is about 6-10 mg. and the liver contains 4-6 mg.

Because of the limited absorption of food folate, only 5-40 micrograms of free folate activity a pears in the urine per day of normal persons on an average diet.

Folic acid acts in enzyme reactions only after conversion to FH_4. There are many metabolic systems requiring folic acid, but the two reactions, the impairment of which causes significant clinical manifestations, are thymidylate synthesis and histidine catabolism. The first, thymidylate synthesis, is a preliminary step in the synthesis of DNA. An interference in this reaction leads to *megaloblast formation* which is the characteristic haematological finding in folic acid deficiency. Interference with histidine catabolism has no serious effect, but provides the basis for a useful diagnostic test. In folic acid deficiency, there is increased excretion in the urine of formiminoglutamic acid (FIGLU), which can be eassily detected. Normal persons excrete little or no FIGLU.

Clinical Aspects of Deficiency

Folic acid deficiency disturbs normal erythropoiesis due to the reason already stated, with the result that the pro-erythroblasts give rise, not to the normoblasts, but to the megaloblasts which may mature to megalocytes. The most characteristic cell in the blood is the intermediate megaloblast about 12-20 microns in size.

Causes of Deficiency

1. Malnultrition
2. Malabsorption e.g. tropical and non-tropical sprue.
3. Increased requirements.
   (a) Some haemolytic anaemias.
   (b) Malignancy
   (c) Pregnancy
4. Inhibition of folic acid reduction by pharmacological agents. e.g. anti-convulsants.

Symptoms of Folic Acid Deficiency

The symptoms most often found are glossitis, diarrhoea, and weight loss, which may also be found with vitamin B_{12} deficiency. The most striking difference is that, with folate deficiency, the neurological signs of damage to myelin do not appear. However, sleeplessness, irritability, forgetfulness are sometimes found and these may be related to disordered cerebral metabolism.

Relation of Folic acid to Vitamin B_{12} in Therapy

The therapeutic effect of folic acid on the vitamin B_{12} deficiency syndromé has certain peculiarities which must be kept in mind. Folic acid will correct the haemopoietic and gastrointestinal manifestations of vitamin B_{12} deficiency but neurological complications may continue to progress with disastrous results. The explanation for this, strictly speaking is not known. However, a reasonable deduction has been made on the basis of biochemical evidence and various theories have been put forward.

(1) Folic acid requires vitamin B_{12} for its own metabolism and can immobilize traces of this important vitamin which may be present in the tissues thereby participating an acute and sudden shortage. There is no evidence that this occurs in normal people or those who are not vitamin B_{12} deficient.

This indicates that in pernicious anaemia, folic acid is haematologically efficient and if the patient is not entirely vitamin B_{12} deficient, no neurological complications will arise.

Further evidence is provided by Bok *et al.,* (1958) who found that when folic acid caused a haematological response in pernicious anaemia, the serum vitamin B_{12} was decreased considerably below the pretreatment values.

(2) Certain metabolic processes in the body require both folic acid vitamin B_{12}. Drill, (3rd ed.) states "when one of two vitamins essential in different phases of deoxyribonucleotide synthesis is limiting, large doses of the nonlimiting vitamin probably (1) increase the efficiency with which the limiting vitamin is utilised in deoxyribonucleotide synthesis, and (2) divert portions of the remaining supply away from those metabolic systems in which it functions singly. Thus, it may be supposed that folic acid treatment of vitamin B_{12} deficiency tends to enhance deoxyribonucleotide synthesis through "mass action" while further depleting other systems of vitamin B_{12}. If vitamin B_{12} has an essential function in neural tissue, these circumstances could aggravate or precipitate the onset of neurological symptoms."

Side-effects

Folic acid is regarded as non-toxic in man.

A very few examples of sensitivity reactions with skin rashes, malaise and bronchospasm have been reported. Some volunteers in a recent study, experienced sleep disturbances and gastrointestinal symptoms. However, these side-effects have been seriously questioned and folic acid is usually considered a drug safe even in doses several times higher than the usual therapeutic levels.

Effect of Folic Acid in Man

In man, folic acid produces euphoria, increased appetite, decreased basal oxygen consumption in pernicious anaemia patients (no change in normal subjects), an increase in the percentage of total calories derived from carbohydrate, an increase in specific dynamic action, an increase in faecal nitrogen, and an increased nitrogen retention. The results suggested that in patients with pernicious anaemia, cirrhosis of the liver and idiopathic steatorrhoea, folic acid increases the absorption of nitrogen from the gastro-intestinal tract and decreases the deamination of amino-acids by the liver. Folic acid also increases human serum cholinesterase activity.

Requirements

The requirements appear to be 0.5-1 mg. daily.

Therapeutic Uses

It is believed that the sole indication of this vitamin is in folic acid deficiency and the therapeutic effects are due to reversal of the deficiency state.

Dosage

Various authorities differ on the dose of folic acid which needs to be administered in different conditions.

In pregnancy, there is almost universal agreement about the desirability of a folate supplement as prophylaxis.Estimates of the dose needed vary however, and amounts between 50 and 5000 micrograms have been prescribed.

In spite of prophylactic treatment, megaloblastic anaemia may develop and in these cases, adequate high doses (ranging from 10-30 mg. daily) may become necessary.

The danger of precipitating neurological complications may be avoided if low parenteral doses (0.1-0.2 mg) are used as a confirmatory diagnostic procedure. These low doses will cause a full haematological response in folate deficiency but not in Vitamin B_{12} deficiency.

Adequate doses have to be given in the other conditions (already enumerated above) where there is a deficiency of folic acid. The dose should naturally be higher when there is reason to believe there is malabsorption.

Folic acid may protect against anaemia and leucopenia produced by x-radiation.

Also, high doses have been found to have a beneficial effect on the granulocytopenia following sulphonamide therapy.

VITAMIN B_{12} AND INTRINSIC FACTOR

Vitamin B_{12}

Vitamin B_{12} also known as cyanocobalamin, crystallizes as dark-red nodules or prisms, the colour being due to a cobalt containing pigment. Cyanocobalamin belongs to the group of cyanocobamides, which it is believed, do not occur naturally, but arise only from the degradation of cobamide coenzymes. Exposure to light converts cyanocobalamin to hydroxycobalamin and the reverse takes place in the dark.

Sources

Vitamin B_{12} is unique among vitamins in that it is synthesised *only* by microorganisms, which may be growing in soil, water, intestine and rumen. In man, it is synthesised in the bowel but this is not absorbed and the faeces therefore contain a large amount of Vitamin B_{12}.

The naturally occurring cobalamins in food are bound to protein and it is usually believed that they are inactive metabolically until split by heat or proteolysis. However, it is possible that complete breakdown of food is not necessary for Vitamin B_{12} absorption and various intermediate digestion products containing B_{12} may be formed and absorbed as such.

Rich sources of cobalamins are organ meats e.g. beef or lamb liver, kidney, heart and bivalves (clams, oysters). Moderate amounts are found in nonfat, dry milk, sea foods (crabs, salmon, sardines) egg yolk and muscle meats.

Metabolic Functions

The cobalamins are involved directly or indirectly in all known metabolic systems in man. They are essential for growth, normal nutrition, normal haematopoiesis, normal production of epithelial cells (including those of the gastro-intestinal tract) and for the maintenance of myelin throughout the nervous system.

Cobalamins are necessary for nucleoprotein synthesis and therefore are required wherever cells reproduce themselves. As the bone marrow is a highly active and rapidly regenerating tissue, it is obvious that deficiency of vitamin B_{12} is reflected in abnormal haematopoiesis. The biochemical system concerned is the deoxyribosyl and thus DNA synthesis, the impairment of which accounts for magaloblastic erythropoiesis.

It is interesting to note that in the absence of adequate quantitities of cobalamin, folate may be trapped at a certain level, thus resulting in a functional folate deficiency even with adequate ingestion and absorption of folate.

Absorption

The average diet contains 5-30 micrograms of Vitamin B_{12}. Vitamin B_{12} is absorbed by two separate machanisms depending on the quantity of the Vitamin to be absorbed.

(1) Physiological or Intrinsic Factor Mechanism

Dietary vitamin B_{12} is freed from protein in the stomach and small intestine under the influence of gastric acid and various enzymes. The free vitamin B_{12} is then attached to the intrinsic factor of Castle secreted by the gastric fundus. This vitamin B_{12} intrinsic factor complex passes down to the ileum where it attaches to receptors on the ileal surface, the process requiring calcium and/or magnesium and a pH higher than 6. The vitamin remains in the ileal mucosa for several hours and is then transported via the blood stream to the liver for storage. About 1-4 micrograms is absorbed by this machanism.

Intrinsic factor is also concerned with the intestinal absorption of cobalamins other than cyanocobalamin.

(2) Mass-action or Diffusion

This mechanism operates in the presence of large quantities of vitamin B_{12} and can probably occur along the entire length of the intestine. Absorption by this method is much more rapid and is important in that, some vitamin B_{12} from foods rich in the substance *e.g.* liver, may be absorbed even in the absence of intrinsic factor. Also, oral therapy of pernicious anaemia by use of large quantities of Vitamin $_{12}$ may be useful.

Factors Enhancing Absorption

(1) d-sorbitol } probably by stimulating increased
(2) food } secretion of intrinsic factor.

Factors Reducing Absorption

(1) Large amounts of oral intrinsic factor concentrate (probably by competing with B_{12}-laden intrinsic factor for ileal receptors).

(2) Large amounts of sorbitol (by producing diarrhoea).

(3) Phytates and disodium edetate (are calium-chelating agents).

Transport

In the blood, Vitamin B_{12} is attached mainly to an $\propto$ 1-globulin, which carries it to the tissues and especially to the liver. This transport protein called transcorrin probably facilitates the uptake of Vitamin B_{12} by maturing erythroid cells. A small amount in the blood is free or loosely bound.

As already mentioned, absorption is delayed in the ileum and peak plasma levels are reached 8-12 hours after ingestion of physiological amounts.

Normal plasma concentration of Vitamin B_{12} is about 450 pg (micromicrograms)/ ml.

Fate and Excretion

The liver is the main storage organ and contains 50-90% of the body's stores which are on an average 4-5 mg. in a normal adult.

It is is believed that no catabolism of Vitamin B_{12} occurs in man and loss is only by excretion. Exretion is mainly via the biliary tract and to a slight extent in the urine.

Vitamin B_{12} is secreted (about 3-7 micrograms daily) into the alimentary tract, mainly in the bile, but some in gastric and pancreatic juices. Of this, all except about 1 microgram is reabsorbed via the intrinsic factor mechanism. Thus, there is an active enterohepatic circulation of Vitamin B_{12}. The unabsorbed portion together with the amount synthesised by the colon is excreted in the faeces (about 8 micrograms).

The small amount of Vitamin B_{12} is not bound to plasma protein may be excreted in the urine (about 0-0.25 micrograms daily).

Clinical Aspects of Deficiency

The clinical manifestations of cobalamin deficiency are those of:

(1) Ineffective haematopoiesis — giving rise to megaloblastic anaemia.

(2) Inadequate maintenance of epithelial cells of alimentary tract — giving rise to gastrointestinal symptoms including glossitis, dyspepsia.

(3) Inadequate myelin synthesis — giving rise to diverse neurological abnormalities with degenerative changes of the dorsal and lateral columns of the spinal cord and peripheral nerves.

Clinically, there is no relation between the degree of neurological damage and the degree of haematological damage probably because of the variable folate intake of individuals. A high folate level corresponds to little haematological damage and vice versa.

Causes of Deficiency

(1) Inadequate dietary intake — tropical nutritional anaemia — (approximately 1 microgram must be absorbed from the diet for minimum requirements.)

(2) *Intestinal malasorption* — probably the most common cause of Vitamin B_{12} deficiency

(a) Pernicious anaemia.

(b) Sprue, idiopathic steatorrhoea.

(c) Total gastrectomy.

(d) Intestinal stasis due to any cause — stricture "blind loop" syndrome, anastomoses, diverticula etc.

(e) Diphyllobothrium latum infestation (fish tape worm).

(f) Organic disease of the bowel wall.

(3) *Increased requirements* — This type of deficiency is seen mainly in pregnancy and naturally, is more frequent in twin pregnancies.

(4) *Failure of utilization in the tissues* — a few cases of megaloblastic, macrocytic anaemia occurring during the adminstration of anticonvulsant drugs have responded to Vitamin B_{12} through the majority need folic acid). Possibly, the anti-convulsant agent interferes with the utilization of Vitamin B_{12}in the tissues.

A Vitamin B_{12} deficiency state can only develop if and when the large body stores are depleted. As the daily requirement is only 1 microgram, several years may elapse before the development of deficiency symptoms following gastrectomy or stoppage of adequate treatment in penicious anaemia.

Diagnosis

The most useful method of confirming Vitamin B_{12} deficiency is the microbiological assay of the serum Vitamin B_{12} level. Normal subjects have levels over 150 micromicrograms per ml. Patients with symptomatic deficiency have levels below 80 micrograms per ml.

The Schilling test is useful in determining the mechanism of Vitamin B_{12} deficiency.

The determination of the erythrocyte transketolase activity may become an important test to differentiate between Vitamin B_{12} deficiency and folate deficiency. Transketolase is of particular interest as it is the first red-cell-enzyme abnormality to have been reported which is exclusive to Vitamin B_{12} deficiency and does not occur in folate deficiency. Erythrocyte transketolase activity is found to be raised in megaloblastic anaemias due to Vitamin B_{12} deficiency and normal in macrocytic anaemia due to folate deficiency. Potential application of this test has yet to be evaluated.

These tests however should be supplementary to the conventional diagnostic procedures viz.

(1) Careful dietary history.

(2) Examination of blood and bone marrow smear.

(3) Tests for gastric free acid after histamin stimulation.

(4) Radiological examination of the gastro-intestinal tract.

(5) Tests to rule out folic acid deficiency.

Simultaneous differential diagnosis and therapy can be provided by a "therapeutic trial" where 1 microgram of cyanocobalamin is administered parenterally daily for 10 days. This will produce a haematological response only in Vitamin B_{12} deficiency whereas doses in excess of 10 micrograms daily may produce a haematological response in patients with folate deficiency.

Dosage

Initial dosage of Vitamin B_{12} depends on the severity of the anaemia, and the presence of complicating factors such as infection and neurological lesions. The response to therapy will determine subsequent doses.

The objectives of treatment are

(1) the gradual replenishment of depleted stores.

(2) the maintenance of adequate intake to balance daily losses.

There are many satisfactory procedures for initiating treatment. A regimen of 200 micrograms three times a week gives complete clinical remission fairly quickly. However, intensive treatment must be continued for 6 weeks for repletion of body stores. In most cases, maintenance by means of monthly injections of 100 micrograms is customary, though even higher doses have been advocated. At this dosage, the plasma Vitamin B_{12} level remains normal for a month.

In patients with severe neurological damage, more intensive therapy has been advocated by some authorities e.g. 1000 micrograms daily for one week or more.

Other authorities have claimed that such high doses are not of significant advantage and have advocated 1 microgram per day in uncomplicated cases, the presence of neurological complications necessitating 30 micrograms per day for 5-10 days. (Goodman and Gilman, 1967).

Careful and frequent examination of the patient's blood and physical signs is important to establish whether medication is adequate. Unless the mean corpuscular volume returns to normal, the patient is not protected against further neural damage. The erythrocyte count should be kept over 4.5 mill/c.mm.

Oral administration in high doses — 1000 micrograms or more given once a week have caused haematological remission, but it is not definite whether this form of treatment repletes body stores.

Toxicity

Bicknell and Prescott (1953) found no toxic effects even with excessive doses of Vitamin B_{12} and state that there are no known contra indication to its use. However, Vitamin B_{12} injection has reported to have given rise to anaphylatic shock and death in one case. Other reports have suggested that very high doses of Vitamin B_{12} may give rise to utricarial type reactions.

Therapeutic Uses

Vitamin B_{12} is indicated in Vitamin B_{12} deficiency states but has also been recommended for various neuropathies, liver diseases, skin disorders, allergies, as a tonic and a growth stimulants in children.

Intrinsic Factor

Intrinsic factor is believed to be a glycoprotein or mucopoly saccharde and has yet not been isolated in pure form. In man, it is formed probably exclusively in the fundus and body of the stomach by the peptic chief cells.

Intrinsic factors has two important properties:

(1) The ability to bind Vitamin B_{12}.

(2) The ability to enhance absorption of Vitamin B_{12} from the ileum — this is a specific, unique property of intrinsic factor.

Intrinsic factor production is stimulated by

(a) D-sorbitol

(b) Food

(c) Insulin

(d) Corticosteroid

(e) Thyroid hormone.

4

Erythrocytic Production & Destruction

In considering the regulation of hemopoiesis, one has found it necessary to study isolated components of the system and the effect of a variety of manipulations thereon. Valuable information has been derived in this fashion, but it is evident that the hemopoietic system must be considered as a whole, since interplay between the various component parts is an important consideration in the regulation of any one of these parts. I shall attempt to develop a model for erythropoiesis, but one in which interaction between other compartments of the hemopoietic system is taken into account. The basic structure of the erythropoietic system consists of four compartments: the pluripotent stem cell, the erythroid committed stem cell, the differentiated erythroid precursors, and the circulating red cells. The pluripotent cell is shared with the myeloid and megakaryocytic systems, and interplay between these will affect erythropoiesis. Finally we have become aware of the importance of ecology on the growth of cells, and in this respect marrow structure and microenvironment assume an increasingly important role.

THE PLURIPOTENT STEM CELL

For many years it has been evident that the differentiated erythroid compartment is not self-sustaining, but is continually fed from a precursor compartment. Studies on transplantation chimeras, together with clinical observations on the Ph^1 chromosome in chronic myelocytic leukemia, pointed to the fact that the stem cell was pluripotential. During the past several years, mounting evidence has accumulated, indicating that there are two functional, if not morphologic, levels, of stem cells, one pluripotent and one already committed to a given line of differentiation. In the case of erythropoiesis, the latter but not the former is erythropoietin (EP) responsive. Evidence for these two levels of stem cells derives from the work of a number of laboratories. Perhaps the most cogent evidence for the existence of two levels of stem cells are studies in which it has been demonstrated that the pluripotent stem cell compartment in large measure is in G_0 whereas the committed cell is predominantly in cycle. Thus Morse *et al* (1979a, b) observed that hydroxyurea (OHU), a rapidly metabolized agent selectively lethal hemopoietic cells in S will directly affect the committed but not the pluripotent compartment in the hypertransfused animal. Rickard *et al* (1970a) noted that when OHU was given to donors, the numbers of mycloid cells found in tissue culture, colony forming cells (CFC) were reduced but the numbers of transplantable colony forming units (CFU) were relatively

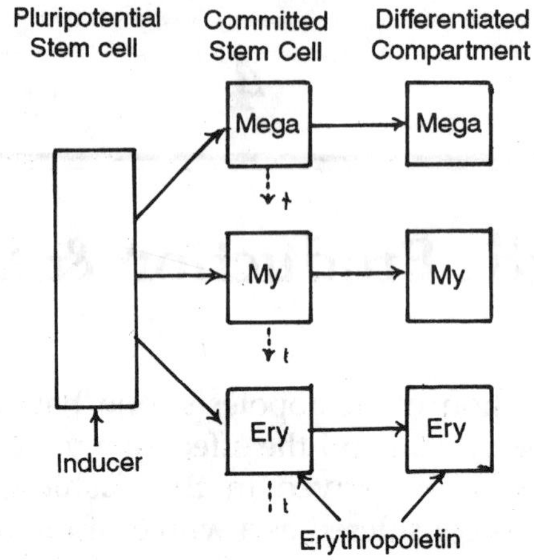

Fig. 4.1. A schematic model of hematopoiesis. Meg—megakaryocytic, MY—myelocytic, ERY—erythropoietic. Dashed line and cross indicate cell death.

unaffected. Similar results have been obtained by Iscove *et al* (1970) using ^{3}HTdR. Thus the CFC appear to arise from a committed compartment in cycle but the CFU arise from the more primitive and resting pluripotent stem cell. Worthy of note, as will be discussed in more detail later, are the interrelationships between the committed and pluripotent compartments. Thus, if an agent is administered that affects the committed compartment, e.g., hydroxyurea, ^{3}HTrD, vinblastine, etc., restoration of that compartment will be accomplished in part through differentiation from the pluripotent compartment. This in turn will lead to a change in the numbers of pluripotent cells of CFU. Hence in experiments designed to evaluate the pluripotent compartment and in which drugs are used, oservations must be limited to the first few hours, since later effects may be abscopal rather than direct.

The factors regulating the pluripotent cell are poorly understood and only recently have come under intense examination. It has been clear from the early experiments of Brecher and Cronkite (1951) on radioprotection in parabiotic animals that pluripotent cells circulate in the blood stream. More direct evidence from transplantation experiments was presented by Goodman and Hodgson (1962). Kretchmar (1969) recently has suggested that the circulating CFU are in a dynamic equilibrium with tissue CFU and lodge to grow where a favourable microenvironment presents itself. Whether, in addition, the committed stem cells are in a similar state of flux cannot be stated, although recent experiments in our laboratory suggest that this may be the case. Thus in mice receiving whole-body irradiation whilst one hind leg is shielded, erythroid recovery in the limb occurs in the absence of CFU proliferation. Further, massive erythroid hyperplasia is seen in the spleen of animals recovering from phenylhydrazine anemia in the absence of CFU proliferation. These observations may of course reflect migration and subsequent

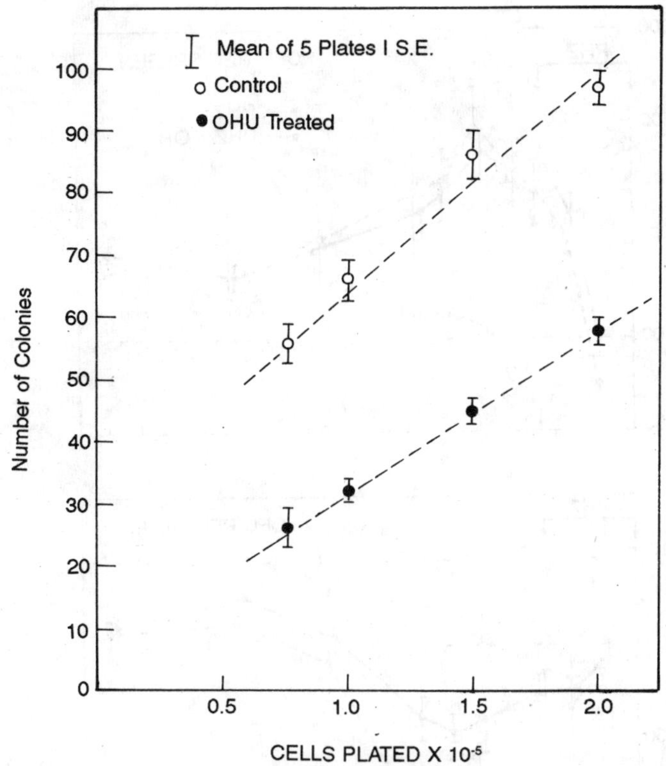

Fig. 4.2. The number of in *vitro* colonies derived from bone marrow cells of normal and hydroxyurea treated mice.

differentiation of CFU, but the magnitude of the response raises the question whether committed cells in addition are migrating.

No hormonal-mechanisms have been described for the regulation of pluripotent stem cells, and it would appear that humoral factors are not operative at this level. What, then is responsible for the maintenance of homeostasis within this compartment? Aside from the aforementioned tissue-blood equilibrium, which in turn reflects ecology, one might suggest a short-range cell-cell type of regulation. Several studies appear pertinent in this respect. Goodman and Shinpock (1968), Goodman and Grubbs (1970), and more recently McCulloch and Till (1970) observed that parental thymocytes and to a much more restricted degree F_1 thymocytes, when transplanted into F_1 hybrids, accelerated the recovery of both CFU and erythropoiesis in the recipient spleens. No effect was detectable in the bone marrow or in splenectomized recipients, suggesting a short range interaction as a consequence of the lodging of chvmocytes in splenic tissue. Further, McCulloch and Till (1970) noted a more rapid recovery of CFU when cyclophosphamide was administered shortly before irradiation and transplantation of parental marrow into F_1 hybrids. From these experiments, it was suggested that recognition at a cellular level played an important role in the initiation of cell division in the pluripotent stem cell and that modification of cell surfaces by drug might also prove to be a stimulus to the

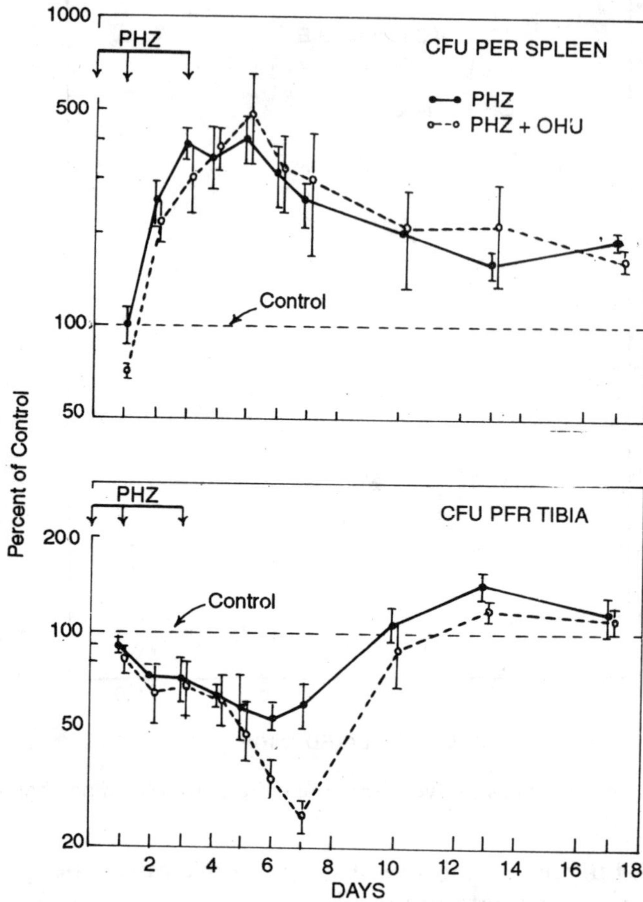

Fig. 4.3. Changes in splenic and tibial CFU in mice given phenylhydrazine (PHZ) alone or in combination with hydroxyurea (OHU). Each point represents the group mean, based on the percent of control, ± 1 SEM. of 8-27 mice.

growth of CFU. The notion that recognition at a surface level is of importance is further suggested by the work of Cudkowicz and Stimpfling (1964), on the role of the H-2 surface antigen in governing stem cell growth.

It seems plausible that short range cell interaction is the governing mechanism for pluripotent cell homeostasis, but we would like to raise the question whether this is stimulatory, as suggested by the authors above, or inibitory, perhaps analogous to contact inhibition *in vitro*. Germane to this question are observations in our laboratory on the behaviour of stem cells in irradiated animals and those recovering from severe anemia. Several years ago, Stohlman (1961) observed that when erythropoietin was given immediately before or after sublethal irradiation, recovery of erythropoiesis was accelerated; when erythropoietin administration was delayed for a period of 24 to 48

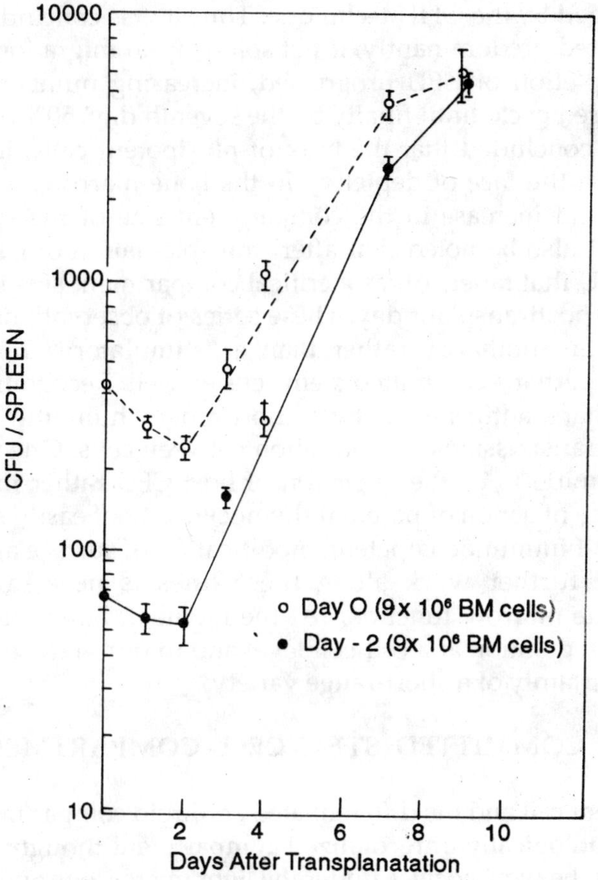

Fig. 4.4. The growth curve for splenic CFU in animals transplanted with aliquots of bone marrow either on the day of or 48 hours after irradiation. Day after the transplant refers to the day after the primary transplant.

hours a much more limited effect was noted. It was proposed that these results might reflect removal of feedback inhibition by differentiation with EP of cells damaged by irradiation but still surviving, i.e., sterile cells incapable of growth. More recently Shadduck *et al.* (1970) noted that, although the plating efficiency was lower, the growth curve of splenic CFU was more rapid when transplantation of bone marrow into lethaly irradiated recipients was delayed for 48 hours. In these experiments, the same bone marrow inoculum was given to groups transplanted immediately or 48 hours after irradiation. Thus host factors were clearly responsible for the differences. While migration and ecology might account in part for these results, differences in growth regulation appear to be implicated. At about the same time, Rencricca *et al* (1970) studied the pattern of response in animals in which severe anemia was produced by phenylhydrazine. In these animals, erythroid hyperplasia developed in both spleen and marrow. As the erythroid response developed, the CFU in the bone marrow decreased whereas those in the spleen increased (Fig. 4.3). The increase in splenic CFU was not accompanied by proliferation of CFU is situ, as judged by the OHU technique. Thus it was concluded that the increase in splenic CFU occurred predominantly, if not solely, from migration. In contrast, in the bone marrow, as depletion of CFU progressed, increasing numbers of the remaining pluripotent cells entered cycle until finally by the seventh day, 50% of the cells were in S and it was therefore concluded that the bulk of pluripotent cells, in the bone marrow were in cycle. Thus in the face of depletion in the bone marrow, the CFU entered cell division. In contrast, an increase in the compartment size of the spleen inhibited cell proliferation. It might also be noted that after transplantation of CFU, there is a rapid growth of splenic CFU that tapers off as a critical compartment size is achieved at about the seventh to eighth posttransplant day. These series of observations appear to us to be better explained by an inhibitory rather than a "stimulatory" relationship between pluripotent cells and perhaps committed stem cells as well. Recognition of cells through surface contract, perhaps antigenic, or by a short range "humoral" mechanism, might well account for the transmission of information between cells. One would envision the role of cyclophosphamide to be the depletion of host CFU rather than modification of cell surface. The mode of action of parental thymocytes is not easily reconciled in such a hypothesis, although if immunocompetent, modification of surface antigen may provide the answer. Clearly further work along these lines is necessary for our overall understanding of bone marrow function. At the moment, however, the date available favour a short-range regulation at a cell-cell level and in our view involves inhibition, if not by contact then certainly of a short-range variety.

THE COMMITTED STEM CELL COMPARTMENT

Between the pluripotent cell and the differentiated erythroid compartment (pronormoblast, etc.), there is a morphologically unrecognized compartment thought to be mononuclear cell that may appear to be lymphocytes under the light microscope and that are committed to differentiation along erythroid lines Whether de-differentiation to a pluripotent cell also occurs is moot, but cannot be discounted. In the case of red cell production, it is this cell that is erythropoietin-responsive. This compartment is normally in cycle but with a variable generation time (T_G). Accordingly, it is in significant measure self-sustaining, but there is substantial evidence to indicate that in the face of severe demand or after injury, e.g. from irradiation or cytotoxic agents, influx from the pluripotent compartment is necessary to support erythropoiesis adequately.

The mechanism of action of erythroprotein in relationship to cell cycle kinetics has been the subject of extensive studies. Lajtha (1967) suggested that EP could differentiate only cells in G_O; this in turn triggered other G_O cells into cycle where they were no longer available for differentiation. Thus, he speculated, compartment depletion was averted. In the light of more recent data, this view no longer seems tenable. Schooley (1965) and more recently Fogh (1970) noted that hypertransfused animals have an increasing erythroid response with successive doses of EP that could not be accounted for by an effect of EP on the differentiated compartment. This they termed recruitment, but, in fact, it appears in large measure to be a manifestation of the variable G_1 in the committed compartment. Morse, Rencricca and Stohlman (1970a,b) gave EP to animals with erythroid aplasia secondary to hypertransfusion, and at various intervals thereafter administered hydroxyurea. The simultaneous administration of OHU with EP reduced the erythroid response. Thus one may infer that a portion of the population responding to EP was in cycle and in S; this does not appear to be compatible with Lajtha's thesis that only G_O cells respond to EP. As the interval between the administration of EP and OHU was increased, there was a proportionally greater reduction in the erythroid response. A second dose of OHU resulted not in an additive but rather a synergistic effect. The greater effect of OHU when given at increasing intervals after EP indicated that the relationship of the mean cell generation time (T_G) to the mean time spent in DNA synthesis (T_S), that is T_S/T_G, was changing. Two explanations are possible; either T_G was shortened relative to T_S or T_S was prolonged. The latter seems incompatible with our current concepts of DNA synthesis and moreover appears to be an illogical response to a stimulus. We infer, therefore, that T_G was shortened in the response to EP and that this was accomplished most likely through a variable G_1. We further conclude that due to a variable G_1, T_G varies in the committed erythroid cell from a minimum of perhaps 10 hours to a maximum of 30 hours—the latter being seen in erythroid aplasia secondary to hypertransfusion. A corollary to this thesis is that the erythropoietin response is associated with shortening of G_1. These time estimates are in remarkable agreement with conclusions that Kretchmar *et al* (1970) reached in constructing a computer model, which also assumed a variable G_1 and T_G. From the data above we have suggested that EP is effective throughout cycle with, perhaps, the exception of T_M.

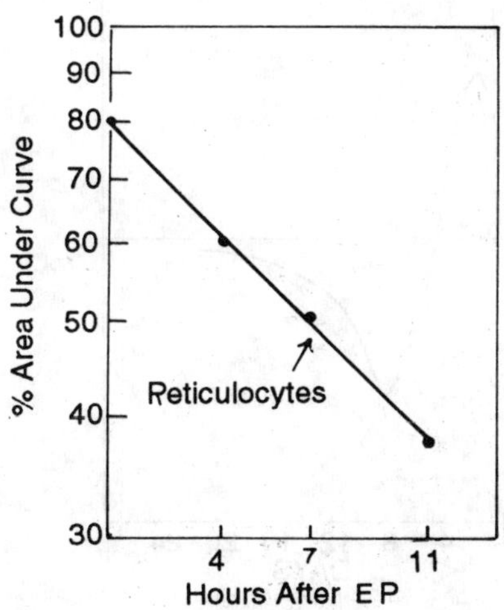

Fig. 4.5. Areas under the reticulocyte curve are compared to the area obtained in EP-treated control animals.

We cannot comment on the possibility raised by Kretchmar *et al* (1970) that EP must be present during both G_1 and S to be effective. After severe stimulation, depletion of the committed compartment in significant measure appears to be averted by influx from the pluripotent compartment. Whether there are additional "braking" forces within the committed compartment awaits further study.

Perhaps worthy of note is the concept of stem cell competition. Clearly if we are correct in assuming apluripotential cell that supports myeloid, megakaryocytic, and erythroid development each with its different demands, there must be some mechanism to adjudicate the priorities. That there is such an interlocking relationship appears clear. Hellman *et al* (1970) have recently summarized their findings. They used endotoxin to judge myelopoiesis and ^{59}Fe to evaluate erythropoiesis. After irradiation injury, they demonstrated preferential differentiation along myeloid or erythroid lines as a function of the interval after irradiation. When marrow from irradiated donors was transplanted into irradiated recipients within the first several days after irradiation of the donor, the ratio of myeloid/erythroid surviving fractions favoured myelopoiesis. As the interval between irradiation and transplantation was lengthened, their ratio reversed. The same kind of effect was seen with drugs—e.g., cyclophosphamide. Morley, Bennet and Stohlman (1970b) reported that the severity of neutropenia in polycythemic mice irradiated with one leg shielded was less than that in normal mice and that myelopoiesis appeared to recover earlier. It is clear therefore that there is an order of priority at the stem cell

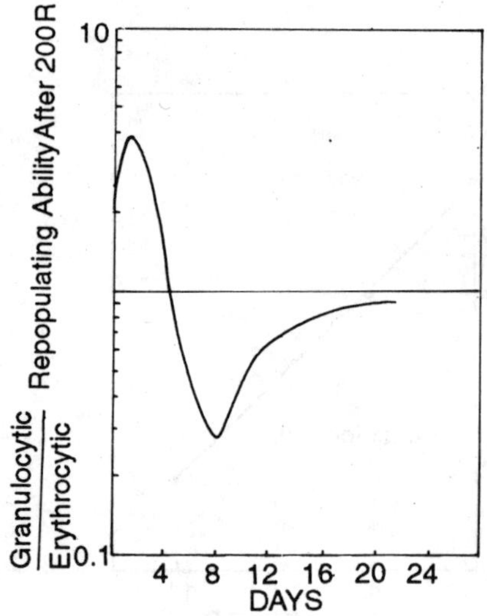

Fig. 4.6. Ratio of survival fractions measured by the granulocytic and erythrocytic repopulating ability following 200 R.

level, but the mechanisms affecting the parameters are unknown. Finally, it might be noted that interpretation of studies in which slit-dose irradiation has been used may well require modification in light of these considerations.

THE DIFFERENTIATED COMPARTMENT

For our purposes, we may consider the differentiated compartment as consisting of two subunits: the proliferating compartment of the marrow, and a storage compartment. Maturation occurs in both. Once cells have been differentiated from the committed compartment into the proliferating compartment of the bone marrow, an obligatory but variable time delay occurs, during which maturation proceeds. In our view, the critical function of maturation in the erythroid cell is hemoglobin synthesis. Erythropoietin initiates this and, we feel, also governs the rate of hemoglobin synthesis. This is predominantly programmed at the time of differentiation, but there is also evidence that EP may affect differentiated cells still capable of nucleic acid synthesis (Stohlman *et al* 1968). As maturation proceeds, the cells go through a variable number of divisions. The generation time of differentiated cells even in the stimulated marrow appears to be fixed at about 10 hours in the rodent and perhaps somewhat longer in man. There may be a further decrease in the generation time after stimulation by perhaps up to 20%, but this is not of major importance in the response to erythroid demands. In view of the relatively fixed generation time, the rate of hemoglobin synthesis becomes an important determinant in the numbers of divisions that will ensue between differentiation and final maturation.

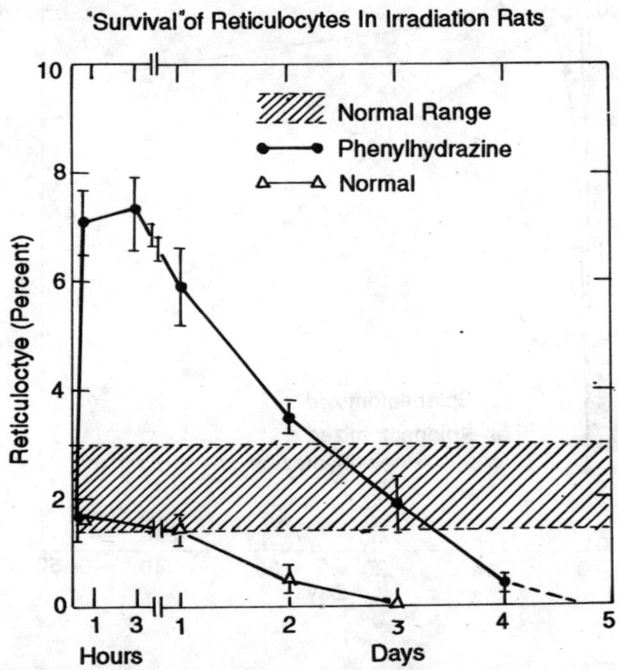

Fig. 4.7. Blood containing 40 per cent reticulocytes was collected from rats responding to a phenylhydrazine-induced anemia. This blood was transfused into irradiated animals and the survival of reticulated cells determined.

The cessation of "nucleic acid and ultimately protein synthesis is thought to be due to interaction between intranuclear hemoglobin and nucleohistones, which also leads to nuclear condensation. The concentration of hemoglobin is critical in this process, and it is thought that a cytoplasmic hemoglobin concentation of ~ 20% is necessary to achieve the cessation of nucleic acid synthesis. Equilibrium exists between the intranuclear and cytoplasmic hemoglobin through nuclear pores. Intranuclear hemoglobin may arise from in situ synthesis, trapping during division, or migration through these nuclear pores. Once nucleic acid synthesis has ceased, the existing RNA governs further hemoglobin synthesis in the late polychromatophilic normoblast and reticulocytes until RNA breakdown is complete, at which point hemoglobin synthesis stops. There is also an interval between cessation of DNA synthesis and enucleation, the governing forces of which are not understood. There are no data on this point, so that we cannot say whether the time for the latter is fixed or variable. Since other parameters of erythroid differentiation are variable, one might suggest that the interval between cessation of nucleic acid synthesis and enucleation is also variable.

Under steady state conditions, at the rate of hemoglobin synthesis is relatively constant. It nevertheless may be altered by a number of variables. For example, in iron depletion, the lack of availability of iron becomes a rate-limiting factor; in the stimulated

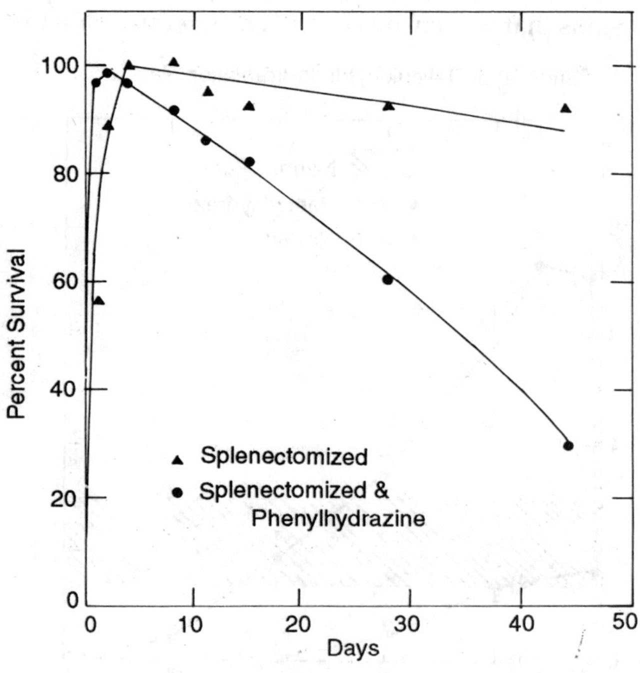

Fig. 4.8. Survival of red cells produced in response to severe anemia induced by phenylhydrazine in splenectomized as compared with intact animals. Phenylhydrazine given on Days 0, 1, 3, and ^{59}Fe on Day 5. Days on abscissi refer to days off ^{59}Fe. Each point represents the mean of 5 animals.

animal hemoglobin, synthehsis is accelerated. Thus, the obligatory time delay for proliferation and in turn the bone marrow transit time are in fact variables rather than being fixed; so also in the compartment that we have chosen to label "Storage," i.e., the late polychromatophilic and reticulocyte compartment. The latter may be conceptually viewed as analogous to the storage compartment for neutrophils. Normally the reticulocytes are released at a time when maturation is almost complete. There is relatively little RNA remaining, and hemoglobin synthesis is almost finished. However, when erythropoiesis is stimulated, reticulocytes are released earlier. In 1962, Stohlman, Moores and Brecher demonstrated that the reticulocyte may be released as much as 24 hours earlier in the stimulated as compared with the normal animal. Similar data were also reported by Stryckmans *et al* in 1968. More recently, these observations have been once again confirmed by Ganzoni *et al* (1969). Thus, the early release of reticulocytes is a part of the response to severe anemia. It is clear, however, that its importance in restoring the red cell mass is limited since it buys only a single day's worth of red cells.

It is well established that macrocytes are produced in the severely stimulated animal. Macrocytosis appears to be a compensatory mechanism to produce large numbers of red cells rapidly. Contributing to the macrocytosis is the early release of reticulocytes, which are larger than adult cells. However, since the bulk of reticulocytes are mature within 24 to 48 hours, simple arithmetic leads to the conclusion that this alone cannot acount for the observed macrocytosis. The more imporant mechanism appears to be the acceleration of hemoglobin synthesis, which, in the face of a relatively fixed generation time, results in a skipped terminal division and the production of large cells. Evidence for this has been reviewed extensively in the past. There is substantial evidence to indicate that the macrocytes produced under these conditions are short lived. The

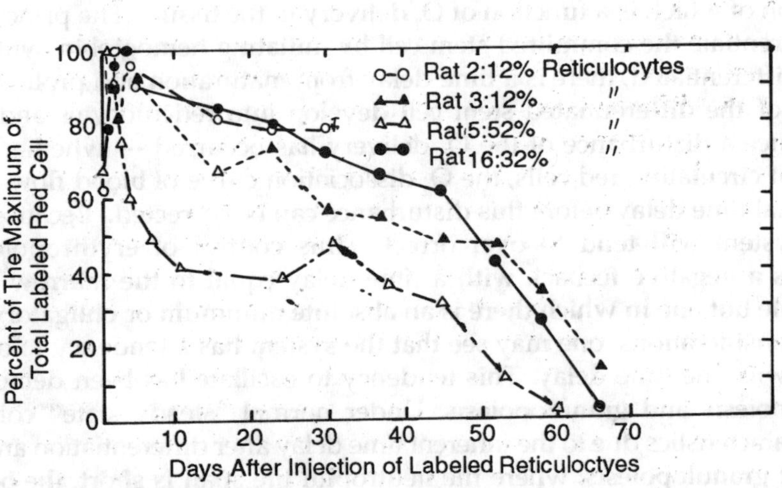

Fig. 4.9. The percent of the maximal value of total circulating labeled red cells versus the time after the autotransfusion of labeled reticulocytes in 4 rats with reticulocyte levels ranging from 5 to 15 per cent after exposure to low oxygen pressure.

mechanism of hemolyis is unknown. In our experience, splenectomy did not alter the survival of these macrocytes. More recently, Ganzoni *et al* (1969) and Robinson (1970) have reported similar experiences, Ganzoni *et al* (1969) further suggested that macrocytes were not removed from the circulation in to but rather portions of the cells were removed. Thus, fragmentation of the macrocyte led to a cell of approximately normal size, which continued to circulate. We cannot exclude this as a possibility, particularly membrane fragmentation, but it does not appear to be of major importance in returning the cell size distribution to normal. Stryckmans *et al* (1968), using single cell autoradiography, demonstrated short lived macrocytes. Had fragmentation been the important mechanism for the removal of macrocytes, these investigators would have observed a decrease in the mean grain count, but not in the proportion of labeled cells. In contrast, they observed a decrease in the proportion of labeled cells but not in mean grain count. Their data as well as those from other laboratories suggest that the bulk of the macrocytes is removed within the first several days to a week after a pulse stimulation. The recent report of Robinson (1970) suggests that the short-lived characteristics of the cells produced in response to erythroid demand are a continuum from bone marrow to peripheral blood. Unable to account for the entire early labeled stercobilin by destruction of peripheral red cells, he proposed that there is substantial ineffective bone marrow erythropoiesis. It is clear from a number of studies that there is a direct correlation between the severity of erythroid stimulation and the degree of hemolysis. Whether ineffective erythropoiesis is the end stage product of such severe erythroid stimulation or in fact is seen in some measure even after mild stimulation remains to be determined.

MAINTENANCE OF THE STEADY STATE

Red cell production is generally thought to be controlled by the hormone erythropoietin, the production of which is a function of O_2 delivery to the tissue. The principal action of EP is to differentiate the committed stem cell by initiating hemoglobin synthesis. Once the cell has differentiated, there is a time-delay from maturation and proliferation before the progeny of the differentiated stem cell develop into reticulocytes and mature red cells. Thus once a disturbance of the O_2 delivery has occurred — whether a change in the number of circulating red cells, the O_2 dissociation curve of blood flow — there will be a substantial time delay before this disturbance can be corrected. Because of this time delay, the system will tend to overcorrect. Thus control of erythropoiesis may be considered as a negative feeback with a time delay equal to the marrow transit time, itself a variable but one in which there is an absolute minimum or obligatory time delay. From these considerations, one may see that the system has a tendency to oscillate with a period of twice the time delay. This tendency to oscillate has been demonstrated for both erythropoiesis and granulopoiesis. Under normal "steady state" conditions, the oscillatory characteristics due to the inherent time delay after differentiation are dampened. In the case of granulopoiesis, where the neutrophil life span is short, the bone marrow granulocyte reserve acts as a "brake" on the oscillatory tendency. As the latter is depleted, for example, in mild bone marrow failure, increasing oscillation is observed and has been recently demonstrated experimentally (Morley *et al* 1970). Although there is some variation in the time of reticulocyte release, the magnitude of this would appear to be

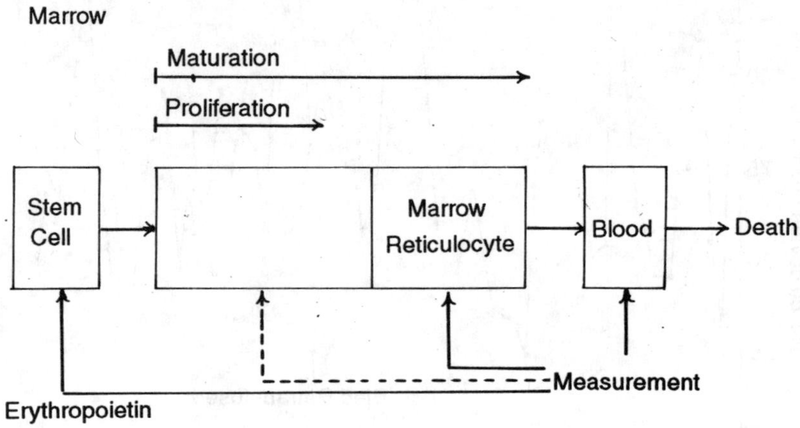

Fig. 4.10. A model for erythropoiesis showing feedback relationship with peripheral blood.

insufficient to provide adequate dampening of the oscillatory characteristics of red cell production. The red cell, however, has a long life span and the production rate is small relative to the number of circulating red cells. To put it another way, the transit time. T_M, is short compared to the total life span T_E. This relationship of T_M/T_E is thought to dampen oscillations of the total red cell mass. However, as T_E is shortened, as in hemolytic anemia, and the relationship of T_M/T_E altered, oscillation would be expected to become more prominent. That this is the case has been demonstrated experimentally by Orr *et al* (1968).

If one considers the reticulocyte as a subset of the total circulating red cell mass, one can see that the tendency for the reticulocyte mass to oscillate will be greater than is the case of the total circulating red cell mass. The reticulocyte has a short life span, T_{ER}, as compared to T_M, and one might therefore anticipate that the relationship of T_M/T_{ER} would not provide effective dampening of oscillations. To test this hypothesis, Morley and Stohlman (1969) bled dogs 0.2-0.5 ml three times a week and measured the absolute numbers of circulating reticulocytes (Fig. 4.11). In six of the eleven dogs studied, there was clear cut periodicity. The period of cycles was ~ 14 days, which would be consistent with a bone marrow transit time of seven days. This is in good agreement with previous estimates of bone marrow transit time for the dog. Further, the phase of cycle was changed 180° by the pulse stimulation of a limited phlebotomy of 1.5% of the total body weight. The latter suggests that the periodicity relates to EP production. Another example of periodicity in the red cell production is the recovery from irradiation injury.

These data indicate that erythropoiesis rather than being a true steady state is in a controlled state of sustained oscillations. Further, the tendency to oscillate may be of importance in interpreting experimental results particularly where the relationships of T_M/T_E or T_{ER} are altered, e.g., in hemolytic anemia, recovery from irradiation injury, bone marrow failure, and the like.

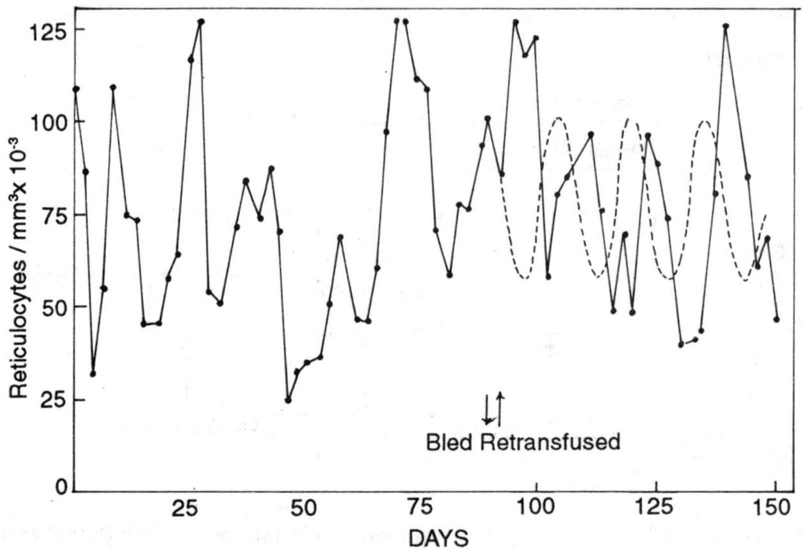

Fig. 4.11. Serial reticulocyte counts showing a reticulocyte cycles. As indicated by the arrows, this dog was bled and 3 days later was retransfued. The dashed line is an extrapolation of the reticulocyte cycle present before bleeding. The experimental procedure seemed to shift the phase of oscillation approximately 180^0, but did not affect the period of oscillation.

THE ECOLOGY OF HEMOPOIESIS

In today's world, ecology has become fashionable, not only in political considerations concerning our total environment, but also in the consideration of the control of hemopoiesis. In addition to the previously described cell-cell interaction, the relationship of hemopoietic cell to the environment in which it lodges is of enormous importance in its subsequent growth characteristics. The question is frequently raised of the relevance of many studies in mice, where splenic hemopoiesis is substantial, to that in man, in whom significant hemopoiesis in the spleen is seen only under pathological conditions. The answer to this question would appear to lie with environmental considerations. The adult marrow is encased in a rigid-structure, which in the mouse is almost entirely red marrow. There is little capacity for expansion; the spleen serves as an alternative expandable site of hemopoiesis. In contrast, in man and other higher order mammals, much of the bone marrow in the adult has reverted to yellow marrow, which serves as a potential reserve area to meet increased demands should it be required. The question appears to me to be how is this programmed, and why does the spleen in man fail to provide adequate support for hemopoiesis when the bone marrow is inadequate for the task, e.g., in chronic hemolytic anemia.

Clearly, the considerations above point to the importance of stromal structure and environment to hemopoiesis. Experimentally, these relationships are best illustrated by the studies of McCulloch *et al* (1965), who noted that the genetically anemic mouse SL/

SL^D has a normal pluripotent hemopoietic cell as judged by transplanation, but that the splenic microenvironment could not support normal growth of the pluripotential cell of this strain or its normal coisogenic litter mate. The nature of the defect is unknown, but clearly it establishes the importance of microenvironment. Patt and Maloney (1970), have recently reviewed their observations on the effect of mechanical removal of bone marrow from rabbits. These workers observed that regeneration of hemopoiesis could not occur in the absence of bone marrow structure. In their experimental model it was necessary for bone marrow structure and in particular trabeculae, to be reestablished prior to the onset of differentiating hemopoiesis. The injection of pluripotent hemopoietic stem cells into the evacuated cavity of the rabbit femur did not produce active hemopoiesis. These studies indicate that once the marrow has been mechanically disrupted and a coagulum is formed, a connective tissue matrix develops; this is followed by trabecular bone deposition and finally marrow formation. They further suggest the regeneration stems from mesenchymal cells of the connective tissue of the Haversian canals. Fliedner *et al* (1970), have suggested that pulsatile blood flow, neurally regulated, within the rigid structure of the bone is required for the fine regulation. It may be further suggested that change in flow and the resulting changes in local environment may be of major importance in the regulation of the response to hemopoietic demand.

The reason for evolution of yellow marrow in the higher order animals is unknown. Crosby (1970), reviewed the experiences of his laboratory, where they have observed the growth pattern of marrow after subcutaneous implantation. Both red and yellow marrows passed through an initial period in which there was proliferation of primitive cells, cancellous bone formation, the appearance of sinusoids, and finally active marrow. Thereafter marrow derived from a fatty source reverted to yellow marrow; active hemopoiesis persisted in that derived from red marrow. The control of such programing has yet to be defined. However, it does enable us to view bone marrow aplasia from two standpoints: *(1)* the failure of the pluripotent stem cell; *(2)* the failure of the supporting structure or bone marrow environment. Thus, in myelofibrosis one might suggest that reversion of red to yellow marrow or a breakdown in the environmental programing may be responsible for the evolution of the fibrosis and the failure of hemopoiesis to thrive.

Microenvironment and cellular ecology are, as can be seen from the above, of enormous importance in the response to increased erythroid demand. In rodents, migration of hemopoietic cells to sites with favourable environmental conditions, e.g., the spleen, is of critical importance; in man, expansion is into yellow marrow. In man, however, compensation in the latter fashion is limited; understanding of the programming of marrow structure and the environmental features of that structure together with an insight into the environmental characteristics of the spleen, which prevent colonization in man, is clearly of clinical and biologic significance.

THE LIFE SPAN OF THE RED CELL

The life span of the red blood cell is shortened in a number of disease states, and for this reason its measurement may be helpful in a variety of clinical situations (Berlin 1964;

Berlin *et al* 1959). Red cell survival studies may be essential to detect the presence of hemolysis, particularly when it is mild or moderate in degree, or in the presence of coexistent disease that may suppress reticulocytosis or render other commonly used indicators unreliable. In principle, serial measurements of red cell survival may be used to detemine the response to therapy in various hemolytic states, but the prolonged

Table 4.1
Historical Development

	DIRECT
1911	Todd and White: Cross transfusion in cow
1919	Ashby: Cross transfusion in man
1946	Shemin and Rittenberg: ^{16}N-labeled glycine
1953	Ebaugh, *et al.*: ^{51}Cr *in vitro* labeling
1954	Cohen and Warringa: Diisopropylfluorophosphate (DFP)
	INDIRECT
	(Rate of Synthesis)
1950	Huff, *et al.*: Plasma and red blood cell iron turnover
	(Rate of Catabolism)
1937	Watson: Fecal urobilin
1963	Coburn *et al.*: Carbon monoxide
1968	Barrett *et al.*: Bilirubin-^{14}C

Table 4.2
Red Blood Cell Life Span

	DIRECT METHODS
Cohort lavels	Glycine—^{15}N, ^{14}C, ^{3}H
	Radioiron—^{59}Fe (^{53}Fe)
	DFP + radioactive DFP
	Seleno-methionine
Random labels	Immunological marker
	DFP—^{32}P, ^{3}H, ^{14}C
	^{51}Cr (^{50}Cr)

INDIRECT METHODS

1. Plasma radioiron clearance and red blood cell radioiron uptake
2. Carbon monoxide excretion
3. Bilirubin production

sampling times required by conventional methods have usually precluded their use for this purpose.

The principal historical landmarks in the development of methods for measuring red cell life span are indicated in Table 4.1. In general, the life span of the red cell can be deduced from (1) survival curves of isotopically tagged erythrocytes, following either *in vivo* or *in vitro* labelling; (2) a calculation of the rate of red cell synthesis, using radio-iron; and (3) measurements of the rates of excretion of various catabolic products of the heme moiety of hemoglobin. These methods may also be classified as follows:

(1) direct—i.e., determination of the survival curves of cells tagged by either

a. cohort labels—which label a small population of cells of approximately the same age either prior to, or immediately after, their entry into the circulation; or

b. random labels—which label red cells irrespective of their age.

(2) indirect—from the rate of synthesis of red cells (ferrokinetics) or the rate of elimination of hemoglobin catabolites.

The cohort methods, with one exception, depend on the labeling of the red cell by biosynthetic incorporation of a precursor into hemoglobin. In addition, they require that the precursor specific activity decrease rapidly so that labeling is essentially complete soon after precursor administration. This is conceptually summarized by the phrase "flash labeling." The net result is that only a small fraction of the circulating cells of approximately the same age are labeled. If these survive for a definite period of time, generally designated as the potential life span, the curve of specific activity of hemoglobin resembles that in Figure 4.12 labeled *glycine.*

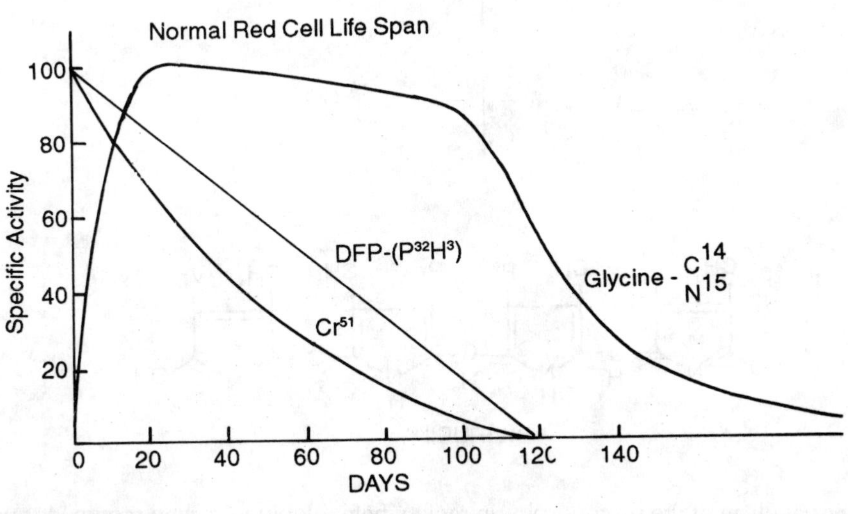

Fig. 4.12. The specific activity of red cells in normal subjects after labeling with glycine, DFP, or ^{51}Cr.

Random labels, on the other hand, attach to mature circulating erythrocytes irrespective of cell age. Labeling may be carried out either *in vivo* or *in vitro*. The age distribution of the labeled cells is the same as that of all the circulating red cells. In normal subjects, the survival curve shows a linear decrease. If, as in the case with ^{51}Cr labeled cells, there is loss of label by elution from intact surviving cells, the survival curve will depart from linearity and resemble that shown for ^{51}Cr in Figure 4.12.

While all methods for determining red cell survival depend on the implicit assumption of a steady state, the indirect methods are particularly dependent on this assumption. Thus they are applicable only when the total red cell volume is constant, or where the rate of change of the total red cell volume is known. The steady state requirement is most obvious when red cell survival is determined from ferrokinetic studies, since in this situation the rate of red cell destruction is calculated from studies that, in fact, measure the rate of red cell synthesis. This approach was initially developed by Huff *et al* (1950), who utilized the rate of disappearance of radioiron from the plasma, and its subsequent reappearance in circulating red cell, to calculate, the rate of red cell

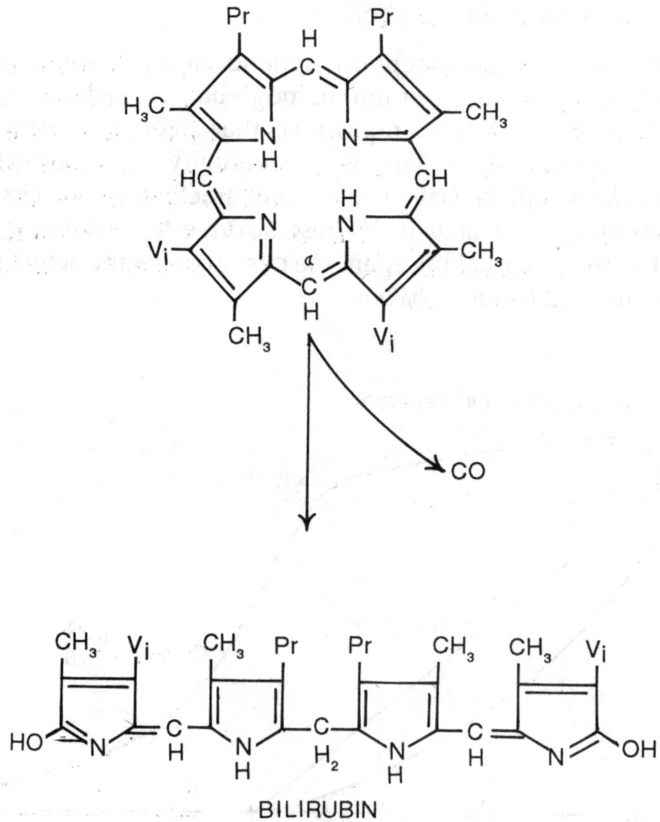

Fig. 4.13. The catabolism of the protoporphyrin moiety hemoglobin to carbon monoxide and bilirubin. The reactions are quantitative, so that one mole of CO and one mole of bilirubin are produced for each mole of heme degraded.

synthesis. If the total red cell volume is known, then the mean red cell life span can be calculated from the rate of red cell synthesis, provided a steady state exists between red cell synthesis and destruction.

Carbon monoxide and bilirubin are the two catabolic products of hemoglobin metabolism that are excreted quantitatively. Both in theory and in practice their production rates can be used to measure the rate of red cell destrucion, and hence, in the steady state, the life span of the red cell. Their use to measure the red cell life span is recent and not widespread.

The only endogenous metabolic source of carbon monoxide is from the catabolism of iron protoporphyrin-protein compounds, i.e., hemoglobin and heme enzymes. One mole of carbon monoxide is excreted for each mole of heme catabolized. Coburn, *et al* have developed methods, for the measurement of the rate of excretion of carbon monoxide and have deduced the red cell life span from these measurements.

Until recently, there were only three ways to measure the rate of bilirubin production: (1) the diversion of bile to the exterior through a tube in the common duct, (2) diversion of bile into the renal pelvis and hence into the urine, and (3) the measurement of fecal urobilinogen. Because the first of these methods, has limited application in clinical medicine, there are very few reported measurements. The second has been used only in the dog. The first two methods measure total bilirubin production directly, whereas the third method requires the quantitative conversion of bilirubin to urobilin followed by the quantitative excretion of urobilin in the feces. It is, in fact, the oldest of the indirect methods, of estimating the red cell life span. At present it appears that in most individuals, the measured fecal urobilinogen excretion accounts for only 50% to 70% of the theroretical or experimentally measured rate of bilirubin production. The chemical methods involved require considerable skill. In three normal individuals who have been studied over a prolonged period of time, there appears to be considerable fluctuation in fecal urobilinogen excretion. It must also be recognized that fecal urobilinogen may be markedly reduced as the result of variation in the bacterial flora following antibiotic adminstration and may be virtually absent in bile duct obstruction or even increased in the blind loop syndrome.

In order to avoid the long sampling time required by both the cohort and random label methods, we have investigated the possibility that a measurement of the bilirubin production rate in conjunction with a measurement of the total red cell volume could be used to calculate the red cell life span. This requires the measurement of

1. the rate of disappearance of labeled bilirubin from the plasma after its intravenous administration,
2. the serum unconjugated bilirubin concentration, and
3. the total red cell volume.

Sampling time is of the order of 24 to 48 hours. This method is applicable at all levels of plasma bilirubin concentration, both conjugated and unconjugated, and remains valid in liver disease.

The following methods, all previously described in detail, are used. Bilirubin is labeled biosynthetically using either ^{14}C- or ^{3}H- labeled δ-aminolevulinic acid as the precursor. The labeled bilirubin is injected intravenously as the bilirubin-albumin complex and the rate of disappearance from the plasma of the isotopically labeled bilirubin determined. The unconjugated bilirubin is extracted from the plasma by the solvent separation system of Weber and Schalm (1962) and counted in a liquid scintillation spectrometer. The plasma bilirubin concentration is determined by the same extraction procedure. The total red cell volume (TRCV) is determined by the method of Gray and Sterling (1950) as modified by Read (1954).

The bilirubin production rate is calcuated from the product of the plasma unconjugated bilirubin pool and the turnover rate of this pool. The pool size is determined from the initial volume of distribution of a tracer dose of labeled bilirubin and the plasma unconjugated bilirubin concentration. The turnover rate of the plasma unconjugated bilirubin pool is calaculated from the rate of disappearance of labeled bilirubin from the plasma.

Figure 4.15 shows a representative clearance of labeled bilirubin from the plasma. In all normals and patients studied for at least 24 hours, the plasma bilirubin disappearance could be described as the sum of three exponentials, i.e., $P(t) = A_1e^{-a1t} + A_2e^{-a2t} + A_3e^{-a3t}$, where P(t) is the plasma bilirubin specific activity. If UCBR is the plasma unconjugated bilirubin pool (in mg), the bilirubin production (BRP) is given by the following:

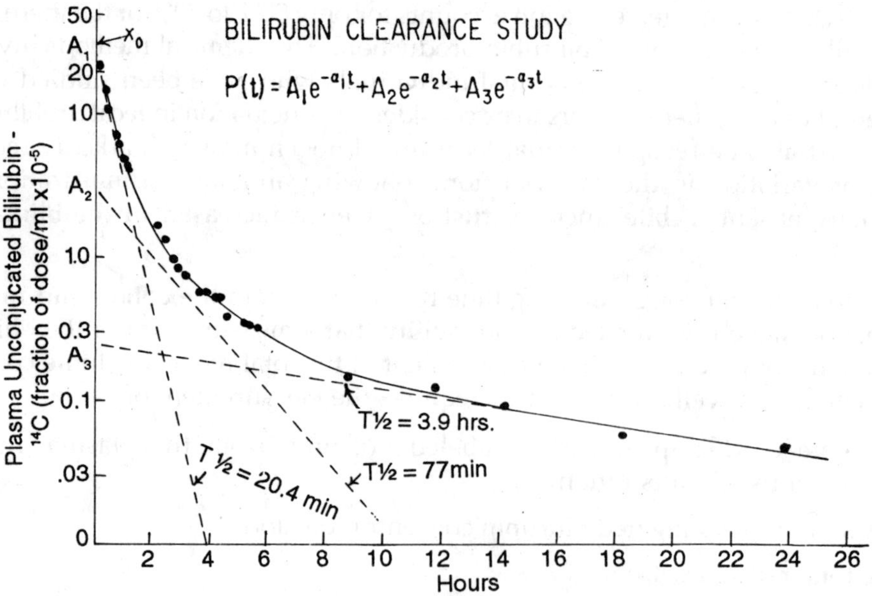

Fig. 4.15. The clearance of labeled unconjugated bilirubin from the plasma in a normal subject. The solid curve represents a computer fit of the data to a sum of 3 exponential functions. Dashed lines are the individual exponential components.

$$\frac{UCBR}{\frac{A_1}{a_1} + \frac{A_2}{a_2} + \frac{A_3}{a_3}}$$

where $A_1+A_2+A_3 = 1$, UCBR = (IVDBR) × (plasma bilirubin concentration), and IVDBR = initial volume of distribution of bilirubin.

The red blood cell life span can be calculated by the following line of reasoning. Since the catabolism of 1 ml of red cells that contains 330 mg of hemoglobin gives rise to 12 mg of bilirubin, then $\frac{(1-x)\,(BRP)}{12}$ = cc of RBC catabolized per day. (1-x) is the fraction of bilirubin production that is derived from circulating red cells. If the total life span red cell volume and the ml catabolized per day are known, then mean (RBCLS) = $\frac{TRCV}{\text{ml RBC catabolized per day}}$. The value of x that we have used is based on other studies of the origins of bilirubin and will be discussed more extensively later.

Tabel 4.3. shows the date from 19 studies done on 13 normal volunteers. The ^{51}Cr RBC t½ for these subjects was in the range generally recognized as normal. The mean calculated RBCLS was 107 days in men and 94 days in women. The values in the males

Table 4.3
Determination of Red Blood Cell Life Span in Normals from Radio-Bilirubin Clearance

Group	*Number*	*Mean RBCLS* (Days)*	*^{51}CR RBC t½ (Days)*
Males	11	107 ± 12	29.4 ± 2.1
Females	BRP = 8	94 ± 11	30.1 ± 4.0
Total	19	101 ± 13	29.6 ± 2.9

* Mean ± SD.

Table 4.4
Red Blood Life Span in Normal Man: A Summary of the Previously Published Data

Method	*Number*	*Mean (Days)*
Glycine	3 male	118
Ashby	87 male	117
DFP	31 male	122
	6 female	114
^{53}Cr Extinction Point	37	113

are approximately 10 to 15 days less than the anticipated 120 days. This discrepancy is somewhat greater in the females. There is some support from other studies that also indicates a shorter RBCLS in the female. It must be recognized that the usually quoted figure of 120 days represents the mode, not the mean, of the survival of the labeled cohort and does not take into account the presence of some random destruction of circulating red cells, which occurs even in normal individuals.

In four studies in patients with Gilbert's syndrome and two with the Crigler-Najjar syndrome, the RBCLS determined from the bilirubin clearance was the same as in the normals, indicating that (1) hyperbilirubinemia *per se* need not shorten the RBCLS, and (2) hyperbilirubinemia *per se* does not invalidate this method (seeTable 4.5). In five of these six patients with hyperbilirubinemia, indpendent measurements of the RBCLS were normal. Tabel 4.6 shows that the RBCLS as determined by the bilirubin method was reproducible at intervals ranging from 1 to 12 months.

Table 4.5
Influence of Serum Unconjugated Bilirubin Concentration (UCBR) on Determination of Red Blood Cell Life Span from Clearance of Radio-Bilirubin

Number	*Mean UCBR Concentration (mg%)*	*Mean RBCLS (Days)*
19 (Normals)	0.40	101
4 (Gilbert's)	1.51	98
2 (Crigler-Najjar)	21.36	119

Table 4.6
Reproducibility of BR-^{14}C Clearance Studies for Measurement of Mean Red Blood Cell Life Span

	Mean RBCLS (Days)		*Interval*
Subject	*Study 1*	*Study 2*	*(Months)*
SB	88	87	1
CK	86	84	1
MW	102	111	1
GM	103	111	1.5
JL	117	108	3.5
DR	94	88	11
KD	123	113	7
DF	63	61	12

In Figure 4.15, the RBC life span as derived from bilirubin production (RBCLS BR) is compared with a ^{51}chromium RBC t½. In two instances the RBCLS BR was normal, but the ^{51}Cr t½ was decreased. Both of these patients had an increasing TRCV during the chromium study, so that the RBC ^{51}Cr t½ (as ordinarily measured) is "falsely" decreased. In the lower left hand square, there are three points where the ^{t51}Cr t½ is considerably greater than expected on the basis of the bilirubin data. In two this was due to an increased BRP resulting from ineffective erythropoiesis; for the third there is no apparent explanation. In 35 of the 40 studies, there was excellent agreement between the two methods.

Figure 4.17 shows the relationship in nine patients between RBCLS as derived from bilirubin production and the red cell life span measured with tritiated diisopropyl flurophosphate (DFP -^{3}H). This shows excellent agreement when the red cell life span is less than 80 days. For the three patients with a RBCLS of 80 days or greater, the DFP method yields a red cell life span approximately 10 to 15 days longer than the bilirubin production method. This difference is similar to that observed in the normal males. The difference between the RCBLS BR and a measured RBCLS (^{3}H-DFP) in the normal individual must be due to either an underestimation of the red cell life span by bilirubin or an overstimation of the RBCLS by glycine, DFP or Ashby methods. It is thought that at least a part of the difference can be attributed to an overestimate of the mean RBCLS by the cohort or random label methods. This stems from the following lines of reasoning.

Almost without exception, the red cell life span is finite in all the species studied. That is, each cell has a finite or potential life span. In addition, in all species studied, some of the cells are destroyed randomly, i.e., without regard to age. The result is that a calculation of the *mean red cell* life span requires determination of two quantities, the finite or potential life span, and the rate of random destruction.

When labeled glycine is used as a precursor, a cohort of highly labeled cells is produced. Because of continued availability of labeled precursor, there is subsequently further labeling of red cells. This has the effect of producing an apparent increase in the potential life span, of the order of five days when the red cell life span is normal. In addition, as a result of continued red cell labeling the midportion of the hemoglobin specific activity curve should continuously rise for several months after glycine administration (see fig. 4.18). That it does not do so indicates that there must be some random destruction of red cells.

What is the evidence for random destruction of red cells when DFP is used to measure the RBCLS ? If it is assumed that 0.2% of red cells are randomly destroyed each day, then as Figure 4.19 shows, this would be difficult to detect when labeled DFP is used due to the inherent scatter in the data. If this quantity of random destruction is added to the usually assumed catabolism of .85% per day associated with a 120 day red cell life span, the mean red cell life span becomes 112 days.

Very few direct measurements exist of the quantity of random destruction of red cells in man, and hence of the mean red cell life span. Even a small rate of random destruction of red cells in the normal will be significant for purposes of calculating the

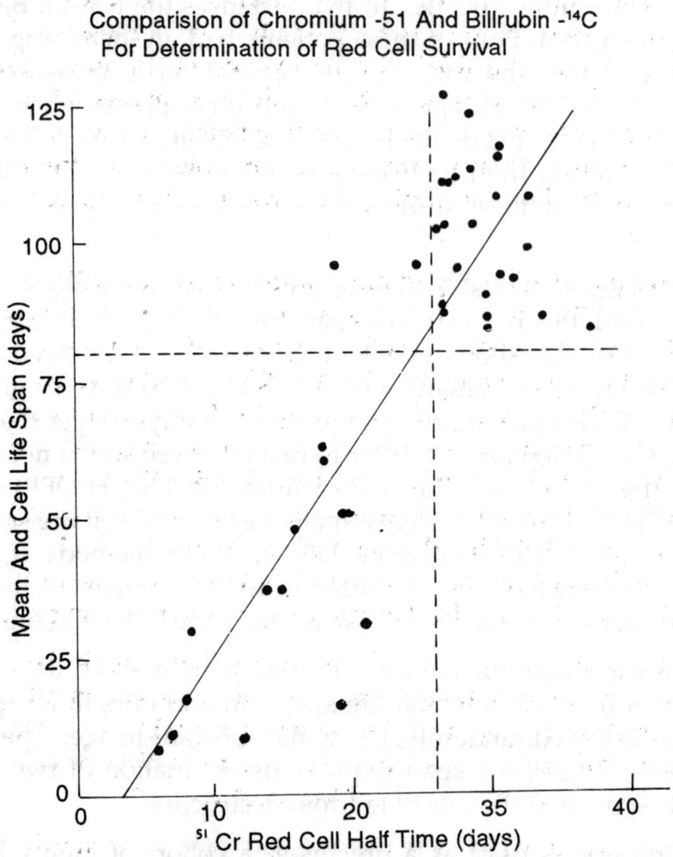

Fig. 4.15. Comparison of red cell life span determined from bilirubin clearance (ordinate) with red cell ^{51}Cr t½ (abscissa). Dashed lines represent lower limits of normal for the two methods.

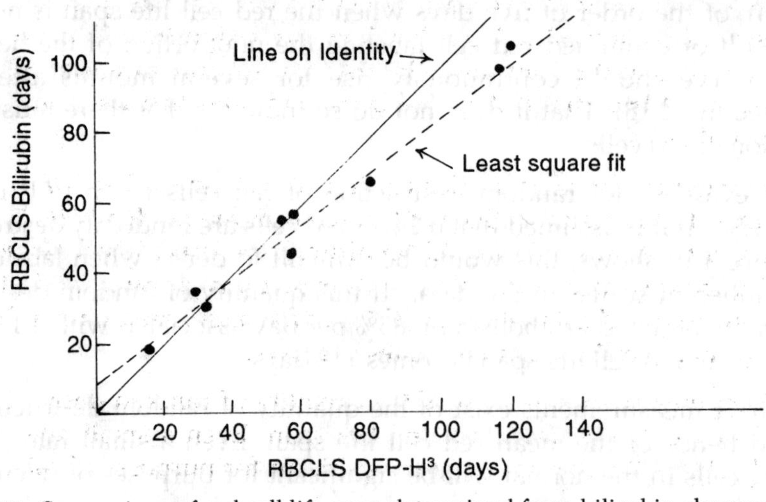

Fig. 4.16. Comparison of red cell life span determined from bilirubin clearance and DFP-(^3H).

mean RBC life span. Continued availability of precursor also leads to an overestimation of RBCLS when glycine is used as a label. Thus the usually quoted value of 120 days for the normal RBC life span is probably greater than the true mean RBCLS. Let us now consider the possible sources of error in the bilirubin method for estimating red cell survival. If one mole of bilirubin and one mole of carbon monoxide are produced per mole of heme catabolized, and if both are excreted quantitatively, the measured BRP and the measured CO excretion should be the same when expressed as moles/day. The data of Coburn *et al* (1966) and more recently of Coltman and Dudley (1969) both yield similar values for the rate of excretion of carbon monoxide and are similar to the measured rate of bilirubin production (Table 4.18). In five subjects, a measured BRP was in good agreement with a simultaneously measured CO excretion. These observations lead to the conclusion that the bilirubin production as measured by the disappearance of labeled bilirubin from the plasma is accurate.

The calculation of RBCLS from the measured rate of bilirubin production requires the following assumptions: (1) that a fixed fraction (80 to 90%) of the total bilirubin is derived from the catabolism of senescent red cells, (2) that all hemoglobin degradation yields bilirubin quantitatively, and (3) that all bilirubin derived from red cells passes

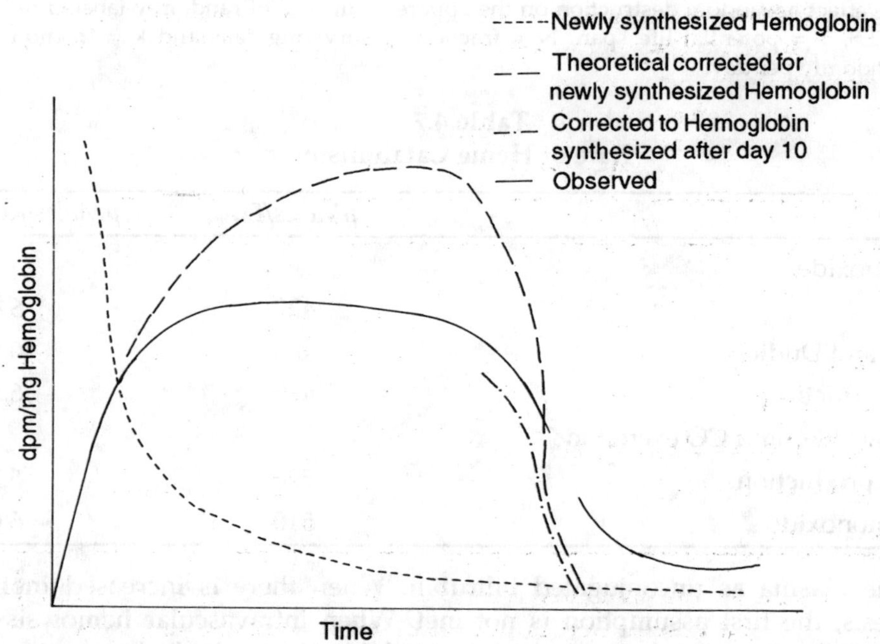

Fig. 4.17. The specific activity of hemoglobin after administration of labeled glycine. Solid curve represents data from a typical experimental study. Since labeled hemoglobin is produced for months after injection of labeled glycine, the specific activity of circulating hemoglobin should continue to rise during this period. That it in fact achieves a plateau suggests that some random hemolysis is occurring.

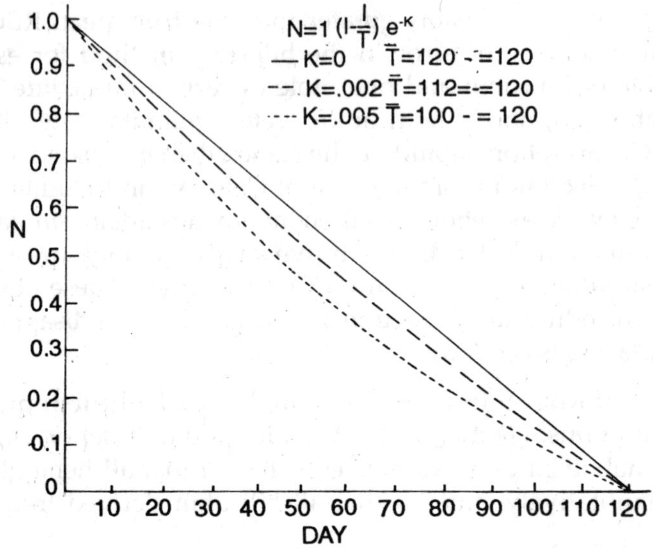

Fig. 4.18. The effect of random destruction on the apparent survival of randomly labeled red cells. T = mean RBCLS, T = potential life span, N = fraction of surviving cells and k = fraction of cells destroyed randomly per day.

Table 4.7
Rate of Heme Catabolism

	μMoles/Day	*μMoles/KG/DAY*
Carbon monoxide		
Coburn	437	6.42
Coltman and Dudley	483	6.60
Bilirubin production	495	6.50
Simultaneous BRP and CO excretion		
Bilirubin production	520	6.76
Carbon monoxide	510	6.63

through the plasma as unconjugated bilirubin. When there is increased ineffective erythropoiesis, the first assumption is not met. When intravascular hemolysis yields more hemoglobin than can be bound by haptoglobin, hemoglobin is excreted in the urine without conversion to bilirubin. With these two exceptions the assumptions appear valid.

The calculation of the red cell life by the bilirubin method requires that the fraction of the total bilirubin derived from circulating red cells be known. At present, this has been determined from studies of the glycine early labeled peak. After administration of glycine, two peaks of incorporation of isotope into bile pigment are found. The first, at 3 to 5 days, is designated as the early labeled peak and the second, at 90 to 130 days, the late peak.

Tabel 4.9 shows the measurement of the amount of isotope in the glycine early labeled peak, as calculated by the method of London *et al* (1950) in 9 studies in this laboratory, and the normals in the literature as summarized by Watson (1965). The ratio between the amount of bilirubin derived from the catabolism of circulating red cells to that derived from all other sources has generally been taken as the same as the ratio between the amount of isotope in the late peak as compared to the early labeled peak. Based on this assumption, the data indicate approximately 80 to 90% of the bilirubin produced is derived from circulating red cells and the remainder from all other sources, i.e., ineffective erythropoiesis and the catabolism of a number of hepatic heme enzymes, myoglobin and other heme proteins. It appears that at least three-fourths of the 10 to 20% not derived from circulating red cells is associated with ineffective erythropoiesis, i.e., it is derived from developing red cells in the bone marrow. The ramainder, approximately 5% of the total, is derived from all other sources. None of these numbers is known with a high degree of precision. All must be considered to be first approximations that rest in particular on the assumption that the precursor specific activity is the same at all times for all sources of labeled bile pigments. This assumption, though fundamental, has not been adequately tested. Despite this objection, the measurement of the amount of isotope in the glycine early labeled peak represents the best available indpendent method of estimating the value of (1-x) in our equation for calculating RBCLS. The value assigned to (1-x) is thus the principal uncertainty in the bilirubin method for determining red cell survival.

We have assumed that 85% of the plasma bilirubin turnover is derived from the catabolism of hemoglobin in senescent red cells and 15% derived from other metabolic sources. This 15% value is approximately midway between the range of measurements reported from the glycine early labeled peak, but is less than the 20% calculated by Gray, Neuberger and Sneath (1950). Coburn *et al* (1966) calculated a value of 26% from their studies with carbon monoxide.

Schwartz (1967) and Barrett *et al* (1966) have demonstrated that the early labeled peak consists of two components, a constant nonerythropoietic fraction and a second, variable component that is proportional to the erythropoietic rate. The latter fraction presumably results from ineffective erythropoiesis. The nonerythropoietic component, being constant, becomes a progressively smaller fraction of total bile pigment production as the erythropoietic rate increases. Application of this concept to our own data implies that the value of (1-x) should increase with increasing erythropoietic rates. Excellent agreement is obtained between the bilirubin and DFP data in patients with shortened red cell survival, using 0.85 as the value of (10—x). The above line of reasoning suggests that a smaller value, perhaps .80 to .75, should be used in the normal. This would result in a value of RBCLS in normal subjects closer to that derived from DFP-^{3}H studies. Experimental work concerning this point is being pursued.

Table 4.8
Glycine Early Labeled Peak Studies

*Subject Normals**	*Diagnosis*	*P/U Ratio*	*RBCLS (Days)*	*Early Labeled Peak (%)*
Normals		0.7—1.4	—	6—20
1.	Normal	0.70	120	10.5
2.	Normal	0.67	120†	10.0
3.	Normal	0.74	109	10.1
4.	Acute intermittent porphyria	1.07	109	7.6
5.	Gilbert's syndrome	0.95	58	13.3
6.	Autoimmune hemolytic anemia	3.90	< 35	—
7.	Paroxysmal nocturnal hemoglobulinemia	0.79	< 20	—
8.	Lead poisoning	0.21	99	42.9
9.	Primary refractory anemia	0.09	90	78.2

* C.J. Waston (1965).

† Assumed.

The BR or CO methods cannot be used in diseases in which the glycine early label peak is disproportionately increased. These are diseases in which ineffective erythropoiesis is increased, and are tabulated in Table 4.9. It is believed that these diseases are readily recognized and should pose no particular problem.

Table 4.9
Diseases with Increased Ineffective Erythropoiesis

1.	Pernicious anemia	4.	Thalassemia syndromes
2.	Erythropoietic porphyrias	5.	Refractory (sideroblastic) anemias
3.	"Shunt" hyperbilirubinemia syndromes	6.	Lead poisoning

One of the interesting consequences of the equation for BRP which follows,

$$\mathrm{BRP} = \frac{1}{\frac{A_1}{a_1} + \frac{A_2}{a_2} + \frac{A_3}{a_3}} \text{ (plasma volume) (serum BR conc.)}$$

is the predictive value of the serum bilirubin concentration. In the normal, the plasma volume as measured with ^{51}Cr-labeled red cells and venous hematocrit varies from 32 to 44 ml/kg with a fluctuation about the mean of about ± 15%. In disease it rarely goes much below 26 ml/kg or above 60 ml/kg (Berlin *et al* 1952); k_e is the fraction of plasma bilirubin irreversibly cleared from the plasma per unit time; $k_e = \frac{1}{\frac{A_1}{a_1} + \frac{A_2}{a_2} + \frac{A_3}{a_3}}$ and has a range of .009 to .023 min^{-1}

in 13 normal subjects (Berk *et al* 1969). Bilirubin production can increase 8- to 10- fold in the absence of transfusions. Thus, in comparison to BRP, the range of values for the plasma volume and for k_e (when the liver is normal) are quite small. As a result, the serum bilirubin concentration can be considered to be directly proportional to bilirubin production.

In 12 individuals studied twice at intervals ranging from one month to six years, the ratio of k_e at the first sudy to k_e of the second study was 1.08 with a range of 0.85 to 1.38. In a group of six patients in which k_e was measured from the clearance of a tracer dose of bilirubin ($k_e{}^{14}C$) and then from a loading dose of unlabeled bilirubin (k_eBR) (2 mg/kg of body weight), the average of the ratio of k_eBR to $k_e{}^{14}C$ was 1.06. These studies suggest that k_e can be considered a constant in any given patient. Hence within the limits imposed by methodology, a change in the serum bilirubin concentration is a good indicator of an equivalent change in bilirubin production rate and thus of a change in the mean red cell life span. The exceptions remain to be determined. Certainly changes in k_e will occur in acquired liver disease, but how rapidly is not known.

Since the range of values that k_e and plasma volume take in the population is small, a serum unconjugated bilirubin concentration has diegnostic value. A serum bilirubin above 3.5 mg% is almost invariably associated with a decrease in k_e below the range of normal, and hence is indicative of liver disease. When the total red cell volume is normal, a serum unconjugated bilirubin belwo 0.7 mg% is normal and the probability of either active liver disease or of hemolysis is low. For the anemic patient, an unconjugated bilirubin value below 0.7 mg% is not necessarily normal and this level should probably be scaled downward proportionately to the total red cell volume. A serum unconjugated bilirubin concentration between 0.7 and 3.5 mg, admittedly a large range, indicates that either (1) liver function is impaired (k_e is reduced), (2) the RBCLS is shortened, or (3) a combination of both is present. It is not difficult to detect a decrease in k_e. Each patient with a decrease in k_e will have four-hour plasma retention of bilirubin after intravenous administration of either a tracer dose or of a loading dose of bilirubin that is greater than 12%.

A significant limitation to the use of the serum BR concentration as an indicator of hemolysis is the necessity for precise measurement. In our laboratory, this is accomplished by repeated measurements of up to 10 samples of plasma obtained during a period of 24 hours. The standard deviation of these determinations has an average value of 0.09 mg%, which in the normal represents a fractional standard deviation of approximately 25%. The standard error of the mean is .02 mg%, so that the fractional standard error of the mean is only 5%. The extent to which the fluctuations about the mean are physiologic, as opposed to methodologic, remains to be determined. Nevertheless, given small standard deviations obtained from our serial measurements, we are confident that changes in the mean bilirubin concentration of ± 0.5 mg% are physiologically significant. Interpretation of these small changes in other laboratories will depend on reproducibility of the serum bilirubin measurement.

5

Hormones Involved in Erythropoiesis

Two levels of hormonal action on erythropoiesis exist. One control, primary in nature is exerted through erythropoietin (erythropoiesis-stimulating factor, ESF). The other involves the action of the so-called orthodox hormones of adeno-hypophyseal target organ origin. Included in this latter group are the principles of the anterior pituitary gonadal, adrenal cortical and thyroidal axis. In this regard, there is growing evidence that the sex and adrenal cortical steroids and the thyroid hormones evoke their stimulatory effects on red cell formation, at least in part, by increasing production of the ESF, probably through actions exerted on both kidney and liver. It is the purpose of this chapter to describe some of our contibution in areas of investigation involving both the ESF and the sex steroids.

ERYTHROPOIETIN (ESF)

Features and Mechanism of Action

It is now recognized that the glycoprotein principle ESF is a prime regulator of erythropoiesis in higher organisms. Current estimates of its molecular weight are in the vicinity of 60,000 to 70,000. It is found in elevated quantities in the plasma, lymph and urine of animals subjected to hypoxia as well as in oxygen-deficiency states in man. Findings suggesting that it is involved not only in "panic" or "emergency" erythropoiesis but in the normal day-to-day replacement of red cells include: (1) its presence in the plasma and urine of normal human subjects, (2) the existence of a sex difference and a diurnal fluctuation in the amount of ESF excreted in the urine, and (3) the observation that an almost complete cessation of erythropoiesis may be induced in normal mice by the injection of anti-ESF serum.

The primary target site of ESF is the hematopoietic precursor element (ESF-committed cell) that it causes to differentiate into the earliest recognizable members of the nucleated erythroid cell series. The mechanisms by which the ESF induces the differentiation of hematopoietic precursor cells have been examined in two types of *in vitro* systems: (1) adult mammalian bone marrow cell and (2) mouse fetal liver cells. The *in vitro* marrow cell studies indicate that the ESF exerts a stimulatory effect on heme formation and this is preceeded by and dependent on the synthesis of a specific RNA assembly. Thus the ESF stimulated the formation of at least six types of RNA in rat bone marrow cells studied *in vitro*. These included rapidly labeled fractions that sedimented at 150, 55 to 65, 45 9,6 and 4 S. It seems possible that the 28 S and 18 S rNAs detected were formed from the stimulated 45 S RNA. The observation that the ESF increased the rate of both r and t RNA formation lends added weight to the contention that erythroid cell differentiation is associated with considerable hemoglobin synthesis. In addition the initiation of specific erythroid functions by the ESF implies the production of some forms of mRNA. It is of interest that an enhancing action on ALA synthetase activity has been reported in the spleens of plethoric mice injected with the ESF and in rabbit bone marrow cell cultures to which the ESF has been added. Like the 5β-H sterioid metabolites the ESF may function in part as a physiologic derepressor of ALA synthetase, a rate-limiting enzyme in the production of heme.

Synthesis of hemoglobin proceeds at a low rate in fetal liver cells obtained from mouse fetuses approximately 10 to14 days old. Addition of the ESF to the culture system at this time markedly increases the rate of hemoglobin production. This response to the ESF is apparently dependent on a period of early and one of relatively late RNA transcription with an intervening phase of DNA replication. Morphological studies suggest that the augmented production of hemoglobin caused by the ESF is also attributable to an increase in the numbers of hemoglobin-synthesizing element that developed from precursor cells.

Model of Stem Cell Replication and Differentiation

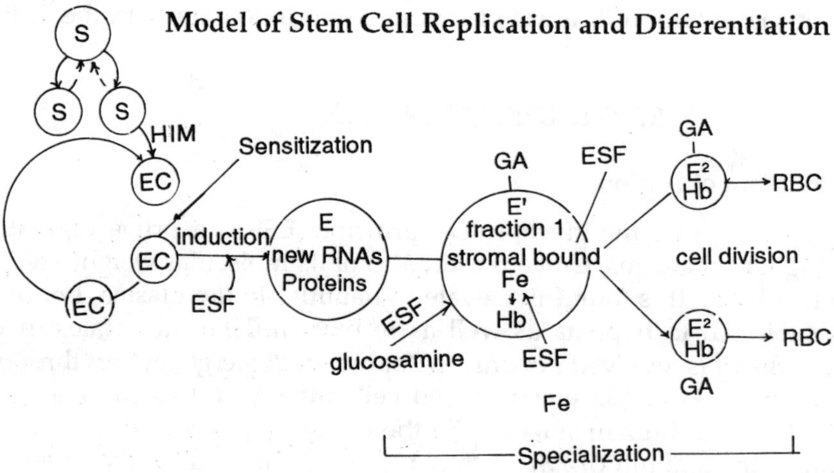

Fig. 5.1. Mechanism of ESF action (s) on erythropoiesis.

S — Primitive stem cell ("colony forming cell") (dotted lines indicate possible negative feedback of stem cells on their own replication).

EC — Erythropoietin-committed cell (forms from S under possible influence of special "Hematopoietic Inductive Microenvironment" ("HIM") (Trentin 1970).

EC' — Sensitized EC (stippled are a represents hypothetical attachment site of ESF).

E — First stage of RBC differentation (induced by ESF).

E^1, E^2 — Later stages of RBC development (may also be influenced by ESF).

Fe — Iron transport into cell (stimulated by ESF).

GA — Cellular materials labeled by glucosamine (enhanced by ESF).

Three phases of differentiation of the ESF-committed stem cell have been postulated: (1) *Sensitization:* this is a mechanism that renders undifferentiated ESF-committed cells inducible or competent to become erythroid elements. Because this phase is markedly inhibited by actinomycin-D, it appears to require DNA-dependent RNA synthesis. It is conceivable that the sensitization may involve production of a short-lived mRNA needed for the formation of an attachment site on the cell surface for the ESF. (2) *Induction:* This action might occur at the cell surface or following entrance of the ESF into the undifferentiated cell. The first subcellular site of action of the hormone has not as yet been identified. Its precise location must await the development of methods that would make possible the isotopic labeling of high purity ESF and then tracing it in the target cells by electron microscopic autoradiographic procedures. At a subcellular site, probably the nucleus, the ESF might serve a derepressor, in the light of the Jacob-Monod concept, thus initiating the transcription of genetic information leading to cell differentiation. (3) *Specialization:* Here specific biochemical and morphological features of the definitive erythroid cell line become unfolded. These changes could arise as a result of the induction of a variety of RNAs essential for the transport of iron into the cell, the incorporation of glucosamine into the acid soluble stroma and soluble cell components, and the production of hemoglobin. These concepts are depicted in Figure 5.1.

The ESF In Nonmammalian Species

It would seem likey that an ESF operates in most if not all classes of the Subphylum Vertebrata. Thus it has been shown that the erythropoiesis-stimulating factor appearing in the plasma of the frog (*Rana pipiens*) and in the bird (Japanese quail, *Coturnix coturnix japonica*) after bleeding is effective erythropoietically in the species from which it is derived but not in the mammalian assay. On the other hand, mammalian ESF does not appear to stimulate erythropoiesis in the frog or bird. This supports the view that class specificity of the ESF exists among the Vertebrata. Further evidence for this contention is provided by findings indicating that although mammalian ESF is rendered inactive by neuraminidase, avian ESF is not destroyed by this enzyme nor is it inhibited by antibody to human urinary ESF. Thus it would appear that although erythropoietins exist in the various classes of the vertebrates, they differ somewhat in their basic structure.

Work in our laboratory has shown the existence of an ESF in the plasma of the gourami fish (*Trichogaster trichopterus*) subjected to bleeding. These fish, when starved, exhibit a marked depression in RBC counts, hematocrit and hemoglobin values as well as in the percent RBC radioiron incorporation and in total circulating RBC volume. Such fish may be used as sensitive test animals for determining the effects of fish ESF. Thus a single injection of 0.15 ml of plasma from bled anemic gouramis to fish with suppressed erythropoiesis due to starvation resulted in a highly significant increase in the rate of radioiron incorporation into the circulating red cells of these animals, an effect not shared by normal gourami plasma. Although the gourami responds to mammalian ESF, approximately 80 times as much of this hormone, on a body weight basis, is required to stimulate erythropoiesis in the gourami as compared to the response in the posthypoxic polycythemic mouse. It is conceivable that all vertebrate erythropoietins possess a common biologically active core but that slight diifferences in attached chemical groupings are responsible for the class specificities described. The administration of very large doses of one type of ESF might produce an effect in another class despite the existence of physiologic class specificity.

Biogenesis of the ESF

The kidney is now acknowledged to be the major site of production of the ESF. The importance of the kidney in this regard was first described by Jacobson *et al* (1957, 1959) who showed that bilateral nephrectomy markedly suppressed the ability of rats to produce the ESF when subjected to various forms of hypoxia including hemorrhage, lowered oxygen pressures, or cobalt treatment. That this decrease in ESF production could not be attributed to the toxicity of the retained wastes was shown by the fact that bilateral ureteral ligation, which resulted in a degree of uremia equivalent to that seen after nephrectomy, caused only a slight reduction in the amount of ESF induced by cobalt administration. It is of interest that of all types of human anemias studied, only those associated with renal disease exhibited either little or no ESF in plasma assays.

Despite the persuasive evidence that has been marshalled to support a renal origin of the ESF, past attempts to extract this principle from the kidney have not been altogether successful. It seemed possible that this inability to detect really significant amounts of ESF even in the kidneys of animals exposed to hypoxia, at least in quantities equivalent to those present in plasma, was due to (1) a true absesnce of the factor in kidney tissue, (2) a tenacious binding of the ESF to subcellular particles, rendering it nonextractable with the usual isotonic media employed (Contrera *et al* 1965), (3) the presence of an inhibitor to the ESF in renal extracts, or (4) the possibility that an activator or precursor of the ESF existed in renal tissues. In 1966, our laboratory reported on the extraction of a factor from the kidneys of hypoxic rats that, when administered intraperitoneally alone, was not erythropoietically active but, when injected intravenously alone (unpublished) or when incubated with normal serum, resulted in the production of the ESF. This principle was named the Renal Erythropoietic Factor (REF) or more recently Erythrogenin. Fractionation procedures have been employed to determine the subcellular location of erythrogenin. In a typical experiment, kidneys were obtained from adult female rats made hypoxic by exposure to 0.45 atmospheres of air for 19 hours. Subcellular fractionation procedures were now employed for obtaining the nuclear, heavy-mitochondrial, light-mitochondrial, and microsomal fractions. Each of these particulate fractions was now suspended in 0.02 M phosphate buffer (pH 6.8) or in distilled water (not below pH 6.0) and subjected to centrifugation at 37,000 g for 30 minutes. The supernatant fluid derived from each extract was assayed for erythropoiesis-stimulating activity both before and after incubation with normal rat serum (NRS) that had been dialyzed against ethylenediamine tetraacetate (EDTA). This dialysis procedure prevents the operation of an ESF-inactivating system present in the incubation mixture that is apparently cation-dependent. A minimum of 5 adult CF-1 female mice (25 to 30 gm), rendered polycythemic by discontinuous exposure to hypoxia, were used to assay the various extracts. The criterion of erythropoiesis employed was the percent incorporation of ^{59}Fe into the circulating RBC. In some instances the radioiron incorporation values were converted into international units of the ESF by reference to the dose-response curve for assay mice injected with the International Reference Preparation (IRP) of ESF

Table 5.1
Erythropoiesis-stimulating Activity of Hypotonic Extracts of Subcellular Fractions of Rat Kidneys, after Incubation with Saline or Normal Serum

Material Assayed		*Percent RBC-^{59}Fe Incorporation (Mean ±IS.D.M.)*
Saline		0.96+/-0.24
Serum		1.43+/-0.30
0.05 IU ESF		6.49+/-0.92
0.20 IU ESF		14.06+/-1.87
	Extract+saline	*Extract+serum*
Nuclear extract	1.47 ± 0.36	2.19 ± 0.33
Heavy-mitochondrial extract	0.87 ± 0.21	1.32 ± 0.35
Light-mitochondrial extract	1.97 ± 0.39	8.94 ± 1.63
Microsomal extract	0.66 ± 0.13	9.64 ± 1.08
Soluble fraction	2.33 ± 0.62	3.01 ± 0.49

This assay is sufficiently sensitive to detect quantities as small as 0.02 to 0.05 units of the ESF.

Table 5.1 shows that no erythropoietic activity was found in extracts of the nuclear and heavy-mitochondrial fractions either before or after incubation with EDTA-dialyzed normal rat serum. However, it will be noted that although extracts of the light-mitochondrial and microsomal fractions were inactive erythropoietically when administered alone to the assay mice, highly significant quantities of the ESF were produced following incubation of these extracts with dialyzed rat serum. Dialyzed normal rat serum administered alone exerted little or no effect in the assay mice. Studies of the kinetics of the erythrogenin-serum system have suggested that erythrogenin is an enzyme that converts a serum substrate (erythropoietinogen) into the active form of the ESF. That it is actually the ESF that is generated in the erythrogenin-serum incubation system is supported by findings indicating that inhibition of the generated erythropoiesis-stimulating activity occurs on addition of anti-ESF globulin to the incubation mixture.

Current Procedure for Extraction of Erythrogenin from Rat Kidneys

1. Kidneys are removed immediately following exsanguination, Decapsulated, weighed and minced.

2. Tissue is homogenized in cold 0.25 m sucrose (10 mg/ml) with potter-elvehjem homogenizer as follows :

   A) The tissue is first homogenized with a loose-fitting pestle which has its diameter reduced 3/8-1/2 mm by grinding against a stone. *The mixture should appear homogeneous at the end of this step.*

   B) The mixture is Re-homogenized using the standardized pestles. *The duration of this step is dependent upon the state of the mixture after step 2A.*

3. The homogenate is centrifuged at 5,500 × g for 10 minutes and the precipitate is discarded.

4. The supernatant fluid is re-centrifuged at 30,000 × g for 35 minutes. This supernatant fluid is discarded.

5. The precipitate is mildly homogenized in the presence of 1-2 drops of cutscum (Detergent) and distilled water (2 ml/gm) while in the centrifuge tubes.

6. The resulting mixture is frozen for 48 hours.

7. On the day of the assay the mixture is thawed and centrifuged at 37,000 × g for 35 minutes.

8. The supernatant contains erythrogenin and should possess 9-13 mg of protein/ml.

Fig. 5.2. Procedure for extraction of erythrogenin from kidneys.

Some laboratories have reported difficulty in demonstrating erythrogenin in renal tissue. This may be attributed to several causes. A too vigorous initial homogenization of the kidneys may induce the release of factors that destroy or inhibit the generated ESF. A second possibility is the use of homogenizing media with a pH of 5 and below that is destructive to erythrogenin. Another cause stems from the inability of some assays to detect consistently ESF activity ranging from 0.05 to 0.1 IRP units. The potencies of most of our renal extracts, in the amounts generally given, fall within this range.

Feedback Relations in the Erythrogenin-Erythropoietinogen-ESF System

We have reported an inhibitory influence exerted by the ESF on its own production. In these experiments, several groups, each comprising six adult rats were established. The rats in Group 1 were subjected to continuous hypoxia corresponding to 0.45 atmospheres of air for 5 hours and bled immediately thereafter. Group 2 was given one intravenous injection of 15 IRP units of human urinary ESF and exsanguinated 5 hours later. Group 3 was injected intravenously with 15 IRP units of ESF just prior to a 5-hour period of hyposia and bled immediately following the termination of the hyposia. The plasmas derived from these 3 groups were pooled of separately and assayed for their ESF content in exhypoxic polycythemic mice. Each mouse received 0.2 ml of plasma intraperitoneally and the erythropoietic response was estimated in terms of percent RBC radioiron incorporation.

For determination of substrate levels, plasmas were first dialyzed against 0.005 M disodium-EDTA before the incubation procedures were begun. Plasma samples containing ESF were treated with anti-ESF (Supplied by Dr. John C. Schooley, University of California, Berkeley) prior to their incubation with erythrogenin. The amount of anti-ESF employed was twice that required to neutralize the erythropoietic activity of the plasma sample. The excess anti-ESF in the plasma was removed by the addition of a serum containing goat anti-rabbit gamma globulin (GARCG) prepared in goats immunized with a gamma globulin fraction of normal rabbit serum. In a sense, this goat anti-serum serves as an anti-anti-ESF.

Figure 5.3 indicates that exposure to hypoxia for five hours resulted in the appearance of considerable ESF in plasma and that, along with this rise, relatively high levels of plasma substrate for erythrogenin were noted (Group 1). The rats that had given 15 IRP units of ESF showed approximately 0.2 units of ESF activity per 0.7 ml of plasma at 5 hours after administration of exogenous ESF (Group 2). Substrate activity in these rats was no different from that observed in plasma samples from untreated rats. Of particular significance was the observation that the ESF levels in plasma from rats receiving both exogenous ESF and exposure to hypoxia (Group 3) were not significantly different from

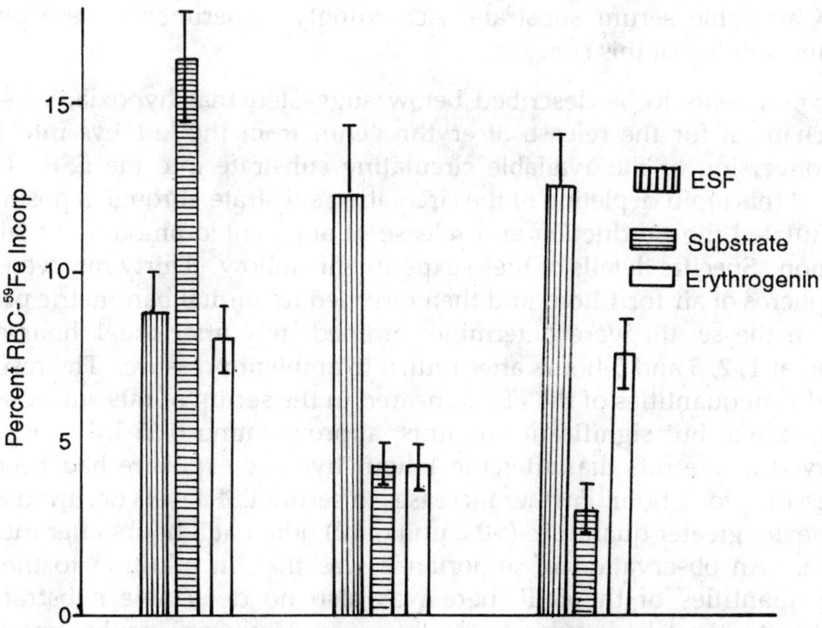

Fig. 5.3. Effect of exogenous ESF on endogenous ESF, plasma substrate and renal erythrogenin levels in rats exposed to hypoxia. The ESF and substrate activity of plasma as well as the erythrogenin levels in the kidney were determined in exhypoxic polycythemic mice and expressed as RBC-^{59}Fe incorporation values. Vertical lines through tops of bars (mean values) indicate ± SEM.

those seen in rats given only the ESF (Group 2). It is also apparent that injection of exogenous ESF just prior to exposure of the rats to hypoxia, caused a marked reduction in substrate levels (Group 3) when compared to those in rats receiving only hypoxia (Group 1). Although renal erythrogenin values were elevated by hypoxia, no inhibitory effects on these levels occurred as a result of administration of exogenous ESF before exposure to the low oxygen pressures. A negative feedback action of the ESF on its own production is thus established. This mechanism apparently operates through an ability of the ESF to decrease the production and/or the activity of plasma substrate.

Changes in Circulating Levels of ESF and Substrate Following Exposure to Hypoxia or Injections of Exogenous Erythrogenin

A fact that impressed us in our studies on the biogenesis of the ESF was that although various types of hypoxia resulted in elevated levels of erythrogenin in the kidney, the increases noted were not of sufficient intensity to account for the associated large amounts of circulating ESF evoked by the same stimulus. In addition, other of our observations indicated that only relatively small quantities of the ESF were produced on incubating erythrogenin with normal samples of serum obtained from a variety of mammalian forms. Findings such as these suggested that the major limiting factor in the production of large amounts of ESF under both *in vivo* and *in vitro* conditions was the quantity of available serum substrate. Accordingly, experiments were performed to determine the validity of this concept.

The experiments to be described below suggested that hypoxia, by serving as a trigger mechanism for the release of erythrogenin from the kidneys into the plasma, caused a conversion of the available circulating substrate into the ESF. Moreover, it appeared that this rapid depletion of the circulating substrate, through a positive feedback action, stimulated the production and release of augmented amounts of substrate into the circulation. Specific details of these experiments follow. Thirty rats were exposed to 0.45 atmospheres of air for 1 hour and then returned to normal barometric pressure. The ESF levels in the serum were determined immediately after the 1 hour exposure to hypoxia and at 1, 2, 3 and 5 hours after return to ambient pressure. The results indicate that insignificant quantities of the ESF appeared in the serum of rats subjected to 1 hour of hypoxia. Small but significant amounts, approximating 0.05 IRP units/ml serum, were observed in the rats that after the 1 hour hypoxic exposure had been at normal oxygen pressures for 1 hour. Further increases in serum ESF levels occurred after 2 and 3 hours with even greater quantities (>0.2 units/ml) noted at 5 hours after interruption of the hypoxia. An observation of importance was that, in addition to the absence of significant quantities of the ESF there was also no detectable substrate in serum immediately after the 1-hour subjection to hypoxia. However, incubation of this 1-hour hypoxic serum with normal rat serum resulted in the generation of significant quantities of ESF, suggesting the presence of increased amounts of erythrogenin in the circulating blood at this time.

We interpret these results as follows: (1) the inability to detect the ESF immediately following a 1-hour subjection to hypoxia is probably the result of an insufficient quantity

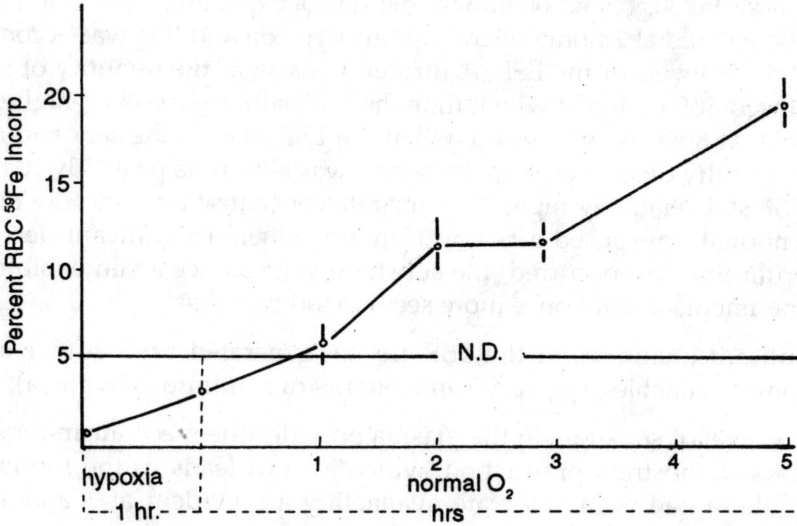

Fig. 5.4. Effect of a 1-hour exposure of rats to hypoxia on the ESF content of the serum during this hypoxic period and during 5 hours after return to normal oxygen pressures. Ordinate indicates the RBC-radioiron incorporation values in assay exhypoxic polycythemic mice, each receiving 1.0 ml of the various sera. ND—nondetectable. Vertical lines through points (mean values) indicate ± 1 SEM.

of substrate in the plasma, (2) the further drop in the level of free substrate, as a result of its reaction with erythrogenin, appears to constitute the trigger mechanism for the appearance of increased amounts of the substrate during the subsequent 5 hours of exposure to normal oxygen pressures. Apparently, sufficient amounts of erythrogenin to engender production of the ESF are probably also present in the plasma during the 5-hour posthypoxia period, (3) finally, the results demonstrate conclusively that once triggered, the events leading to ESF formation attain completion independent of the original hypoxic stimulus.

Additional results in accord with a feedback role of both the ESF and the serum substrate were derived from studies on rats exposed continuously to hypoxia (0.45 atmosphere of air). Ten groups, each consisting of four rats, were established. Determinations of ESF and of serum substrate were made after 0, 15, 30 and 45 minutes and following 1, 2, 3, 5, 8, 10 and 15 hours of hypoxia. For this purpose, in each of the 10 groups, 1 ml of serum was incubated with 1 ml of saline for 1 hour and assayed for its ESF content. In addition, 1 ml of serum after treatment with anti-ESF to eliminate the ESF present and then with GARGG to rid the serum of excess anti-ESF was tested for its substrate content. This was determined by incubating this treated serum with 1 ml of eythrogenin (derived from 0.5 gm hypoxic rat kidney) and then assaying the incubation fluid for the quantity of ESF generated. Each assay mouse received an intraperitoneal injection of 2 ml of each of the mixtures tested. Figure 5.5 shows that the ESF was not detectable at any of the time intervals examined during the first hour of hypoxia. Although substrate levels were normal at 15 minutes of hypoxia, they decreased to non-detectable levels at the 30, 45 and 60 minute periods of exposure. Significant amounts of the substrate were noted at 2 hours of continuous hypoxia and this was accompanied by a marked rise in the levels of the ESF. A further increase in the quantity of substrate in the serum occurred at 5 hours, at which time the ESF values were even higher than they were at 2 hours. At 8 hours of hypoxia, when the ESF level in the sera had attained its maximum the quantity of sutbstrate in the serum was also at its peak. By 10 hours, with the levels of ESF still relatively high, the substrate concentration had now decreased to that found in normal unexposed rats. By 15 hours, when a significant decrease in the quantity of serum ESF had occurred, the substrate values once again exhibited a rising trend. The experiments, would once more seem to indicate that:

1. significant quantities of the ESF are not generated until sufficient substrate becomes available (e.g., at 2, 5 and 8 hours of continuous hypoxia),

2. a low level of substrate in the plasma provides the mechanism for subsequent increased substrate production, which in turn leads to the formation of the ESF; these nadirs in substrate availability are evident at 1 and 10 hours of continuous hypoxia,

3. the fluctuations that occur in the ESF levels in animals exposed continuously to hypoxia (Camiscoli and Gordon 1970) are due most likely to variations in the production and/or availability of the substrate.

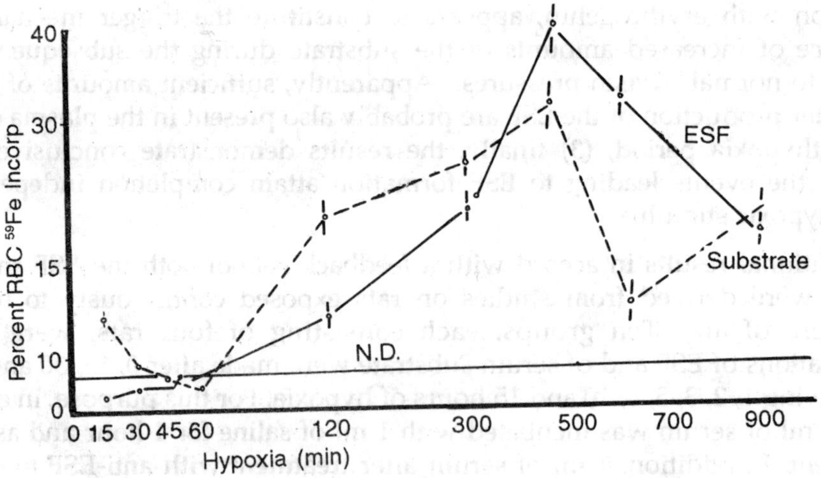

Fig. 5.5. Effects of continuous exposure of rats to hypoxia on the ESF and substrate content of the serum. Ordinate represents the RBC-radioiron incorporation values in assay exhypoxic mice, each receiving 1.0 ml serum for ESF or 1.0 ml serum for substrate assays. ND—nondetectable. Vertical lines through points (mean values) indicate ± 1 SEM.

Thus as shown in Figure 5.5 the attainment of elevated levels of ESF corresponding, for example, to 1.5 to 2.0 units per ml of serum at 8 hours of continuous hypoxia, is followed by a precipitous decline in substrate activity. Thus it seems again that the negative feedback action of the ESF on its own production is mediated through a decrease in the availability of substrate. When the ESF levels descend (e.g., at 15 hours), this feedback effect is no longer operative and a resumption of substrate production ensues. Similar mechanisms appear to operate in ESF production in fetal lambs rendered anemic by injection of phenylhydrazine.

It became of interest to determine whether the effects of hypoxia of ESF and substrate production could be simulated by increasing the level of erythrogenin in the blood through its direct intravenous administration to normal, nonhypoxic animals. To this end, six groups of 4 adult rats were used to study the time sequence effects. Five ml of erythrogenin fluid (obtained for 2.5 gm of hypoxic rat kidney) were injected intravenously into each of the 24 rats. Determination of ESF and substrate levels were made at 5, 10, 20, 60, 120 and 180 minutes following administration of the erythrogenin. The methods employed for estimating ESF and substrate values were similar to those outlined for the continuous hypoxia experiments described above. The data are graphed in Figure 5.6. It will be observed that serum obtained from rats at 5 minutes after erythrogenin injection contained no detectable ESF; substrate was present at this time in the amount found in normal untreated rats. At 10 minutes after erythrogenin injection, the serum possessed detectable amounts of ESF and approximately normal quantities of substrate. Observe that at 20 minutes following erythrogenin administration, both the ESF and substrate were absent. At 60 minutes, although no ESF was present, a rise in substrate level had become evident. At 2 and 3 hours after erythrogenin injection, the substrate level had risen appreciably, and this was paralleled by rise in the circulating level of ESF. These experiments may be interpreted to men that

1. **direct instillation of erythrogenin into the venous blood results in generation of a small amount of ESF,**
2. **the rapid generation of the ESF temporarily depletes the plasma of substrate; again the lowering of substrate provides the trigger mechanism or production of relatively large quantities of substrate which leads to enhanced formation of the ESF,**
3. **the amount of ESF formed is directly correlated to the plasma substrate content, i.e.., substrate levels apparently constitute the major rate-limiting factor in ESF biogenesis,**
4. **although it seems that a single intravenous injection of erythrogenin is sufficient to engender ESF production for at least 3 hours after its administration (provided adequate amounts of substrate are available), the possibility cannot be precluded that endogenously produced erythrogenin also enters into the formation of the ESF at the second and third hours. We hope to resolve this problem in donor rats deprived of their kidneys.**

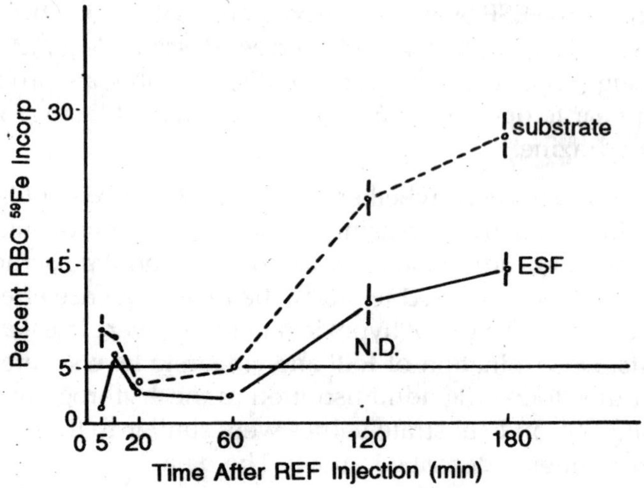

Fig. 5.6. Influence of a single intravenous injection of erythrogenin on the ESF and substrate content of the serum of rats. Ordinate represents the RBC-radioiron incorporation values in assay exhypoxic polycythemic mice, each receiving 1.0 ml serum for ESF or 1.0 ml serum for substrate assays. Vertical lines through points (mean values) indicate ± 1 SEM.

Our concept for the biogenesis of the ESF and the feedback roles of the ESF and the serum substrate is depleted in Figure, 5.7. We envision hypoxia, the fundamental erythrocytogenic stimulus, as triggering the release of erythrogenin from its site of production the kidney. Erythrogenin interacting with the substrate (erythropoietinogen) either in the plasma, the kidney or both, results in the formation of the ESF. The rise in ESF levels does not proceed unchecked. After attaining peak values, the ESF exerts an inhibitory effect on its own formation through a suppressive action on the production and/or release of the substrate. ESF formation is thereby curtailed until it attains a value sufficiently low to permit a resumption of stubstrate production. This in turn results in a further generation of the ESF. Eventually, the increased numbers of circulating red cells that result from enhanced ESF production act in an inhibitory capacity on the synthesis and/or availability of renal erythrogenin and suppression of ESF formation.

The precise nature of the feedback relations of erythrogenin and the substrate to the biogenes is of the ESF remains to be explored. In particular, the question whether the liver is actually the source of the substrate requires attention. In addition, it is obvious that a full comprehension of these feedback relations must await the development of procedures that will permit simultaneous detection of erythrogenin in the kidney and plasma as well as substrate and ESF levels in response to a variety of erythropoietic stimuli and depressants.

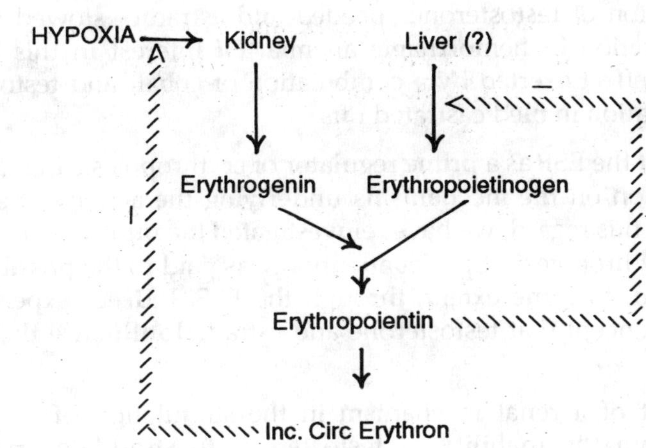

Fig. 5.7. Scheme for biogensis of the ESF.

SEX STEROIDS

In 1941, our laboratory demonstrated that testosterone stimulated and estradiol inhibited erythropoiesis in castrated and in hypophysectomized rats. It was also shown that, whereas injections of equine gonadotropin resulted in significant increases in red cell numbers in normal and hypophysectomized male rats, females treated with the same preparation exhibited either no change or a decrease in circulating red cell numbers. These results were interpreted to mean that both exogenous and endogenously produced androgen served as a potent stimulus to erythropoiesis in the rodent. The criteria for erythropoiesis-stimulating activity employed were increases in peripheral red cell numbers, hemoglobin concentration, and reticulocytosis. Similarly, in both male and female hypophysectomized rats injected with testosterone, the posthypophysectomy bone marrow hypoplasia was significantly repaired, with the numbers of erythropblasts considerably increased and vacuolization much less marked. On the other hand, the fatty hypoplasia characteristically seen in the marrows of hypophysectomized rats appeared to be intensified by estradiol injections; fewer nucleared erythroid elements were also evident in the marrows. Findings reported by Crafts (1946) and by Van Dyke *et al* (1954) were in general agreement with the contention that testosterone was a potent stimulator of red cell production in hypophysectomized animals. Similarly, the opposite effects exerted by androgens and estrogens on erythropoiesis suggested that the sex dimorphism in red cell counts observed among representatives of the Class Mammalia and Aves was attributable to the differential actions of the sex steroids in the two sexes. Subsequent studies indicated that the sex hormones were concerned with recovery from the anemia induced by hemorrhage in rats. The evidence upon which this conclusion was based included the facts that:

1. bled male rats regenerated their red cells more quickly than bled females,
2. recovery from anemia occurred more slowly in castrated males than in spayed females, and

3. administration of testosterone speeded and estradiol slowed the rate of red cell regeneration in hemorrhagic anemia. Of interest in this study was the synergistic effect exerted by a combination of cobalt and testosterone on red cell regeneration in bled castrated rats.

The acceptance of the ESF as a prime regulator of erythropoiesis in higher organisms has refocussed attention on the mechanisms underlying the actions of sex steroids on red cell production. In this regard, we have reinvestigated the influence of several steroids and derivatives on erythropoiesis. Special attention was paid to the possibility that these actions were mediated, to some extent, through the ESF. Indeed, experiments will be cited to support the concept that testosterone and estradiol influence the production of the ESF.

The involvement of a renal mechanism in the stimulation of erythropoiesis by androgen is seen from the inability of testosterone to stimulate erythropoiesis in nephrectomized mice. Attempts were made to determine the renal mechanism forming the basis for the enhancing effects of androgens on erythropoiesis. In this connection, we have investigated the possibility that the renal erythrogenin-erythropoietinogen-ESF axis is involved in this action.

Experiments with Testosterone

We have already reported that administration of testosterone results in an increased production of the ESF in rats, mice, rabbits and tamarins. A description of only those studies performed in mice will be given here. Adult female Ha/ICR Swiss mice (25 to 30 gm) were injected intramuscularly once every 7 days with 5 mg long-acting testosterone cyclopentylpropionate (TCP; "Depo-testosterone," Upjohn Co.) in 0.25 ml suspending medium. Another group of mice was given the same schedule of TCP injections but, in addition, were exposed to hypoxia (10 per cent oxygen) for 30 hours just before they were killed. At various time intervals after initiation of TCP treatment, the mice were exsanguinated and their plasmas tested for erythropoiesis-stimulating activity in mice rendered plethoric by intraperitoneal injections of homologous red cells. Percent incorporation of radioiron into circulating red cells was employed as the erythropoietic criterion.

Table 5.2 indicates that erythropoiesis-stimulating activity became apparent in the plasma of the mice by the fourth day after initiation of TCP treatment. This activity was maintained until the eighth day following which it decreased, with markedly lowered values evident on days 10 and 12 (3 and 5 days, respectively, after the second injection of TCP). Mice given the same schedule of TCP injections but, in addition, exposed to hypoxia before sacrifice displayed at 8 and 12 days considerably greater plasma ESF activity than could be ascribed to the additive effects of TCP and hypoxia given separately. Fried and Gurney (1965) have obtained essentially similar results.

The capacity of plasma from testosterone-injected animals to stimulate erythropoiesis cannot be attributed to the presence of residual androgen in the plasma samples for the following reasons: (1) erythropoietic activity of the plasma diminished with continued injections and with increased dosages of administered testosterone, (2) administration of

Table 5.2
Erythropoiesis-stimulating Activity of Plasma from Mice given Androgen (TCP) and/or Subjected to Hypoxia

Group	*Day plasma obtained*	*Percent RBC-^{59}Fe Incorporation (Mean ± 1 S.E.M.)**
Donor mice given	0	0.2 ± 0.03
TCP only	2	0.4 ± 0.04
	4	3.4 ± 0.06
	6	4.1 ± 0.05
	8	4.0 ± 0.05
	10	0.8 ± 0.06
	12	0.6 ± 0.05
Donor mice given	2	5.2 ± 0.4
TCP and hypoxia	4	8.2 ± 0.06
	8	11.0 ± 0.08
	12	13.5 ± 1.00
Donor mice given hypoxia only		4.1 ± 0.05
Untreated mice		0.2 ± 0.02

* Six plethorized mice were used to assay each sample. Each mouse received subcutaneous injections of 0.5 ml plasma daily for 3 successive days. On the fourth day, they were injected intravenously with 1 μCi ^{59}Fe in 0.5 ml saline and the percent RBC-radioiron incorporation determined 24 hours later.

anti-ESF completely abolished the ability of testosterone to stimulate erythropoiesis in mice and inhibited the erythropoiesis stimulating effects of plasma from testosterone-treated mice. These two studies give additional firm support to the contention that testosterone augments erythropoiesis in rodents by stimulating the production of the ESF.

The possibility was now investigated that the stimulatory action exerted by testosterone on erythropoiesis was mediated through an increased production of renal erythrogenin. Accordingly, the influence of testosterone and hypoxia in the levels of ESF in plasma and on the erythrogenin content of the kidney was studied. Similarly, the mechanisms responsible for the depressive effects exerted by estrogen were examined. In these experiments, adult male rats (250-270 gm) of the Long-Evans strain served as plasma, serum and kidney donors.

Testosterone

Four groups, each comprising 6 rats, were established. Group 1 was given a single subcutaneous injection of 12.5 mg testosterone cyclopentylpropionate (TCP) in 1 ml cottonseed oil. The control group (2) was injected subcutaneously with 1 ml cottonseed oil. The rats of Group 3 received a single subcutaneous injection of 12.5 mg TCP and in addition were subjected to 19 hours of hypoxia (0.4 atmospheres of air) 5 days after the testosterone injection. Group 4 was administered a single subcutaneous injection of the vehicle and 5 days later were exposed to 19 hours of hypoxia. All rats were killed by blood withdrawal on the sixth day following the injection.

Estrogen

Two groups of five rats were employed as donors. Group 5 received a single subcutaneous injection of 5 mg estradiol benzoate (EB) in 1 ml of peanut oil and 25 hours later were exposed to 8 hours of hypoxia corresponding to 0.4 atmospheres of air. The rats of Group 6 were given a single subcutaneous injection of 1 ml of peanut oil and 24 hours later were subjected to 8 hours of hypoxia. The rats of these 2 groups were killed by exsanguination on termination of the hypoxic period.

The bloods of the 6 groups were heparinized, the plasmas collected, pooled and stored at -20^{0}C until used. The kidneys from these 6 groups of rats were also separately pooled and subjected to the already described subcellular fractionation procedure for the extraction of erythrogenin. The incubation procedures for each of the 6 groups consisted of adding 6 ml of erythrogenin-containing fluid (from 3.0 gm hypoxic rat kidneys) to 6 ml EDTA-dialyzed normal rat serum. The incubation were carried out for 60 minutes in a water bath shaken at 37^0 C. In the experiments involving estrogen, two additional incubation were done to determine whether the estrogen had influenced the production and/or activity of the serum substrate. These involved addition of: (1) six ml of erythrogenin from peanut oil-injected hypoxic rats to 6 ml of EDTA-dialyzed serum from nohypoxic rats that had received a single subcutaneous injection of 12.5 mg EB 32 hours previously (Group 7), and 2/ 6 ml of erythrogenin from peanut oil-injected hypoxic rats to 6 ml of EDTA-dialyzed serum from nonhypoxic rats that had been given a single subcutaneous injecion of 1 ml peanut oil (control) 32 hours earlier (Group 8).

The plasmas and erythrogenin-serum incubation mixtures were tested for erythropoiesis-stimulating activity in exhypoxic polycythemic mice. Each of 5 to 6 mice received either 1 ml of plasma or 2 ml of incubation mixture as a single intraperitoneal injection on day 3 following interruption of the hypoxia. They received an intravenous injection of 0.5 μCi ^{59}Fe in 0.2 ml saline on day 5 and were killed on day 7 for determination of the percent RBC-radioiron incorporation. These values were converted into equivalent ESF units by reference to the standard curve for the International Reference Preparation.

Results for the Testosterone Groups

As noted before (Mirand *et al* 1965, the plasmas obtained from the TCP-treated rats (Group 1A) exhibited more erythropoiesis stimulating activity than did that from the controls receiving the vehicle for TCP (Group 2A; see Table 5.3). Exposure to 19 hours of hypoxia resulted in a marked increase in ESF concentration in the plasma (Group 4A).

Table 5.3
Effect of Androgen (TCP) and Bypoxia on Plasma ESF and on Renal Erythrogenin (EG) in Rats

Group	*Donors and materials tested*	*Percent RBC—^{59}Fe incorporation (Mean ± 1 S.E.M.)*	*Mean ESF units/ml plasma or 2/ml of EG-serum incubate*
I.	TCP-treated, nonhypoxic		
	A. Plasma	9.5 ± 1.0	0.085
	B. EG + EDTA-dial. NRS*	7.6 ± 0.5	0.065
II	Oil-treated, nonhypoxic		
	A. Plasma	2.1 ± 0.6	NS †
	B. EG + EDTA-dial. NRS	4.2 ± 0.6	NS
III	TCP-treated, hypoxic		
	A. Plasma	32.7 ± 3.0	1.5
	B. EG + EDTA-dial. NRS	13.9 ± 1.0	0.18
IV	Oil-treated, hypoxic		
	A. Plasma	23.8 ± 2.6	1.0
	B. EG + EDTA-dial NRS	9.2 ± 1.0	0.08

* NRS = normal rat serum.

† NS = not significant.

The plasmas of the rats that were given the combined TCP-hypoxia treatment (Group 3A) displayed an even greater increase in plasma ESF. Erythrogenin activity of the kidneys was significantly greater in the rats receiving TCP (Group 1B) or hypoxia (Group 4B) than in the controls injected with the vehicle (Group 2B). Even greater erythrogenin activity was observed with the combination of TCP and hypoxia (Group 3B) than for either stimulus given alone.

Results for the Estrogen Groups

Table 5.4 shows that the increase in erythropoiesis-stimulating activity in plasma evoked by hypoxia was markedly inhibited by a single injection of EB (cf. Groups 5A and 6A). The suppressive action of estradiol on plasma ESF in rats exposed to hypoxia was not associated with any change in the erythrogenin content of the kidneys (Groups 5B and 6B). Thus incubation of renal erythrogenin from rats subjected to hypoxia with EDTA-dialyzed serum from oil-injected controls resulted in the generation of considerable quantities of the ESF (Group 8). However, one may observe in Group 7 that significantly less ESF was produced when EDTA-dialyzed serum from rats treated with estradiol was employed in the incubation system.

Table 5.4
Effect of Estrogen (EB) and Hypoxia on Plasma ESF and on Renal Erytbhrogenin (EG) in Rats

Group	*Donors and materials tested*	*Percent RBC—^{59}Fe incorporation (Mean ± 1 S.E.M.)*	*Mean ESF units/ml plasma or 2/ml of EG-serum incubate*
V.	EB-treated, hypoxic		
	A. Plasma	8.7 ± 0.7	0.075
	B. EG + EDTA-dial. NRS *	10.6 ± 2.1	0.09
VI.	Oil-treated, hypoxic		
	A. Plasma	28.6 ± 3.9	1.2
	B. EG + EDTA-dial. NRS	9.3 ± 1.3	0.085
VII.	EG (oil-treated, hypoxic) + EDTA-dial, serum (EB-treated, nonhypoxic)	4.3 ± 0.9	NS†
VIII.	EG (oil-treated, hypoxic) + EDTA-dial serum (oil-treated, nonhypoxic)	11.5 ± 1.2	0.11

* NRS = normal rat serum.

† NS = not significant.

These experiments lend additional support to the concept that testosterone stimulates erythropoiesis in rodents through the production of the ESF. It seems probable that this augmented production of the ESF is due to a rise in erythrogenin activity evoked by testosterone. Of interest are the observations that the combination of testosterone and hypoxia evoked greater rises in renal erythrogenin activity and in the plasma ESF than those seen with either stimulus given alone. Based on ESF unitage, it would appear that the increased effects of the combination of testosterone and hypoxia on both erythrogenin and plasma ESF are more likely synergistic than additive in nature.

The results indicate that the inhibitory influence exerted by large doses of estradiol on ESF production in rats subjected to hypoxia is not associated with an alteration in the erythrogenin content of the kidney. Of considerable interest, however, are the findings that incubation of erythrogenin from hypoxic rats with serum from rats given estradiol results in the formation of considerably less ESF than when control serum is used in the incubation system. It would appear likely that the depressive influence exerted by large doses of estradiol of ESF production derives from a reduction in the quantity and/or activity of the serum factor that functions as the substrate for erythrogenin. It may be that estrogen, by depressing some phases of protein metabolism in the liver, e.g., the glutamic-oxaloacetic and glutamic-pyruvic transaminase systems, curtails the formation of the serum substrate.

Experiments with Steroid Metabolites

Sicne a number of steroid metabolites have been shown to stimulate heme synthesis in chick embryo liver cells and in the erythroid cell precursors of the chick blastoderm, a study was undertaken to determine the influence of several of these factors on erythropoiesis in rodents. The structure of these compounds are indicated in Figure 5.8.

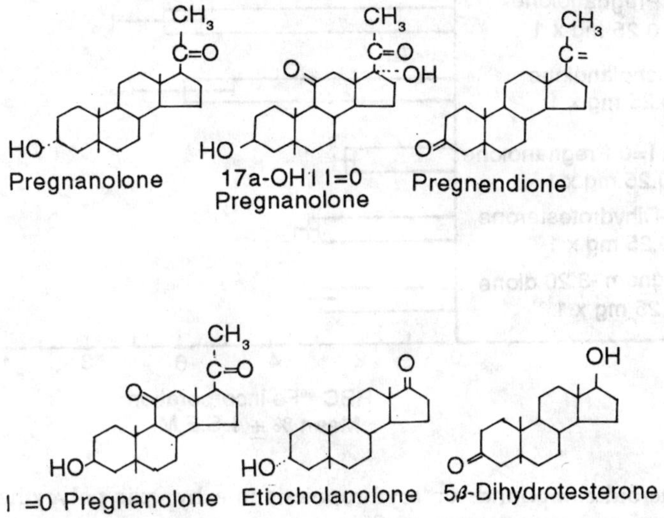

Fig. 5.8. Structure of steroids tested in present study for erythropoietic activity.

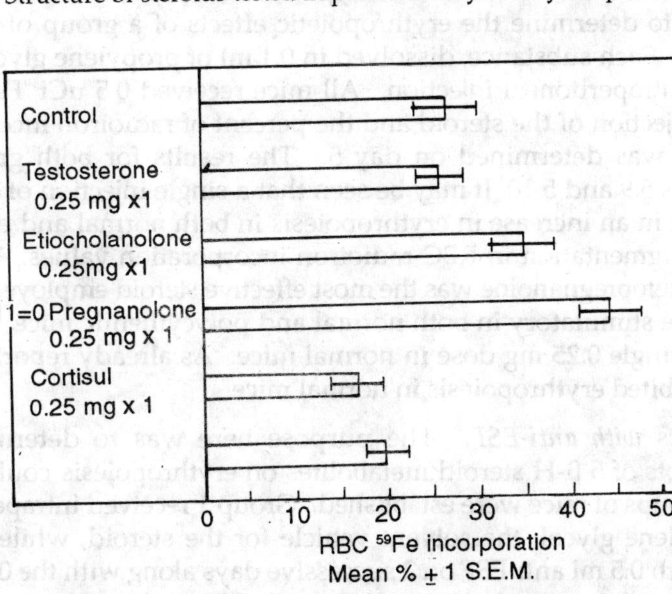

Fig. 5.9. Effects of steroid compounds on erythropoiesis in normal mice. Vertical lines through the tops of the bars represent ± 1 SEM.

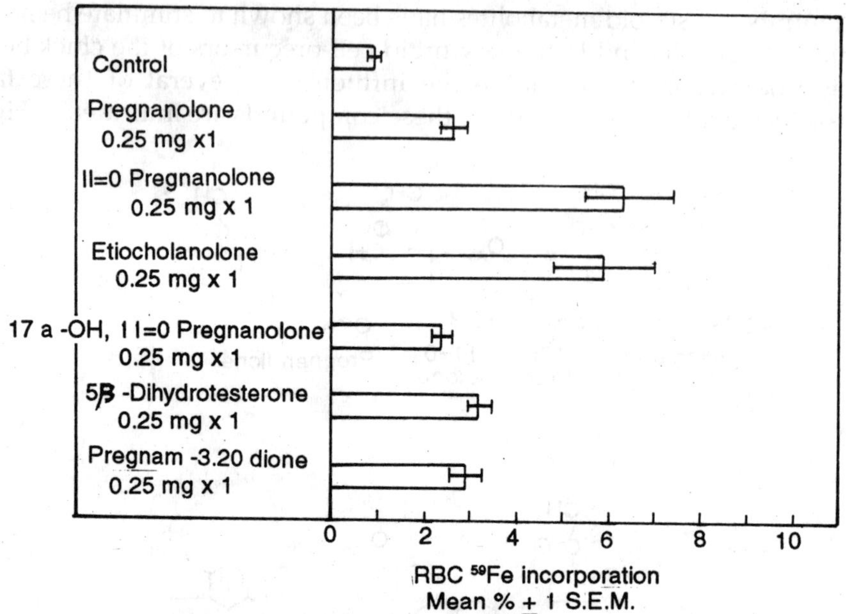

Fig. 5.10. Effects of steroid compounds on erythropoiesis in exhypoxic polycythemic mice. Vertical lines through the tops of the bars represent ± 1 SEM.

Studies in mice. Both normal and exhypoxic mice (adult females of the CF-1 strain) were employed to determine the erythropoietic effects of a group of steroid hormones and metabolites. Each substance, dissolved in 0.1 ml of propylene glycol, was given as a single 0.25 mg intraperitoneal injection. All mice received 0.5 uCi^{59}FeCl_3 intravenously 48 hours after injection of the steroid and the percent of radioiron incorporation into the circulating RBC was determined on day 5. The results for both groups of mice are shown in Figures 5.9 and 5.10. It may be seen that a single injection of a number of these steroids resulted in an increase in erythropoiesis in both normal and exhypoxic mice, as judged by the augmentation in RBC-radioiron incorporation values. These figures also indicate that 11-ketopregnanoine was the most effective steroid employed. Enocholandone also proved to be stimulatory in both normal and polycythemic mice. Testosterone was ineffective as a single 0.25 mg dose in normal mice. As already reported, both estradiol and cortisol inhibited erythropoiesis in normal mice.

Experimtents with anti-ESF. The purpose here was to determine whether the stimulatory effects of 5 β-H steroid metabolites on erythropoiesis could be abolished by anti-ESF. Six groups of mice were established. Group 1 received intraperitoneal injections of 0.1 ml propylene glycol, the solvent vehicle for the steroid, while mice in Group 2 were injected with 0.5 ml anti-ESF on 2 successive days along with the 0.1 ml of propylene glycol. Groups 3 and 4 were administered a single 2.5 mg dose of testosterone propionate and those in Groups 5 and 6 received 2.5 mg of 11-ketopregnanolone. Each mouse in

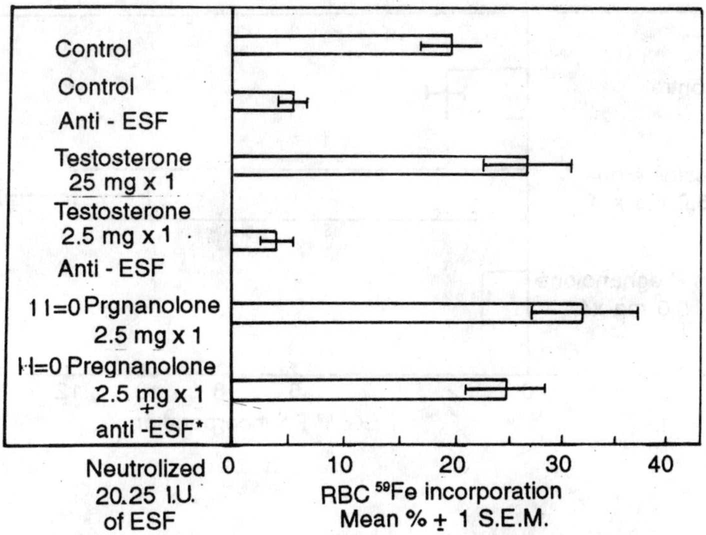

Fig. 5.11. Effects of anti-ESF antibody on the erythropoietic response of normal mice to testosterone and 11-ketopregnanolone. Vertical lines through the tops of the bars represent ± 1 SEM.

Groups 4 and 6 was also injected on 2 successive days with 0.5 ml of anti-ESF. At 48 hours after administration of the steroid, all mice were given 0.5 μCi radioiron and the percent RBC ^{59}Fe incorporation values determined 48 hours later.

Figure 5.11 indicates the influence of anti-ESF serum on the stimulatory effects exerted by steroids on erythropoiesis in normal mice. Anti-ESF markedly decreased erythropoiesis in the normal vehicle injected mice, suggesting once again that normal erythropoiesis is largely under the influence of the ESF. As reported previously, the erythropoiesis stimulatory effect of testosterone was abolished by anti-ESF. However, only a slight, statistically insignificant depressive action was exerted by anti-ESF on the erythropoietic effect of 11-ketopregnanolone. These results support the interpretation that the erythropoietic action of the 5 β-H steroids does not involve ESF mediation.

ESF content of plasma from rats injected with steroids. These experiments were performed to determine the influence of testosterone and 11-ketopregnanolone on the production of the ESF in adult female rats of the Long-Evans strain. The rats were injected intraperitoneally with 5.0 mg testosterone propionate or with 5.0 mg 11-ketopregnanolone daily for 4 days. They were killed on day 5, their plasmas collected, pooled separately, and assayed for ESF activity in exhypoxic polycythemic mice.

Figure 5.12 shows that, as noted before, marked stimulatory effects on RBC-radioiron incorporation values were produced with plasma from testosterone-treated rats. This

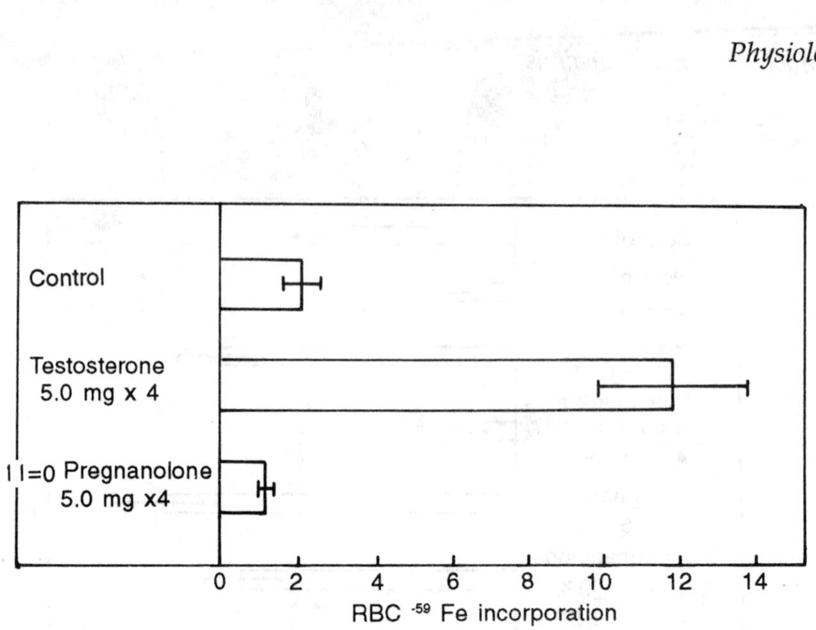

Fig. 5.12. Erythropoiesis-stimulating activity of plasmas obtained from testosterone and 11-ketopregnanolone-treated rats as determined in exhypoxic polycythemic mice. Vertical lines through the tops of the bars represent ± 1 SEM.

plasma activity was due to ESF evoked by testosterone, since we have demonstrated that prior treatment of this plasma with anti ESF resulted in complete loss of its erythropoietic activity (unpublished results). Of importance were the additional observations that the plasmas of rats receiving 11-ketopregnanolone exerted no erythropoiesis-stimulating effects on assay mice. Evidence that the kidney is not involved in the stimulatory effects of 11-ketopregnanolone on erythropoiesis is seen from its inability to elevate the renal erythrogenin levels in rats (Table 5.5). As noted before testosterone treatment caused a significant rise in renal erythrogenin activity.

Table 5.5
ESF-generating Capacity of Erythrogenin (EG) Extracted from Kidneys of Rats Treated with Testosterone Propionate (TP) or 11-Ketopregnanolone (11-K)

Source of EG	*Percent RBC-^{59}Fe incorporation (Mean ± 1 S.E.M.)*
Propylene glycol-treated rats × 4 (control)	4.1 ± 0.9
TP-treated rats-5.0 mg × 4	8.6 ± 0.7
11-K-treated rats-5.0 mg × 4	3.8 ± 0.9

The present studies indicate that at least two different mechanisms are responsible for the erythropoietic actions of steroids and certain of their derivatives. It is now well-known that testosterone stimulates ESF production in rodents and in man. The present studies confirm these findings in testosterone-treated rodents. This concept receives additional support from the ability of anti ESF to inhibit the erythropoiesis-stimulating effect of testosterone. On the other hand, as demonstrated in these experiments, the erythropoiesis-stimulating activity of the 5 β-H pregnane compound, 11 ketopregnanolone, was not associated with increased levels of plasma ESF, a finding that derives further support from the observation that its action was not prevented by anti-ESF. Since 5ß-H C_{19} and C_{21} steroids act to directly stimulate hemoglobin synthesis in cultured chick blastoderms and porphyrin-heme synthesis in chick embryo liver as well as to augment heme production in cultured human bone marrrow cells, it seems probable that the effects of these steroids on erythropoiesis in the mouse are exerted directly on the blood-forming tissues *in vivo*.

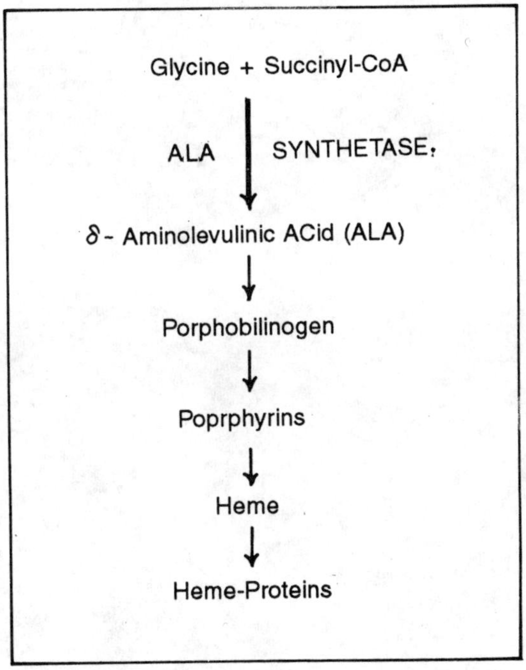

Fig. 5.13. Role of ALA synthetase in the production of heme and hemeproteins.

We have recently shown that 11-ketopregnanolone also stimulates erythropoiesis in transfusion-induced plethoric mice. Since this state is associated with a virtual disappearance of the nucleated erythroid cell compartment, it would appear likely that the primary action of the 5 β-H steroid is exerted directly on the ESF-committed precursor cells, inducing them to differentiate into early erythroid cells. It is also possible that, as for the hepatic and erythroid cell lines of the chick embryo, these steroids induce the formation of δ-aminolevulinic acid (ALA) synthetase in erythroid cell precursors of the mouse, thus leading to increased formation of heme and subsequently of hemoglobin in these elements. It is of interest that the ESF increases δ-ALA synthetase in rabbit bone marrow cell *in vitro,* suggesting the possibility of a similar mechanism of action of the 5 β-H steroids and of the ESF on hemoglobin formation in erythroid precursor elements.

It is hoped that the results obtained with steroids in the present experiments,. particularly the 5 β-H C_{19} and C_{21} metabolites lacking classical sex hormone actions, will stimulate studies of their possible use in indicated refractory anemias in man. Some success has been obtained recently with certain steroids in the treatment of patients with a variety of anemias, and the availability of a group of erythropoietic steroids without masculinizing effects might prove of therapeutic value.

6

Phagocytes

Phagocytes are cells capable of incorporating and, under certain conditions, of digesting inert or living particles. These cells include polymorphs and mononuclear cells, both monocytes and macrophages.

Since 1882, when Elie Metchnikoff discovered the importance of these cells in the resistance of organisms to infectious diseases, it has been shown that the function of phagocytic cells, especially macrophages, is not limited to destruction of infectious agents but also includes numerous immune functions.

Origin

Polymorphs, monocytes, and macrophages originate from bone marrow stem cells (Fig 6.1). In bone marrow cell cultures, macrophage and polymorph clones appear. The quantity of clones produced may be augmented by addition of a serum substance,

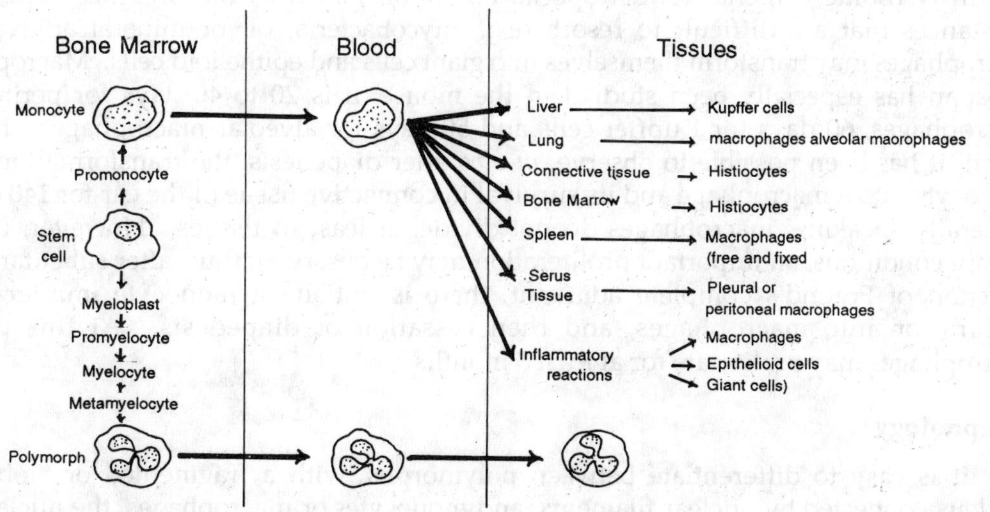

Fig. 6.1. Origin of phagocytic cells.

colony-stimulating factor (CSF). CSF production is increased in inflammatory states and by infection. However, the mechanisms by which preferential monocytosis or polymorph leukocytosis occurs are unknown, despite numerous studies.

Polymorphs

One may distinguish between a proliferation period that lasts 6 days, during which time the stem cells give rise, successively, to myeloblasts, progranulocytes, myelocytes, and metamyelocytes, and a maturation period, which also lasts 6 days, during which time metamyelocytes transform into polymorphs. One defines, by staining granules, neutrophil, eosinophil, and basophil polymorphs. Mature polymorphs exit from the blood vessels by diapedesis into inflamed areas. In the extravascular spaces, polymorphs survive only a few days. In man, 10^{11} polymorphs diasppear each day, largely into the gut and other mucosal surfaces.

Monocytes and Macrophages

The bone marrow origin of monocytes and macrophages is now universally accepted, but it is not yet known whether the promonocyte is the only intermediary between stem cell and monocyte. However, there is no doubt that monocytes are the precursors of mononuclear phagocytic cells found in the tissues. These cells differentiate from monocytes that have crossed blood vessels by diapedesis, in the case of alveolar macrophages found in lungs, histiocytes in the connective tissue, and peritoneal, pleural, and lymph node macrophages. Other monocytes are fixed along liver or spleen sinusoids, giving rise to liver Kupffer cells and to splenic macrophages. Unlike polymorphs, which are rapidly sed after diapedesis, monocytes may persist in the tissues for a long time. When monocytes leave the vessels, they undergo, within a few days, an increase in size and in lysosome content. Under special conditions, such as the presence of foreign substances that are difficult to resorb (e.g., mycobacteria, oil or mineral adjuvants), macrophages may transform themselves into giant cells and epithelioid cells. Macrophage life-span has especially been studied in the mouse; it is 20 to 40 days for peritoneal macrophages, 60 days for Kupffer cells and 50 days for alveolar macrophages. In the rabbit, it has been possible to observe, *in vivo* after diapedesis, the transformation of a monocyte into a macrophage and its survival in connective tissue of the ear for 140 days. Generally speaking, macrophages do not divide, at least in tissues. However, under certain conditions, an important proliferation may be observed; thus, after subcutaneous injection of Freund's complete adjuvant, there is initially a monocyte immigration, maturation into macrophages, and then cessation of diapedesis. At this point, macrophages may proliferate for at least 3 months.

Morphology

It is easy to differentiate between polymorphs, with a fragmented or "lobular" nucleus connected by nuclear filaments, and monocytes or macrophages, the nucleus of which is homogeneous and oval or kidney-shaped. These cells have other distinguishing features.

Hyaloplasm

Very clear differences between polymorphs and mononuclear phagocytes are striking when the living cells are observed under a phase-contrast microscope, or better yet, with scanning microscopy. Ploymorphs have pseudopods, which are cellular extensions. Macrophages manifest characteristic cell membrane movements (waves). These waves are due to a continuous emission of hyaloplasmic veils that may cover half or more of the cell diameter. These "veils" are emitted not only at the point of contact with the substrate but overlay the entire cell surface.

Cytoplasmic Organelles

Mitochondria

At variance with polymorphs, which contain few or no mitochondria, monocytes and macrophages possess mitochondria of variable size.

Endoplasmic Reticulum

Practically absent in polymorphs, endoplasmic reticulum is of variable importance in mononuclear phagocytes. Ribosome density may be very important when macrophages are issued from inflammatory foci or from "immunostimulated" animals.

Golgi Complex

Practically nonexistent in polymorphs, the Golgi complex is fairly prominent in monocytes and macrophages.

Lysosomes

These organelles are particularly numerous and of various size in polymorphs, constituting polymorph granules. In monocytes, lysosomes are rare. In macrophages, their number varies with the immune situation and degree of macrophage activation. In phagocytic cells, these lysosomes contain numerous enzymes and other substances, including cationic proteins, such as lactoferrin. It has been shown that various substances are absorbed by macrophages by means of pinocytic vacuoles formed by hyaloplasmic membrane invaginations. These vacuoles are then transferred to the perinuclear zone. Proteins and proteolytic enzymes that originate in the endoplasmic reticulum cisternae are transferred to the vesicles derived from the Golgi complex, which are called primary lysosomes. Primary lysosomes fuse with pinocytic vacuoles to form secondary lysosomes. These secondary lysosomes may again fuse with pinocytic vacucles or, as we shall see, with a phagocytic vacuole to become a phagosome.

Retractile Structures

Tubules and filaments have been recently demonstrated in macrophages. They play a role in cell motility, since it has been shown that cytochalasin induced alteration of the microfilaments can modify the orientation of cellular organelles and suppress membrane movements.

Other Intracytoplasmic Organelles

Phagocytic cells obtained from inflammatory exudates very often contain vacuoles of variable size. These organelles include not only pinocytic vacuoles but also larger phagocytic vacuoles. In many cases, the phagocytic material is still present and after staining, the inside of the vacuole may appear eosinophilic. In polymorphs, one also finds important amounts of glycogen by electron microscopy.

In summary, phagocytic cells are characterized by a large quantity of lysosomes, pinocytic and phagocytic vacuoles, and numerous membrane extensions.

Study Methods

It is easy to obtain phagocytic cells from animals, but not from man, which explains why most studies of phagocytosis have been performed in the former.

In Vivo

The only method that permits in vivo observation of macrophages or polymorphs consists of creating an inflammatory focus under conditions in which its development may be followed under the microscope. One can, for instance, perforate a rabbit's ear and fix to each side of the ear a glass or transparent plastic slide. If the distance between the two slides does not exceed 20 µm, it is possible to see first, the healing of the wound and, ultimately, the neovascularization of the connective tissue. Inflammation can then be provoked; it is now possible to observe diapedesis of polymorphs and monocytes and to follow transformation of the latter into macrophages. By this means, the same (one) macrophage has been followed for as long as 140 days.

It is also possible to study some macrophage functions, especially uptake of foreign particles, by measuring the rate of blood elimination of carbon or radioactive particles. This method, introduced by Biozzi, Benacerraf, and Halpern, consists of injecting mice intravenously with a carbon suspension and collecting, at regular intervals, the blood from orbital venous sinuses. Photocolorimetry of the samples collected at various times gives the carbon content in systemic blood. It has been shown that elimination of the carbon particles is exponential. The phagocytic index, K, can be calculated as follows:

$$K = \frac{\log C_0 - \log C_t}{t}$$

where C_0 and C_t are serial blood carbon concentrations. This formula does not take into account variations in carbon removal due to alterations in liver or spleen weight that may change after immunostimulating treatments or that relate to age or animal strain. To take these parameters into account, one expresses the results by a corrected phagocytic index:

$$\alpha = \sqrt[3]{K}\frac{W_A}{W_L + W_S}$$

where K is the phagocytic index, W_A represents the animal's weight, W_L is the liver weight, and W_S denotes spleen weight.

This technique examines the ability of macrophages to ingest, not their ability to destroy ingested material. Such an estimation may be performed by intravenous injection with bacteria that are known to be easily ingested and insensitive to serum bactericidal factors. Like carbon particles, the bacteria rapidly disappear from the blood; 2 hours after injection, 90% of bacteria are found in liver and spleen macrophages. At variable intervals, between 0 and 3 hr postinjection, spleen and liver are collected and their bacterial contents are measured. The difference between the number of organ-localized bacteria at 1 and 3 hrs after injection expresses the relative propensity of the liver and spleen macrophages to ingest bacteria. This method is particularly useful in studying the bactericidal potency conferred by immunization against bacteria that proliferate in the macrophages of normal animals.

In Vitro

These methods of studying polymorph or macrophage functions may be applied immediately after cell collection or, for macrophages, after variable times of in vitro survival.

Obtaining Materials

Polymorphs can be obtained from blood or from inflammatory exudates. Macrophages may be obtained only from the same sources but also from organs, organ fragments, and natural body cavities.

Blood

One of the oldest methods involves collecting the buffy coat after blood sedimentation, either spontaneous or accelerated by means of polyinylpyrroli-done or lectins. Of these "buffy" leukocytes, only polymorphs and monocytes adhere to the glass walls; the other cells are eliminated by washing. After a 3-day incubation at 37^0 C, only monocyutes that have transformed into macrophages persist. It is also possible to directly obtain monocytes by centrifugation of heparinized blood in the presence of a concentrated albumin solution or gradients of high molecular weight substances.

Inflammatory Exudates

The injection of protein or glycogen into the peritoneal or pleural cavities produces an inflammatorry exudate within a few hours. Twenty-four hours later, the exudate contain mostly neutrophils; 4 days later, essentially only macrophages are found. One must, however, recognize that macrophages obtained by these methods are not all functionally identical. The frequent use of oil and culture medium for bacteria (such as thioglycollate medium) induces the production of exudates that contain macrophages that have incorporated oil or agarose particles. It has been shown that these inflammatory agents may produce metabolic and functional changes in phagocytic cells. For example, the bactericidal potency of macrophages obtained after agarose injection is much higher than that of macrophages obtained after mineral oil injection.

Rebuck's technique is often used in man. After skin abrasion with a needle, a sterile glass slide is applied to the skin an maintained for variable periods of time. The inflammatory reaction thus provoked features exudation, which is rapidly followed by polymorph and mononuclear cell diapedesis. About 10 hr later, the majority of cell are polymorphs. After 4 days, the majority of cells are macrophages.

Organs or Organ Fragments

It is an old observation that liver or spleen fragments from new born animals placed into a nutritive medium are rapidly surrounded by very mobile macrophages. This phenomenon makes possible the isolation of liver macrophages by two different methods. The first one consists of injecting animals intravenously with very fine iron carbonyl particles. The liver is then perfused, and the perfusion liquid is placed into a magnetic field that retains the Kupffer cells that ingested magnetic particles. Another method, decribed recently, is also applicable to spleen macrophages. It involves fragmenting tissues and incubating them successively in collagenase and trypsin. The cells obtained are put into culture, and an early washing separates out macrophages by means of their glass adherence property. A method for obtaining lung alveolar macrophages consists of rinsing the lungs with physiologic medium intoduced in the trachea. After repeated washings, the liquid contains a suspension of macrophages detached from lung alveoli.

Lastly, it is possible to separate spleen macrophages from other cells by cutting the spleen into small pieces and incubating spleen cells in petri dishes. After 1 or 2 hrs of incubation, followed by repeated washings, spleen macrophages are separated by their adherence porperty from other spleen cells.

Culture

Numerous techniques can be used to obtain macrophages in culture. Macrophages must be maintained in an enriched synthetic medium, such as Parker's or Eagle's, that contains 10 to 15% fetal serum with a pH of 6.8 to 7.2. Serum may be replaced by 2% albumin. At variance with some cell lines that may be maintained in suspension, macrophage can only be kept alive in vitro as long as they adhere to a supporting surface. It is rare, under usual conditions, to observe a significant proliferation of peritoneal macrophages taken from adult animals in vitro. It is possible to observe a certain degree of macrophage proliferation when they are cultured in media that contain supernatants of fibroblast cultures (Virolainen) or chronic inflammatory exudates.

At variance with the majority of cell types, macrophages cannot be separated by use of trypsin or calcium chelator. When one wants to recover macrophages from a culture, it is necessary to culture them on either collagen or coagulated serum. In this setting, collagenase or trypsin may be used to detach cells from their "support." For polymorphs, it is not possible to maintain viability in vitro for more than 24 hrs. The media described above for macrophages can be used for short periods of time, as in the case of macrophages; polymorph functions must not be studied in cells in suspension but only when cells are fixed to culture recipients.

Functions

In addition to phagocytosis, phagocytic cells, particularly macrophages, have several other functions.

Nonimmunologic

Lipid Metabolism

With ^{14}C-labeled fat, it has been shown that macrophages, especially Küpffer cells, ingest and degrade chylomicrons. Macrophages also participate in fatty acid and cholesterol syntheses. It has been shown in experimental arteriosclerosis that macrophages localized in the aortic walls synthesize a significant amount of the cholesterol present in the atheromatous lesion.

Protein and Carbohydrate Metabolism

Because of their high content of hydrolytic enzymes, macrophages are able to degrade proteins (globulins, albumin) and polysaccharides. Protein degradation is variable and relates to the type of macrophage present. This variability may explain why one antigen is destroyed by certain macrophages but not by others. It has also been shown that rat and mouse peritoneal macrophages can synthesize transferrin and β_1C and β_1E globulins. In addition, liver macrophages may synthesize antihemophilic globulin prothrombin and proconvertin.

Other Functions

The "deoxification" function of macrophages is very important. It has long been known that alveolar macrophages are capable of incorporating atmospheric dust. Macrophages are also involved in liver glycuroconjugation. They play a central role in healing processes: macrophages eliminate necrotic cells and foreign bodies from inflammatory foci. Lastly, their role is important to erythropoïesis, because they carry iron to erythrocytic precursors.

Immunologic

The intervention of macrophages and polymorphs in immunologic reactions by means of phagocytosis is well established. Macrophages are implicated also in interferon and antibody syntheses, delayed hypersensitivity, and tumor immunity. In this chapter, we shall examine only aspects that relate to phagocytosis.

Phagocytosis is defined as the property of polymorphs and macrophages to take up and eventually digest (under favourable conditions) inert particles and living or dead microorganisms. The classic three phases in phagocytosis are as follows: an adhesion phase, during which the phagocytic cell comes in contact with the particle; an incorporation phase, during which the particle is absorbed into the cytoplasm; and a third phase, which features alternate possibilities that depend on the functional state of the cell and the nature of the ingested material. The latter may be digested or persist. In

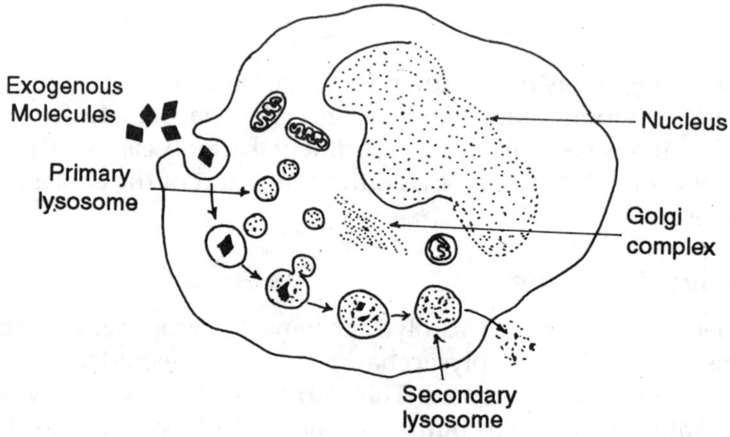

Fig. 6.2 Phagocytosis.

the latter circumstance, living microorganisms may proliferate inside the cytoplasm of macrophages.

Adhesion Phase (attachment)

To make contact with the material to be phagocytased, phagocytic cells must be able to move. This movement is possible only if the cell forms pseudopod (polymorphs) or cytoplasmic veils (macrophages). The adhesion of phagocytic cells to particles is the consequence of various interactions between cellular and extracellular factors. It depends also on the nature of the particles being ingested.

Cellular Factors

Cellular factors are relatively hard to study, because it is always difficult to distinguish between purely cellular factors and the various substances present in the "halo" of the cell surface. All results must be interpreted strictly in relation to the techniques used. We shall see later that the factors that determine adhesion of a particle to phagocytic cells are very different when the cells are in suspension from those that

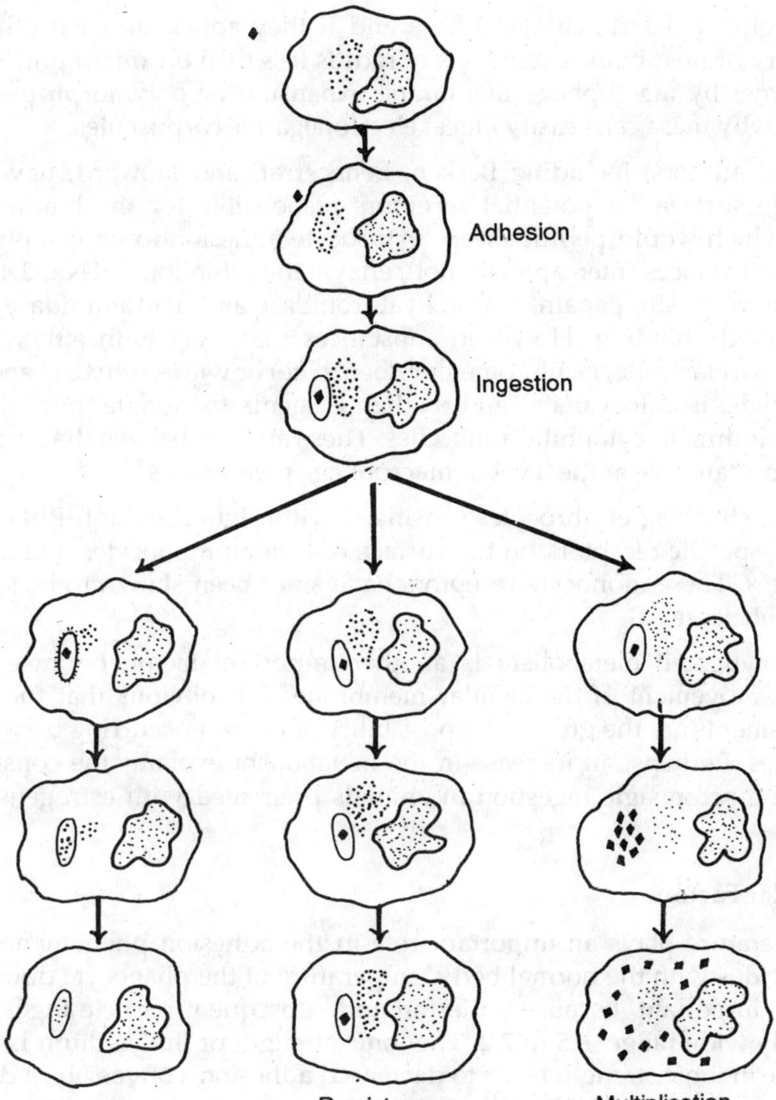

Fig. 6.3. Fate of bacteria after phagocytosis.

apply when the cells are adherent to a surface. It is known that the characteristic movements of the membranes of macrophages are not present when the cells are in suspension. Thus, although it is technically easier to quantify the results when phagocytic cells are in suspension, this experimental condition is very artificial and bears little resemblance to cells that have adhered in vivo.

It has been believed that contact between phagocytes and particles might depend on their respective electric charges (Fenn). Phagocytes and bacteria are electronegative, but whether this charge is uniformally distributed is not known. Pethica has shown that on a theoretical basis, two electronegatively charged cells can come in contact if their respective global electric charge differs and if they adhere to each other through the intermediary of membrane extensions of radius less than 0.1 micro μm. Such conditions are easily met by macrophage membrane expansion or polymorph pseudopods, thus explaining why these cells easily ingest electronegative corpuscules.

Several authors, including Berken, Benacerraf, and Howard, have examined the macrophage surface for potential receptors responsible for the binding of cytophilic antibody, which would permit sheep erythrocyte adhesion to guinea pig macrophages. Reductive substances (mercaptoethanol), enzymatic inhibitors (F1Na, 2,4-dintrophenol), and enzymes (trypsin, papain, lipase, hyaluronidase and neuraminidase) have no effect on the antibody binding. However, substances that react with either free sulfhydryl groups (iodoacetaminde, *p*-chloromercurylbenzoate) or with sulfhydryl and amide groups (formaldehyde, isothiocyanate) and oxidizing agents (periodate, nitrite) are capable of inhibiting binding to cytophilic antibodies. These authors believe that sulfhydryl groups play an important role at the level of macrophage membranes.

Huber, studying erythrocytes sensitized withn IgG-class anti-RhD antibodies, has shown IgG-specific receptors on the surface of human monocytes and spleen and liver macrophages. These monocyte receptors have since been shown to be specific for IgG1 and IgG3 subclasses.

Phagocytic cell metabolism is another important factor, because it controls the continuous movement of the cellular membrane. It is obvious that the more vigorous these movements are the greater the possibility of contact occurring between phagocytes and particles. Perhaps, an increase in the metabolism explains the considerably higher capacity of macrophagic ingestion in animals pretreated with estrogens, endotoxin, or lecithin.

Extracellular Factors

Temperature plays an important role in the adhesion phenomenon. The optimal value coincides with the normal body temperature of the phagocyte donor; pH does not seem to be important, because adhesion and subsequent particle ingestion may occur over a fairly wide range, 6.5 to 7.2. The ionic strength of the medium is also important. An increase in ionic strength leads to decreased adhesion; conversely, a decrease in ionic strength causes enhanced adhesion.

Modifications of the extracellular medium may alter adhesion. Divalent cations play an important role; it is known that in the presence of a calcium chelator, the medium totally suppresses adhesion. Some lipids, like triolein, may augment adhesion, but others may decrease it. Some complement fractions favour adhesion, but this is probably true only in the case of polymorphs. It has been shown by McCutcheon and Vaughan that macrophages may perform phagocytosis without complement, especially when they are maintained in vitro in the absence of serum globulin and when they adhere strongly to a surface. However, even under these conditions, one cannot totally exclude a role of some complement components, because it has been shown that macrophages are able to synthesize β_1C and β_1E globulins.

Antibodies play an important role in the phagocytosis of both bacteria (as opsonins) and viruses, but this phenomenon appears to be less important for macrophages than for polymorphs. In vivo, in the absence of bacteria-opsonizing globulins (axenic animals or newborn pigs), peritoneal and subcutaneous macrophages ingest pathogenic and virulent bacteria.

Furthermore, it has been shown by Wardlaw and Howard that macrophages from the perfused liver are able to phagocytose *Staphylococcus aureus, Bacillus cereus, Coryneabacterium murium,* and *Streptococcus pyagenes* more efficiently in the absence of serum; *Escherichia coli, Pseudomonas pyocyanea,* and *Proteus mirabilis* can also be eliminated in the absence of normal serum. One concludes from all this information that bacteria do not require the presence of antibody to be phagocytosed. However, in particular, for pyogenic bacteria, the addition of antibody considerably enhances phagocytosis. In vitro, macrophages kept in suspension are unable to phagocytose some bacteria (*Salmonella typhimurium* smooth, *Klebsiella pneumoniae*) in the absence of specific opsonins. Conversle, if the same macrophages are maintained, not in the suspension but on a surface (glassslide), bacterial phagocytosis occurs. For some bacteria, such as *Lasteria monocytogenes* and *Mycobacterium tuberculosis,* the presence of a specific antiserum does not significantly modify the adhesion of macrophages to these bacteria. This particular aspect of phagocytosis by cells adhering to a surface is termed "surface phagocytosis."

If, indeed, specific antibodies have an adjunctive effect on the adhesion phase, they do no longer seem as indispensable as previously thought. Moreover, macrophages seem to require less serum protein factors than do polymorphs. It is of interest to consider what portion of the molecule binds to the phagocytic cells to facilitate adhesion. Berken and Benacerraf and, more recently, Huber have shown that the Fe fragment of antibody is responsible for this binding. Abramson has additionally demonstrated that for IgG, the N-terminal part of the Fc fragment is implicated and that the binding occurs only when the disulfide bridge that links the two heavy chains is intact.

Nonspecific opsonins have been little studied in the case of macrophages, and it is unwise to extrapolate to macrophages from findings obtained by studying polymorphs. The only information now available concerns the degree of ingestion, which depends on previous adhesion, when macrophages of peritoneal cavities are stimulated by various substances. It is, however, difficult to dissociate the role of extracellular substances from that of the cell itself. As far as polymorphs are concerned, results must be interpreted with caution because of the particular experimental conditions utilized in these studies.

The adhesion of particles to phagocytes greatly depends on the physicochemical nature of the particles. Here again, it is perhaps too easy to explain adhesion and preferential ingestion of certain particles in the basis of the respective electric charges. It is likely that the surface electric charge does play a role in the initial contact between particle and the phagocytic cell, but a definite conclusion on this point cannot now be stated. It is known that certain substances present on the particle surface may considerably diminish or even inhibit adhesion. One very striking example is that of pneumococcal polysaccharides, which act to suppress phagocytosis of pneumococci by phagocytic cells. Analogous observations are seen for M proteins of streptococci and for smooth walls of salmonellae. It is possible to inhibit phagocytosis of certain bacteria by resuspending them in mucin and to significantly modify particle adhesion by heating or treatment with certain basic polypeptides. An adverse effect of certain detergents has also been demonstrated, both in vivo and in vitro.

A description of the adhesion phenomenon must naturally include a description of erythrophagocytosis. Vaughan has observed that even though macrophages (in suspension) cannot usually phagocytose red cells in absence of the specific antibody, the antobody is not needed for phagocytosis of aged red blood cells. This finding indicates that splenic macrophages do not need opsonins to remove aged erythrocytes from the circulation. It would be important to know the factor(s) on the surface of young erythrocytes that inhibit their phagocytosis by macrophages of the reticuloendothelial system.

The problem of recognition of "nonself" by phagocytes is probably relevant to adhesion. Data on this subject have essentially been obtained with macrophages. Is a given macrophage able by itself to recognize a foreign cell? Experiments on this subject have shown that when red blood cells of various species are incubated with mouse macrophages in the presence of mouse serum, the greater the phylogenetic differences, the greater the phagocytosis. Similar experiments and findings have been performed with human macrophages. Recognition does not occur in the absence of serum factors. Therefore, macrophages must recognize foreign cells with the help of serum constituents.

Ingestion Phase

Ingestion refers to the penetration of inert or living particles in the cytoplasm of the phagocyte. Ingestion is associated with an "invagination" of the macrophage membrane, which then contains the ingested particle. The periphery of this "invagination" next fuses to form a "phagocytic vacuole" also called a "phagosome."

It is known that this phagocytosis phase is dependent on the metabolism of the phagocytic cell. Karnovsky has shown that ingestion is temperature dependent and that it occurs within pH limits of 6 to 8. Ingestion is associated with energy consumption due to a change in macrophage metabolism that occurs during ingestion. One must, however, distinguish between different metabolic machanisms in alveolar and peritoneal macrophages. In the guinea pig, alveolar macrophages expend energy provided by oxidative phosphorylation: for peritoneal macrophages, energy is provided by glycolysis. Some authors have suggested that the ATPase of the macrophage membrane may act as if it is a "mechanoenzyme." Paralleling this energy release, an increase in phospholipid synthesis occurs that maintains the integrity of the macrophage membrane.

Intracytoplasmic Fate of the Ingested Particles

Depending on the nature of the ingested particle and the origin and function of phagocytic cells, there are three possible end points. The particle may be digested, may simply persist, or may proliferate inside the phagocyte.

Digestion

When a living or inert particle enters a phagocytic vacuole, lysosomes come into contact and release their contents. From phase-contrast and electron microscopy, it is now known that, initially, adhesion occurs between lysosome walls and phagocytic vacuole. Lysosome and vacuole walls then fuse. The free communication between the lysosome and the phagocytic vacuole allows lysosomal enzymes to make contact with the ingested particle.

Several factors seem to be responsible for fusion of lysosome walls and phagocytic vacuoles. The low pH within the phagocytic vacuole and changes in the peripheral wall tension of the membrane may play particularly important roles. One readily sees that in the case of biodegradable materials, digestion may occur after contact of the particle with numerous enzymes contained in the phagocytic lysosomes (aminopeptidase, succino-dehydrogenase acid phosphatase, cathepsin, lysozyme, glycuronidase, ribonuclease, deoxyribonuclease, arylsulfatase, lipase, cytochrome C oxidase, cholesterol esterase, galactosidase). Some authors also believe that there are, in addition, bactericidal or bacteriostatic substances in lysosomes. Amano, Gershon, and Ramseier have found isolated substances, chemically poorly defined, that exert a marked bactericidal action. One should note, however, that these results have not yet been confirmed and that the bactericidal activity reported by these authors does not correspond to and that observed in macrophages. It is generally believed that bacterial death may occur within minutes after ingestion: the intravacuolar environment cannot alone explain why bacteria are killed inside the macrophage, at least in relation to pH and enzymatic content.

Even though we do not yet know how macrophages kill bacteria, some information is available for polymorphs. It is known that the bactericidal effect of polymorphs is due to hydrogen peroxide; when glucose is oxidized by the hexose monophosphate shunt, NADPH (nicotinamide-adenine dinucleotide phosphate) is transformed into NADP by NADPH oxidase:

$$2\,\text{NADPH} + O_2 \xrightarrow[\text{NADPH oxidase.}]{\uparrow} H_2O_2 + 2\,\text{NADP}$$

NADH oxidase also promotes transformation of NADH to NAD with release of H_2O_2 and NAD

$$2\,\text{NADH} + O_2 \xrightarrow[\text{NADH oxidase.}]{\uparrow} 2\text{NAD} + H_2O_2$$

The bactericidal effect of H_2O_2 is enhanced by the activity of myeloperoxidase contained in polymorphs. Klebanoff has shown that the bactericidal effect was also enhanced by certain halogens, such as iodine, that were present in significant quantities in polymorphs.

It has also been shown that the H_2O_2 + halogen + myeloperoxidase system is bactericidal at concentrations lower than are necessary when each constituent acts alone or together.

Persistence

This phenomenon is seen whenever the particle cannot be digested by phagocytic cells, despite the presence of lysosomal enzymes. Thus, part of atmospheric dust (carbon, silica, asbestos) may persist throughout the entire life-span of macrophages. Such persistence is observed not only for inert particles; intact bacteria, parasites, and probably viruses may also persist within the phagocyte cytoplasm. This persistence, more precisely an equilibrium between certain microorganisms and macrophages, has important consequences and, in particular, may relate to the origin of latent infection. Another important consequence of persistence of microorganisms inside macrophages relates to therapy. It is well-known that intracellular microorganisms are not only protected from the humoral defense mechanisms of the organism but also from antibiotics. For example, salmonella, brucella, tubercle bacillus, or *Listeria monocytogenes* may persist within macrophages, even when the macrophages are placed into a medium that contains antibiotic concentrations 10 times higher than that shown to inhibit bacteria in vitro. The significance of this observation in clinical infection is obvious. This observation explains why infections should be treated rapidly, by use of high antibiotic doses. It also explains, at least in part, why such infections as brucellosis and tuberculosis often become chronic and difficult to cure.

Multiplication

This phenomenon is seen in the case of macrophages infected by virulent mycobacteria, salmonella, listeria, brucella, pasteurella, some staphylococci, and streptococci. Certain parasites, such as toxoplasma, histoplasma, fungal agents including *Candida guilliermondi,* and numerous viruses can also multiply inside macrophages. Multiplication is the basis of another aspect of virulence of the microorganisms within the phagocytic cell. It is known that some microbes, like pneumococci, are virulent because they are not ingested by phagocytic cells (protected by their polysaccharides). Here the virulence is manifested by the ability of these bacteria, once ingested, to proliferate inside the macrophages. One should note, in addition, that the virulence of salmonellae also relates to their difficult intake (due to the smooth aspect of the bacterial wall) plus their ability to proliferate within the phagocytic cells. These observations underscore the complexity of anti-salmonella immunity.

One wonders why some microorganisms are able to multiply within the cytoplasm of macrophages, which at other times possess a remarkable bactericidal potency. Some have suggested that substances necessary for microorganism multiplication are present within macrophages, namely, erythritol in the case of brucella growth. However, if, indeed, such substances favour the growth of certain bacteria, extrapolation from the culture tube to the macrophage cannot fully be accepted, because this phenomenon relates to the cytotropism of only certain bacteria. In fact, as we have already discussed, when bacteria are enclosed within the phagocytic vacuole, unfavourable conditions for growth are present due to the high concentration of hydrolytic enzymes and especially the acid pH. It is obvious that some bacteria are still able to multiply under these conditions; possibly, the ingested bacteria do not come into contact with lysosomal enzymes or perhaps the vacuolar pH is not always acid. The first possibility can be excluded, particularly for listeria. The second hypothesis remains to be tested. In experiments performed with mouse peritoneal macrophages, it has been observed that bacteria apparently able to multiply within macrophages (*Mycobacterium tuberculosis* H37RV, *L. monocytogenes, Brucella melitensis)* are, indeed, ingested. The ingestion is not, however, followed by disappearance of all lysosomes. The phagocytic vacuole is therefore not readiiy seen. Conversely, bacteria incapable of multiplying inside the macrophage (*Bacillus anthracis, S. typhimuriun* smooth, *Kl. pneumoniae*) are seen within large phagocytic vacuoles, and their ingestion is followed by disappearance of lysosomes. These observations led Fauve to propose that bacterial multiplication inside of macrophages was made possible by an inhibition of release of lysosomal contents. This hypothesis, recently confirmed, explains why certain bacteria may multiply inside macrophage cytoplasm. It seems obvious that because they are not vulnerable to the lytic action of lysosomal enzymes or to the low pH, some bacteria may multiply within the phagocytic vacuole (which has been observed with electron microscopy). In addition, inhibition of release of lysosomal contents into a phagocytic vacuole may also explain why ingested bacteria are shielded from antibiotics that are contained in secondary lysosomes; Bonventre has shown that antibiotics present in the extracellular medium penetrate the macrophage by pinocytosis and then are present in lysosomes. Another consequence of intracellular multiplication is that metabolic products of some bacteria diffuse into the cytoplasm, eventually resulting in macrophage necrosis. This phenomenon has been well demonstrated during phagocytosis of *M.tuberculosis* and *Listeria*; the metabolic cytolysin may lyse lysosomes once the membrane of the phagocytic vacuole has been lysed.

Less well studied have been the factors that influence virus multiplication or nonmultiplication within macrophages. Multiplication has been observed for such viruses as murine hepatitis and ectromelia; as with bacteria, nonpathogentic or less virulent viruses are destroyed, whereas virulent viruses multiply. The multiplication of virus inside macrophages may have great importance to certain viral infections. In the case of ectromelia or murine hepatitis, virus multiplication in Kupffer cells may produce lesions of the liver parenchyma.

It has been shown by Hirsch that eosinophil polymorphs can also phagocytose bacteria. It is noteworthy that eosinophil are heavily represented within exudates of allergic reactions. In vitro, eosinophils are attracted to antigen antibody complexes, especially in the presence of antigen excess. Eosinophils ingest the antigen-antibody complexes, then degranulation occurs. Because the granules contain substances capable of blocking the physiologic action of histamine, serotonin, and bradykinin, it is possible that eosinophils not only protect the tissues and the host by phagocytosing antigen-antibody complexes but also diminish the effects of mediators of the inflammatory reaction.

Phagocytosis may be depressed in certain immunodeficiency states (septic familial granulomatosis. Chediak-Higashi syndrome). Phagocytosis may be decreased by some immunodepressants (corticosteriods, cyclophosphamide, ionizing radiation). However, these agents alter not only the mechanism of phagocytosis but also production of phagocytic cells.

Phagocytosis may be stimulated by a recruitment of phagocytic cells at the level of aggression foci or by activation of phagocytic cells, particularly after injection of various immunostimulants [BCG (Bacillus Calmette-Guerin), bacterial endotoxins, synthetic polynucleotides, bacterial extracts].

7

The Production of Leukocytes

In recent years, there has been a great expansion in our knowledge concerning the rate of production of normal granulocytes, the characteristics if their release into the peripheral blood, their intravascular life span, the "compartments" in which they are found, and the mobilization of these cells in response to various stimuli. Less is known about their ultimate fate but it is known that large numbers are lost into the gastrointestinal, and urinary tracts.

Many unanswered questions concern formation and destruction of leukemic leukocytes. The early popular hypothesis that leukemia was an excessive and more rapid proliferation of myeloid precursors with a failure of maturation has not been substantiated. It was first suggested by Astaldi and Mauri (1953) and subsequently repeatedly confirmed that leukemic cells are not "wildly proliferating" but that some defect leads to persistence of immaturity and in the accumulation of cells. The precise nature of this defect has never been elucidated but the presence of increased numbers of myeloid cells in acute or chronic granulocytic leukemia could theortically result from a number of factors or some combination thereof. These factors might include: (1) an increase in production of leukemic cells due to an enlarged stem cell compartment or other preceersor; (2) a marked prolongation of the intravascular survival time; (3) a decrease in leukemic cell death and cell loss.

In general, it can be said that under normal circumstances granulocytopoiesis is a cell renewal system so that cell production equals cell death. In patients with leukemia in relapse, granulocytopoiesis exceeds cell loss, resulting in an expanding population. However, in certain circumstances, such as in adult acute myelocytic leukemia, this may not be the case, and leukemic cell production may equal cell loss so that the peripheral white blood count remains stable for long periods of time.

Granulocytes in the adult animal or man are produced in the bone marrow where, in normal individuals, there is an orderly progression of division and maturation from the earliest cell, the stem cell, successively through the various cell types to the mature polymorphonuclear leukocytes so that morphologic compartments are identifiable. In leukemia, evidence from cell kinetic studies and from histological examination shows that leukemic cells may be produced in a variety of sites in addition to the bone marrow, i.e. lymph nodes, liver, spleen testes etc.

Both stem cells and the regulation of granulocyte production have for a long time been the subjects for a great deal of work and speculation. Nevertheless, relatively little is known about stem cells particularly in man, although there is a fair amount of information, which has been derived entirely from animal experiments. The stem cell compartment must be able to maintain itself against continued removal of cells for differentiation, to reconstitute itself if depletion occurs, and to increase its rate of cell production on demand. Available evidence suggests that a cell similar to a small lymphocyte may be the common stem cell, although a good case can be made for the monocyte.

Spleen colony studies demonstrate that erythroid, myeloid and megakaryocytic cells are probably derived from pluripotential cells. Bruce and McCulloch (1964) suggested that there are two classes of stem cells : (1) colony-forming cells and (2) cells that may be their progeny and respond to erythropoietin. However, it was subsequently shown that the experimental conditions used, i.e., exogenous and endogenous colonization, probably measure different characteristics of stem cells. Additional support for a common stem cell comes from several reports indicating that a heavy demand for one type of cell diminishes the production of the others. However, cloning experiments using an agar method of tissue culture yield colonies of mixed populations of granulocytic and monocytic cells. Upon recloning, these cells can originate from appropriate individual precursors. These findings are of great interest but do not rule out the single pluripotential cell theory because of the artificial experimental conditions.

In addition to the stem cell compartment, which is self-replicating, there is also a large differential proliferating pool consisting of the myeloblasts and promyelocytes, probably not self-sustaining. There are large and small myelocytes, and these two types of cells represent "subdivisions" of the main pool, the large cells representing a dividing pool supplying cells to the small cell maturation pool. It is not known whether all of these small myelocytes then go on to divide or to mature and enter the next compartment. A key role has recently been suggested for the myelocytes in which it is believed that granulocyte production is expanded by an increase in the number of myelocyte divisions and a shortening of the generation time. This appears to be the most attractive hypothesis at the present and is consistent with most of the known facts.

Maturation occurs in the nonproliferating pool, consisting of metamyelocytes, band forms, and the segmented neutrophils. There is some controversy concerning the most mature cell capable of DNA synthesis and division in the myeloid series in animals, but the evidence in man favours the myeleocyte. DNA synthesis then ceases, but other biochemic and morphologic changes occur in both nucleus and cytoplasm. The maturation of myeloid cells is morphologically characterized by a progressive condensation of the nucleus together with gross changes in the cytoplasm, particularly in the appearance of granules. In the mature cell, the nucleus is pyknotic and the granules become quite prominent.

The biochemical events accompanying maturation are not completely known largely because of technical problems in obtaining adequate numbers of cells at the same level of maturity. However, some data are available from radioautographic studies and despite its technical limitations this approach has yielded important information on the comparative rates of macromolecular synthesis at the various levels of maturation. The rate of DNA synthesis decreases with maturity until the metamyelocyte stage, when it ceases completely. Whether the nucleus of the mature granulocyte can be "reactivated" is unknown. RNA and protein synthesis, like DNA synthesis, also decrease during maturation. Similarly, rates of DNA, RNA, and protein synthesis are significantly reduced in leukemic blast cells. However, there is a major problem in the interpretation of these data obtained by using labeled precursors, i.e., the variation in the rate of catabolism of nucleosides in cells at different levels of maturity. For example, mature cells catabolize thymidine more rapidly than immature cells, which may account for the lower thymidine incorporation into the more mature cells of the myeloid series. Similarly, if a leukemic cell contained more amino acid decarboxylase than its normal counterpart, labeled amino acid incorporation would be reduced and it would be concluded that the rate of protein synthesis was low.

With the completion of maturation, the mature granulocyte enters the so-called "mature granulocyte reserve" of the bone marrow. Though estimates vary, there are probably approximately 2-3 $\times 10^{11}$ granulocytes in this comprtment. Approximately 10^7 to 10^8 cells are released into the blood from this reserve per minute under normal circumstances, but this can be accelerated on increased demand, i.e., infection and in response to agents such as bacterial endotoxin and etiocholanolone. Leukapheresis experiments, particularly in dogs, served to increase our understanding of the bone marrow reserve and clearly indicate that it is the chief source if not the only one for mature granulocytes in the blood. Ordinarily, the release of cells from the bone marrow is a function of the utilization rate of granulocytes. At a given moment, the peripheral blood granulocyte count does not reflect the status of the marrow reserve, but a persistently elevated neutrophil count reflects an adequate reserve and production rate. The marrow provides an adequate reserve to meet demands that may vary greatly and suddenly. The acute depletion of peripheral blood granulocytes occurs during leukapheresis results in marked leukopenia, because the rate of entry of cells is exceeded but, following this, granulocytes rapidly enter the blood and the count rises rapidly. During this phase, it becomes very difficult to induce leukopenia as apparently the rate of entry exceed the rate of removal of granulocytes. Initially, after leukapheresis, there is no obvious evidence in the marrow of an increase in granulocyte production, but within two or three days myeloid hyperplasia becomes quite prominent. Even though myelopoiesis may be prevented with heavy irridiation, the leukocytosis in response to intense leukapheresis still occurs. In one experiment, more than seven times the number of cells in the circulating pool was removed without significantly impairing the acute response.

Leukapheresis studies in man have added little to our understanding of granulocyte production largely because the instruments used do not have the efficiency to achieve adequate depletion of the total blood granulocyte pool. Granulocytopenia could be induced but was usually of short duration. However, the remarkable capacity for myelopoiesis was illustrated in one patient with chronic myelocytic leukemia and an initial white blood count of 76,000 per cmm who was subjected to leukapheresis intermittently for nearly one year. During that period 1.18 $\times 10^{13}$ leukocytes were collected, which, if 10^9 cells can be considered to weigh about 1 gm, would come to 10 kg of tissue. In spite of this, production was able to keep pace with demand and significant leukopenia never occurred. Removal of approximately 5×10^{12} cells in a 5 week interval resulted only in a decrease of the leukocyted count from 256,000 per cmm to 128,000 per cmm. With the daily removal of 2.0 to 3.0×10^{11} cells from patients with chronic myelocytic leukemia, there was a gradual decrease in white blood count that persisted for only a few weeks.

In assessing normal granulocyte production in the bone marrow, the labeling index utilizing tritiated thymidine is very useful and provides and estimate of the number of cells about to divide. Because cells in the dividing and nondividing pools can be detected readily by morphologic criteria, extra information from the uptake of tritiated thymidine by cells in cycle can be used to estimate granulocyte production. However, in leukemia it is impossible to distinguish between cycling and noncycling blast cells on morphologic grounds alone. It was suggested years ago, based on stathmokinetic and lebeling studies, that the proliferative capacity in acute leukemia was very low compared to normal marrow. Gavosto *et al* (1964) reported that the *in vitro* labeling index of blast cells in acute leukemia was in proportion to the size of the cells, but was not related to the phase of the cell cycle. They concluded that the larger cells were the younger ones and that with aging, proliferative capacity was lost. Mauer and Fisher (1966) subsequently suggested that the large leukemic cells comprise a relatively small fraction of the leukemic cells in the marrow (about 12% in the two patients reported) with a labeling index, after a single injection of tritiated thymidine, of approximately 50%. Virtually none of the small cells was labeled. They thought that the large cells were the dividing population, but after one or two divisions these cells became smaller and stopped dividing. The small "nondividing" leukemic cells were, however, capable of reentering the proliferative phase.

In a paptient with acute leukemia following a single injection of tritiated thymidine, 10% of the small blast cells and 75% of the large were labeled. By 24 hours, the labeling index of the large blasts had decreased to 22% and that of the small increased to 20%. During the fourth to the seventh days, an additional nine injections of tritiated thymidine were given, following which 93% of the large cells and 72% of the small cells became labeled. These results were interpreted as suggesting that the only identifiable source of labeled cells for maintenance of the large blast cell population was the small cell compartment.

Although these studies are quite intriguing, one of the difficulties with the concept is that the technique ordinarily used to prepare slides usually results in a great deal of variability in cell thickness even on the same slide. With the evidence that these small cells may re-enter the proliferating pool, the sharp distinction between these two types of cell becomes rather artificial. The studies of Clarkson are consistent with the suggestion that the vast majority of leukemic cells are capable of DNA synthesis, but that cell cycle times vary greatly. Recent studies in this laboratory (Rosen and Perry 1970) indicate that at least in one animal leukemia, the small supposedly non-dividing leukemic cells are readily able to induce leukemia and death upon transplantation to normal animals. Regardless of whether one accepts the presence of a so-called non dividing cell population, or cells in G_0, or in a prolonged G_1, the fact remains that the anti-tumor agents currently in use probably do not affect these cells significantly and it is these cells which are of the greatest concern in the treatment of acute leukemia. In this connection it is of interest to note that in the steady state, only a very small proportion of mouse bone marrow cells are in DNA synthesis. The greater proliferative state of mouse lymphoma accounts for the marked difference in the sensivity of these two cell populations to a variety of chemotherapeutic agents *in vivo*.

Normally, approximately a third of the myeloid cells in human bone marrow are in proliferation, and the average labeling index is about 30%. It has been estimated that approximately one cell per 100 normal granulocyte marrow cells is produced per hour and about four cells per 100 myeloblasts are produced per hour. The mean granulocyte production in normal individuals is approximately 163 × 10^7 granulocytes per kilogram of body weight per day.

There are good data indicating that granulocytic production is moderately increased in acute and chronic granulocytic leukemia. Cell generation times in leukemia are essentially within the normal range or perhaps somewhat longer. Most of the blasts are either nondividing or in a prolonged G_1.

In patients with chronic granulocytic leukemia, granulocyte turnover is usually moderately increased above normal, but may range from 145 × 10^7 granulocytes per kilogram per day to as much as 2.0 × 10^{10} granulocytes per kilogram per day in patients with very high peripheral white blood counts. Rough estimates from our own kinetic data in patients with acute granulocytic leukemia reveal granulocyte production in the range of 5 × 10^8 to 5 × 10^9 granulocytes per kilogram per day.

The observation that a significant proportion of the stem cell population is normally in a testing phase suggests that the output from this pool is probably a function of demand. As indicated above, stem cells have never been clearly identified and there is considerable controversy which cell (s) is the stem cell. In any case, they are probably present in very small numbers; however, Warner and Athens (1964) and more recently Cronkite (1970) consider the myelocyte compartment as the prime source of new cells contributing to the marrow precursor pool. As mentioned above, kinetic data are consistent with this hypothesis. Myelocytes can be divided, on the basis of size, into a small and large cell population and it is quite possible that the small cells may fall into the same type of "nondividing" population as discussed above. The considerations concerning the G_0 cells may also apply above here. It should be mentioned, however, that Morley and Stohlman (1970) who recently studied myelopiesis in mice with shielded marrow receiving x-irradiation, found noevidence of a significant increase in the myelocyte proliferative rate when neutropenia developed.

There has been a great deal of speculation concerning humoral substances that might be responsible for the control of granulocyte production and/or release. Evidence has been presented for a leukopoietic or leukocytosis-inducing factor that has been obtained from the plasma of animals undergoing repeated leukapheresis or receiving bacterial endotoxin, by the study of isolated rat femora and spleens. There are problems in the interpretation of these data, since it is difficult to separate the observed effects due to the postulated factor from effects possibly due to a granulocyte mobilizing agent, such as endotoxin or etiocholanolone.

Materials with "leukopoietin" activity have been reported from plasma and tissues and from the plasma of dogs recovering from drug-induced myelotoxicity. The ability of cells from a shielded leg to form endogenous spleen colonies is increased by exposure of the rest of the body to 250 kv x-rays, whereas the number of transplantable colonies remains unaltered. This suggested regulation by a humoral factor. Recently it has been reported that sera from AKR mice with spontaneous lymphoid leukemia are capable of stimulating colony formation by mouse bone marrow cells. Sach's group reported that mature normal rat granulocytes produce a substance that inhibits the activity of an inducer required for the development of granulocyte colonies from normal hematopoietic cells seeded in soft agar. Rytoma and Kiviniemi (1968) also proposed the mature granulocytes contain and probably produce this specific feedback inhibitor, a granulocyts chalone. Evidence for an antichalone regulating the rate of granulocyte production has also been presented. The chalone and antichalone were partly purified and appear to have molecular weights of 4,000 and approximately 3,000 respectively. Presumably these materials are unrelated to thymidine phosphorylase, an enzyme in the salvage pathway for thymidine. It has been postulated that this pathway may be important in regulating DNA synthesis and cell division. The role of these factors in myeloproliferative states, if any, is impossible to determine at this time and there is little information available concerning the control of leukocytosis due to infection or inflammation. Evidence for a granulocyte mobilizing factor in infection was presented years ago, when it was postulated that a polypeptide, "leukotaxine", could be obtained from inflammatory exudates that increased capillary permeability and induced local migration of granulocytes. Confirmatory work has not been reported. Whether chalones, antichalones or similar substances are involved in cyclical neutropenia or in leukemia is intriguing but presently a matter of speculation. Periodic oscillations of the neutrophils have also been proposed in normal individuals. However, analysis of the reported cases indicates that relatively slight alterations in release of cells from the bone marrow or changes in the marginal pool could be responsible and that it might not involve neutrophil production at all.

If a humoral substance is to be considered in the control of myelopoiesis, the concept must explain the increased granulocyte production seen in response to leukapheresis. Many hypotheses have been proposed, but there is little incontrovertible evidence for any of them. However, in view of the leukapheresis experience there must at least be a feedback loop that reflects the concentration of granulocytes in the peripheral blood. In addition, other factors must affect this control mechanism in order to account for the changes in acute and chronic infection, myeloproliferative disorders, infections associated with leukopenia, alterations of white blood count due to bacterial endotoxin, etiocholanolone, extracorporeal irradiation, etc.

Although a great deal of information is available concerning the prevascular and intravascular life of the granulocyte, relatively little is known concerning its kinetic and ultimate fate once it leaves the blood. The circulation can be considered as a "patrol route" for granulocytes, so that in the event that their "services" are required they can have relatively quick access to the intruder, i.e., infecting organism, foreign body, etc. In the normal individual , the average sojourn of the granulocytes in the periphereal blood is a reflection of two processes, aging and random loss. The mean half-life of all the granulocytes in the blood is approximately six and one-half hours or, in other words, the average time a granulocyte spends in the blood is between 6 and 12 hours. The average sojourn of granulocytes lost by senescence alone is approximately 30 hours and this represents only a small fraction of the total granulocytes in the blood. Granulocytes that have left the vascular tree are thought not to return but they may reenter the circulation from organs such as the spleen and perhaps other sites.

Random loss is probably determined by intravascular factors like commensal organisms, which would tend to mobilize granulocytes, but there have been few studies of granulocyte kinetics in germ-free animals. Granulocyte counts are decreased in germ-free mice, but there is disagreement concerning the size of the postmitotic pool compared to that in conventional mice. However, upon removal of mice from the germ-free environment, the mature marrow reserve decreases and the dividing precursor pool increases. These changes are apparently in response to the appearance of bacteria and other organisms in the gastrointestinal tract, respiratory tract and elsewhere.

There are few data concerning the loss of granulocytes from the body, but some of these studies should be cited. The granulocyte count in the saliva of a normal individual is approximately 1,500 per cmm and this could mean a loss of 10^8 to 10^9 granulocytes per day by this route alone. After an *in vivo* granulocyte label, labeled cells appear simultaneously in oral lavages and in the blood indicating that emigration of these cells from the blood is a random process. In fact, the specific activity in the oral lavages is higher than in the blood, suggesting that the younger cells have a greater capability of migrating to this extravascular site. Another example of random loss is shown by experiments in which newly labeled cells rapidly migrate into induced peritoneal exudates. Similarly, it has been demonstrated that all the granulocytes entering inflammatory exudates were derived directly from the blood. Approximately 10^6 granulocytes per cm^2 of abraded area per hour were mobilized in induced skin abrasions in normal individuals but the cellular content of exudates in patients with acute leukemia in relapse was markedly reduced.

The loss of granulocytes in the urine has been well recognized since Addis proposed the test that bears his name. A normal individual may have approximately 2×10^6 granulocytes in his total 24 hours urinary excretion and in acute glomerulonephritis this may rise fifty-fold. In patients with pyelonephritis, the excretion rate may be as high as 2 to 3×10^7 per day and in cystistis it may rise to more than 10^8 per day.

The pulmonary system is involved in the trapping of leukocytes from the circulation and although it was suggested that very large numbers of cells were removed in the lungs after transfusion, the results are difficult to interpret because of recent work indicating that at least a portion of the cells is only transiently trapped. However, there is no question that significant numbers are removed permanently and enter the alveoli.

In animals that were catheterized, upto 20% of the granulocytes in the blood of the right ventricle were removed during passage through the pulmonary bed. These then may migrate up the tracheobronchial tree to be swallowed, to reenter the circulation, or to disintegrate.

Studies of the rate of loss of granulocytes in the gastrointestinal tract are few, but Ambrus and Ambrus (1959) perfused intestinal loops of dogs *in vivo* and obtained approximately 2×10^6 granulocytes per minute. Granulocytes were found in the stomach, but these studies of gastric loss were only qualitative because most of the cells had degenerated. These investigators also showed that large numbers of cells were removed by the normal liver and spleen. There does not seem to be significant trapping in the spleen normally in man, at least as detected in studies utilizing transfusions of *in vitro* ^{51}Cr-labeled autologous cells, but in patients with leukemia, significant pooling, at least transiently, is observed.

To estimate the numbers of granulocytes that accumulate at sites of infection or injury would be difficult, but obviously from clinical observation it must be very great. Brecher *et al* (1953) first showed that transfused granulocytes migrated in large numbers to infected areas. Recently, it has been demonstrated that large numbers of homologous granulocytes are capable of being mobilized in patients with acute leukemia. Studies of granulocyte kinetics in patients with subacute or chronic infections have revealed total blood granulocyte pools ranging from normal to six times the normal mean, and the distribution between the circulating and marginated pools was similar to that seen in normal imdividuals. The granulocyte turnover rate surprisingly was only slightly increased. There does not appear to be a good explanation for this—except perhaps a purely speculative one—that the normal random loss is curtailed and the cells are channeled preferentially to the area of infection. In patients with acute infection, granulocytes enter the blood from the bone marrow more rapidly, and the cells are younger, but the turnover in the blood does not appear to differ from normal. Animal studies have shown that in acute experimental infections, release from the bone marrow is accelerated with an increased marginated pool and the blood transit time is shortened intially. With clinical improvement, the transit time is prolonged, suggesting a decrease in the mobilization of granulocytes from the bone marrow.

Metabolic Control of Leukocytes

Several authors have pointed out that phagocytosis is a primitive cellular process, the study of which may provide useful correlations between physiological function (ingestion of solid objects by the cell) and metabolic changes that are essential to that phenomenon. Establishment of appropriate systems of suitable phagogcytic cells and particles *in vitro* presents few problems, and for over fifteen years a good deal of data has been assembled, particularly on the metabolic behaviour of polymorphonuclear leukocytes while they are ingesting such objects as bacteria (dead or alive), insoluble starch, or polystyrene spherules.

Measurement of the Uptake of Solid Objects by Phagocytes

All measurements needed for studying metabolic concomitants of phagocytosis could be made with a high degree of precision and accuracy—bar one. That exception has unfortunately been a cardinal one; the measurement of the number of particles ingested by the cells. The methods used to establish such values have been of a different order from those used to determine metabolic intermediates. Further, we have generally lacked data on *rates* of uptake of particles, particularly maximal rates. Instead, the extent of uptake after protracted times has usually been reported. These matters have been discussed recently and will merely be mentioned here. The techniques that may be used for determinations of ingestion are essentially of two kinds: (a) measurement of the disappearance of particles from the medium, (b) determination of particles that have been rendered intracellular. In the first case, if excess particles are provided at zero time to ensure maximal rates of uptake, one must deal with rather small differences between

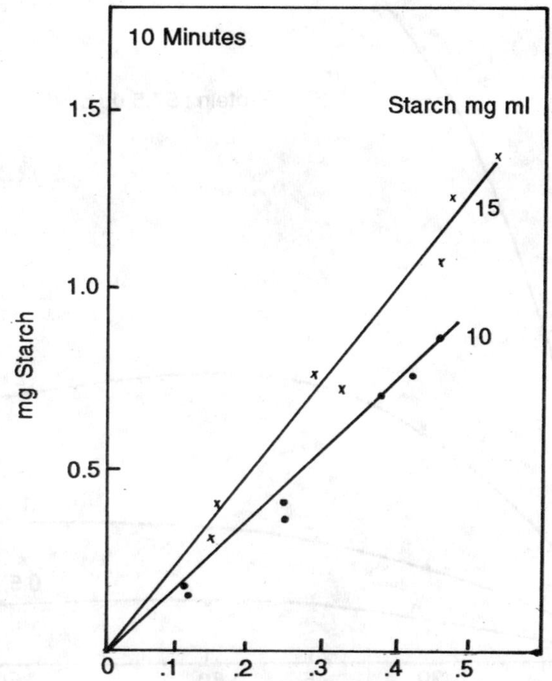

Fig. 7.1. Variation in uptake of labeled starch as a function of the number of cells on the dish. Two levels of starch were examined (10 mg and 15 mg per dish), and the time of incubation was 10 minutes. The abscissa gives the amount of cell protein per dish; the ordinate is the cellular uptake per dish. Guinea pig PMN were used.

large numbers at later times after phagocytosis has occured. If intracellular particles are determined as in b/a happier situation prevails, but it is necessary to separate the cells from excess extracellular particles before the quantification—a process that makes precise timing (and thus establishment of rates) less than optimal.

The actual assessment of particles is usually done by counting under the microscope or, if they are bacteria, by growing them; only rarely have chemical or physical methods been employed. When all this is considered, it is clear that the comment made above concerning the gap between the measurements of ingestion and those of metabolism has some validity. This critique does not at all detract from previous studies where the use of the more approximate measures provide information adequate to the purposes envisaged.

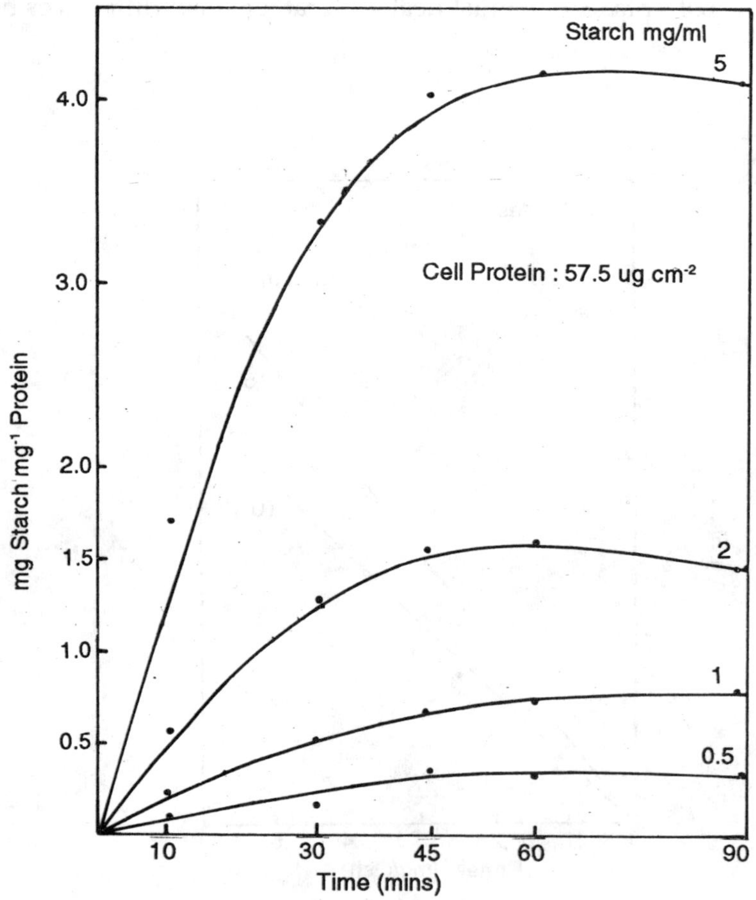

Fig. 7.2. Time curves of uptake of labeled starch and various loads. The volume of fluid per dish was 1 ml. In this experiment, staturation was achieved later than usual. If a plot is made from each curve for the uptake at times up to 30 minutes linearity with load is noted. Normally one uses an excess load. Guinea pig PMN were used.

As the approach to the biochemical basis of phagocytosis becomes more refined, for example in assessing the effect of modifications of the cell membrane on ingestion or in determining the effects of substances that might react rather specifically with cellular components (such as colchicine, which interacts with microtubules), precise measurements of ingestion and especially of ingestion rates become necessary. We have developed and described a method that employs monolayers of cells and radioactive particles. Measurements are made of radioactivity in cells after incubation. The use of such monolayers is not novel; when the cells are in this form they may effectively be washed free of adherent particles and assayed only for those particles that have actually been rendered intracellular. The cells studied by this method up to now have included polymorphonuclear leukocytes, induced peritoneal monocytes, peritoneal macrophages, alveolar macrophages, and eosinophiles. Some of these types have been taken from more than one species, i.e., guinea-pig, mouse, man and rat. Figures 7.1 and 7.2 give some indication of the manner in which the method works. Linearity prevails with respect to the number of cells present, and one may achieve linearity for a given number of cells with respect to the external "load" of particles. Linearity with respect to time may also prevail. The effectiveness of this method and its convenience and rapidity may prove very substantial. For any given particle, one may calculate the kinetic values as one does for enzyme reactions, recognizing, however, that the analogy is not absolute. Deficiencies of the method include limitations in available labeled particles and difficulties encountered in maintaining stable monolayers under some experimental conditions one might wish to use.

Effect of a Modification of the Cellular Surface Charge on Particle Uptake

In early papers, Ponder (1926, 1928) discussed elegantly the effect of such physical parameters as the surface charge on the phagocytic cell and the viscosity of the cytoplasm on ingestion of particles. The charge on the particle also plays a part. The treatment Ponder offered was theoretical. He commented that his results were "singularly unsatisfactory, for they are only of the nature of approximations, they are incapable of experimental verification except in a very general way, and their importance is quite out of proportion to the difficulty of obtaining them." These remarks are perhaps overmodest, for the concepts propounded have stimulated a number of later investigators. Indeed, Ponder's further statement is entirely warranted: "the results, or results like them must ultimately find a place in the complete physical theory of phagocytosis which will some day be developed, together with the fact that they serve to throw some light on the nature of the process of ingestion as it must occur in experiment."

Nowadays the surface charge of whole cells may be measured by electrophoretic means, and that of particles similarly determined. Some methods also exist for altering the charge of cells, and one excursion by our laboratory into this area might appropriately be mentioned here. The polymorphonuclear leukocyte contains a good deal of neuraminic acid, of which about 50% appears to be superficial. This conclusion was reached from the fact that sialidase (neuraminidase) can release maximally about 50% of the total cell sialic acid when it acts on whole cells under optimal conditions. This alters the net charge on the cells by reducing the amount of sialic acid—a negatively charged substance—on the surface. In the past Ginsberg and his collaborators showed that treatment of polymorphonuclear leukocytes with a crude sialidase indeed affected the ability of the cells to phagocytize. The effect may be ascribed to what might have been an interesting inhibition of glycolysis at the level of phosphohexose isomerase or perhaps a transport block for glucose or its glycolytic intermediates above fructose-6-phosphate. The combination of a possible linkage between surface sialic acid, transport, a glycolytic enzyme, and phagocytosis, or some of these, constituted an attractive problem.

With the improved method for assessing the degree of ingestion of particles, we have been led to reexamine the situation. In brief, we found that the removal of maximal amounts of exterior sialic acid by *purified* sialidases had no effect on the ability of the cells to phagocytize starch particles or some labeled bacteria. This confirmed earlier imtimations we had had when we used polystyrene spheres and cells in suspension, where the measurement of particle uptake was performed by counting spherules interiorized.

As a footnote to this observation, we should mention that strenuous efforts to locate the inhibitor of glycolysis that was present in the original filtrate studied by Ginsberg have availed us naught. Our observations were that desialation did not cause significant inhibition in glycolysis or phagocytosis. An inhibitor of phagocytosis was obtained from a crude sialidase by dialysis. We are thus forced to conclude at this point (1) that desialation with consequent decrease of the negative charge on the surface of

Table 7.1
Effect of Desialation of Guinea Pig PMN on Phagocytosis and Glycolysis

*Pretreatment**	*Sialic Acid Released†*	*Uptake‡*	*Lactate§*
Control	0.1 ± 0 (2)	1.40 ± 0.001 (3)	878 ± 9(3)
Purified sialidase¶	3.6 ± 0 (2)	1.30 ± 0.009(3)	ND
Crude sialidase**	4.6 ± 0 (1)	0.28 ± 0.003 (3)	952 ± 17 (3)
Dialyzed crude sialidase***	3.5 ± 0(2)	1.36 ± 0.33 (6)	ND

* 30-45 minute exposure of cells prior to measurement of phagocytosis and lactate production.

† Nanomoles NANA (sialate) mg^{-1} protein. Total acid-hydrolyzable NANA = 9.33 ± 0.002 nanomoles mg^{-1} cellular protein. Number of experiments in parentheses.

‡ mg starch ingested mg^{-1} protein.

§ Nanomoles lactate mg^{-1} protein hr^{-1}. 5 mM glucose in external medium.

¶ Neuraminidase from *V., cholera.*

** Crude lyophilized *V. cholera* culture filtrate.

*** Dialyzed crude *V. cholera* filtrate.

these cells had no effect on the uptake of the particles we used, (2) that desialation does not inhibit glycolysis, (3) that the inhibitor of glycolysis observed by Ginsberg and his collaborators must have been rather specific to the particular strain of *Vibro cholera* that was the source of the sialidase. The substance present in our crude filtrates that was dialyzable and did inhibit uptake apparently had no effect on glycolysis (Table 7.1).

As Ponder pointed out, it is the mutual effect of charge on the phagocytic surface and on the particle surface that has to be considered. The particles that we have used have carried either no, or at best a very small, negative charge. The possibilities are now ripe for more definitive studies in this area because of available modes of controlling more variables than heretofore at the cell surface, of obtaining appropriately charged particles, and of making more precise measurements of uptake.

Dependence of Phagocytosis on Energy-Yielding Metabolic Steps

In a fascinating paper, Fenn (1922) showed that between 30 degree C and 37 degree C, and Q_{10} for phagocytosis was approximately 2. Below 30 degree C, the value was considerably greater than 2 when quartz or carbon particles were used, probably due to changes in the cytoplasmic viscosity. We have previously shown, as others have, that ingestion of particles by white cells does require metabolic steps that yield energy consistent with a Q_{10} of 2. The data for actual uptake were achieved by the older methods

Table 7.2
Guinea Pig PMN Representative Data on Distribution of Engulfed Particles Under Various Conditions

Conditions	*Particles Per cell*					*Experiments*
	0	*1-5*	*6-10*	*11-15*	*>15*	
Aerobic (normals)	1	5	8	8	78	2
Anaerobic	3	5	3	10	79	2
Normal	3	7	9	9	72	4
Iodoacetate (1×10^{-4}M)	16	23	25	9	27	2
Normal	1	10	18	8	63	2
NAF (2×10^{-2} M)	13	35	14	8	30	2
Normal	6	18	2	2	72	3
KCN (1×10^{-3} M)	8	10	2	2	78	3
Normal	3	0	12	16	69	2
Dinitrophenol (1×10^{-4} M)	1	2	6	25	76	2

* Results expressed as percentage of cells containing the designated number of particles.

Table 7.3
Effects of Metabolic Inhibitors on Guinea Pig PMN

Inhibitor	*Concentration mM*	*Percentage Inhibition (a)*	*(b)*
Iodoacetate	0.3	81	97
Fluoride	20.0	76	91
Cyanide	1.0	6	1
2,4-dinitrophenol	0.5	24	4

a. With labeled starch as the particles.

b. With dead tubercle bacilli ($H_{37}R_v$) grown on ^{13}C-glycerol as the particles.

of assessment of particle uptake. The effect of various inhibitors of metabolism on the uptake of particles is illustrated in Tables 7.2 and 7.3 for polymorphonuclear leukocytes. The two Tables offer a comparison between the older and new methods of measurement of ingestion. The former (Table 7.2) certainly yielded the overall fact that inhibition of glycolysis definitely depressed particle uptake, and inhibition of aerobic metabolism apparently did not. The newer method (Table 7.3), in which maximal rates were determined, showed that while this is true overall, some energy does appear to come from oxidative phosphorylation, even more evident with respect to cells from mouse polymorphonuclear leukocytes in Table 7.4. In the mouse, the polymorphonuclear leukocytes are quite perceptibly sensitive to dinitrophenol and, less obviously, to cyanide. These cells presumably depend more heavily on oxidative metabolism to provide energy for the phagocytic ingestion phase than do their couterparts from guinea-pigs—and this fact is borne out by other observations.

Table 7.4
Effects of Metabolic Inhibitors on Mouse PMN*

Inhibitor	*Concentration mM*	*Percentage Inhibition (a)*	*(b)*
Iodoacetate	0.3	56	51
Iodoacetamide	1	63	
Flouride	21	26	30
Cyanide	1.2	0	9
Cyanide	3.6	26	
2,4-dinitrophenol	0.5	69	38

* Two representative experiments.

Whereas phagocytosis in guinea pig *monocytes* elicited from the peritoneal cavity exhibits a dependence on the intactness of the glycolytic cycle, phagocytosis in similar cells from mice shows a very considerable dependence on oxidative phosphorylation, i.e., there is a depression of maximal rates of particle uptake of about 50% in the presence of ordinary concentrations of cyanide or dinitrophenol.

Respiration of Leukocytes During Phagocytosis

In our laboratory and in other's, many measurements have been made of the effect of the ingestion phase of phagocytosis on respiration of the cells. Respiration is a conveniently measurable variable, and its determination leads to some quite intriguing questions. In Table 7.5, we report the effect of phagocytic activity on the respiration of a number of different phagocytes from mammalian sources. The main observation here is that there is a paradox: several cell types that depend heavily on glycolysis to supply energy for the phagocytic process also exhibit a very marked (two-fold) respiratory increase. In those cases, phagocytosis is not significantly inhibited by cyanide or dinitrophenol, and presumably does not require a supply of energy from oxidative phosphorylation. Such cells are the polymorphonuclear leukocytes and monocytes,

Table 7.5
Respiration of Phagocytizing Cells of Different Species

Species and cell type	QO_2* *Resting*	*Phagocytizing*
Guinea pig		
PMN (34)	2.5 ± 0.1	6.2 ± 0.3
Peritoneal monocytes (12)	8.5 ± 0.8	20.8 ± 2.2
Alveolar macrophages (12)	20.4 ± 0.1	25.1 ± 0.1
Rat		
PMN (6)	5.0 ± 0.4	6.5 ± 0.3
Mouse		
PMN (7)	5.7 ± 0.3	12.8 ± 1.5
Peritoneal monocytes (3)	14.5 ± 1.9	25.9 ± 3.9
Peritoneal macrophages‡ (6)	14.5 ± 2.0	16.3 ± 2.8
Human		
PMN (4)	1.1 ± 0.1	2.5 ± 0.3

* Qo_1 = μl O_2 mg^{-1} protein hr^{-1}. Number of determination, in parentheses.

‡ These cells, obtained by peritoneal lavage, were used without settling and spreading on a surface. They are contaminated by lymphocytes to the extent of 30-50%.

particularly of the guinea-pig. A number of other cells, among which one may count the macrophage washed from the peritoneal lining of the mouse and the alveolar macrophage of the guinea-pig, show very little perturbation of respiration during phagocytosis. Here, interference with oxidative metabolism by adding cyanide or dinitrophenol causes rather large depressions of particle uptake. The fact that these cells show little perturbation of respiration during phagocytosis may indicate that they are essentially rather efficient or "close coupled". One might expect that they would also be susceptible to anaerobic conditions whereas the polymorphonuclear leukocytes and monocytes of the guinea pig are not. Why, particularly in the guinea-pig, is there a large burst of respiration during phagocytosis, and what is its function?

Phenomena Linked to Increased Respiration in Polymorphonuclear Leukocytes

Concomitantly with the respiratory increase in phagocytizing polymorphonuclear leukocytes, particularly of guinea pig, rat, and man, we and others have noted an increase in the activity of the hexose monophosphate shunt, which rises from 1% to values of 10% of the total gulcose utilized as the cells pass from the resting state to full phagocytic activity. These data were calculated by application of the concepts and formulae of Katz and Wood (1963) and Berger and Karnovsky (1966). The second, and tremendously important facet of the respiratory increment during phagocytosis in these cells, has to do with production of hydrogen peroxide. This was correctly inferred by Quastel and his collaborators, who studied the oxidation of formate by phagocytizing polymorphonuclear leukocytes, and recognized that the increased conversion of that labeled substrate to CO_2 was probably due to its catalase-activated oxidation in the presence of hydrogen peroxide.

The question of the linkage of the increased respiratory activities to the increased shunt activity has been vexing and we shall not attempt to discuss the many ideas that have been advanced (Karnovsky 1968).

The following summarizes the findings in our laboratory:

1. We believe that an NADH oxidase is responsible for the conversion of NADH produced during glycosis to NAD^+ with the production of hydrogen peroxide. Our evidence rests on the purification of this enzyme and the establishment of its stoichiometry as being $NADH+H^++O_2= NAD^+ + H_2O_2$. In a recent publication, we have shown that there is, certainly in the guinea pig polymorphonuclear leukocyte, more than enough of this oxidase to match the increased respiration during phagocytosis. The question arises how the resptatory increment may be linked to the activation of the hexose monophosphate shunt. We have previously adduced evidence that the excess pyruvate that would result from deficient reduced diphosphopyridine nucleotide could "sop up" NADPH and convert it to $NADP^+$. The latter has been shown to be the controlling component in the operation of the shunt pathway (Beck, 1958). An NADPH-linked lactate dehydrogenase was indeed found to be present in guinea pig cells. However, in our laboratory and elsewhere, this enzyme appears not to be active in cells of human origin, nor in those of rats. In the rat, Reed (1969) has shown conclusively that the

stimulation of the hexose monophosphate shunt was obtained by the following series of reactions in a glutathione "cycle":

(a) $H_2O_2 + 2\,GSH \rightarrow GSSG + 2\,H_2O$

(b) $GSSG + NADPH + H^+ \rightarrow 2\,GSH + NADP^+$

Reed (1969) demosntrated that reaction (a) was catalyzed in rat PMN by glutathione peroxidase. The second reaction (b) was catalyzed by glutathione reductase. The H_2O_2 would, according to our ideas, derive from the activity of the NADH oxidase mentioned above. The $NADP^+$ formed as a result of reaction (b) would stimulate the hexose monophosphate shunt, and would be converted by the reactions of that cycle back to NADPH.

In the guinea pig we had explored the reactions studied by Reed and reached the following conclusions:

1. that there was no significant glutathione peroxidase activity,
2. that a very substantial oxidation of GSH to GSSG could be occurring nonenymatically.
3. that there was a very great excess of glutathione reductase to regenerate $NADP^+$.

In the human PMN we have found rather low values of glutathione peroxidase and more than adequate reductase. The situation for glutathione peroxidase is summarized for the rat, guinea-pig, and human PMN in Tabel 7.6.

Table 7.6
Glutathione Peroxidase Activity*

Particle-Free Supernatant (PFS) of PMN	*GSH Peroxidation†* *Exp.1*		*Exp.2*	
Guinea Pig‡	ND		2.4 ± 0	(2)
Human §	26.9 ± 2.3	(3)	29.3 ± 2.6	(4)
Rat ¶	272.8 ± 14.8	(2)	325.4 ± 11.3	(5)

* Assayed by method of Paglia and Valentine (1967).

† Nanomoles GSH. mg^{-1} $protein^{(PFS)}$ min^{-1} (mean ± se). Rates corrected for nonenzymatic rate, which is 23.0 nanomoles GSH. min^{-1} in the cuvette (1 ml). Number of assays in parentheses. Total PFS protein is about one-half the total cellular protein.

‡ Peritoneal exudate PMN from single animal in each experiment.

§ Peripheral WBC (85-90% PMN) from single patient in each experiment.

¶ Peritoneal exudate PMN from 2-5 animals pooled in each experiment.

Functions of H_2O_2 Formed During Phagocytosis

Klebanoff (1968) has recently given provocative and stimulating demonstrations of the possible role of H_2O_2 in the bactericidal action of leukocytes. He has demonstrated that a system comprised of H_2O_2 a peroxidase and a halide (particularly iodide) constitutes a very effective bactericidal system. Concomitantly with this activity—and perhaps adventitiously—the bacteria are iodinated. The following points might be borne in mind with respect to PMN, at least those of guinea pigs:

(i) They are rich in a specific peroxidase (myeloperoxidase) that is released from a lysosome-like granule during phagocytosis.

(ii) They do produce H_2O_2 during phagocytosis as discussed above.

(iii) They are reputed to concentrate iodide but in any case contain enough chloride to allow the system suggested by Klebanoff to work.

(iv) There are competing pathways for the H_2O_2—which might allow for some regulation of its level—especially since there appears to be a difference between "nascent" H_2O_2 produced, for example by oxidase activity (e.g., NADH oxidase,

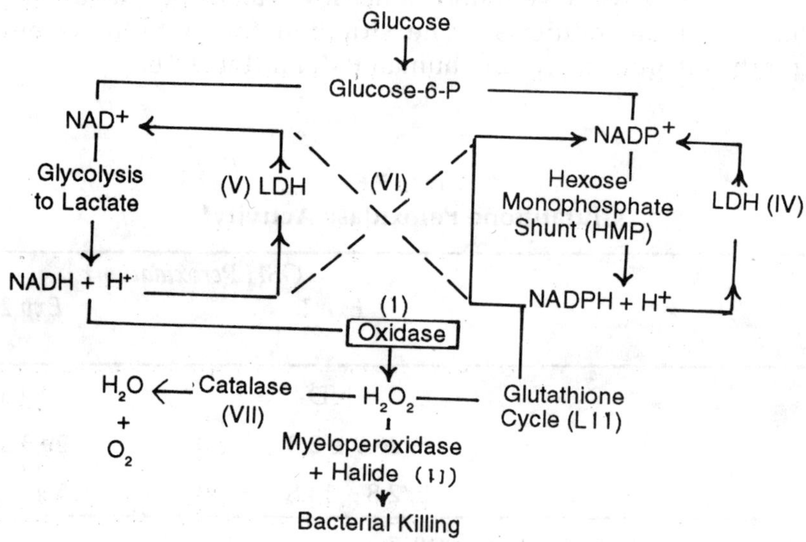

Fig. 7.3. Fates of hydrogen peroxide in polymorphonuclear leukocytes. The peroxide is generated from NADH by an oxidase (Reaction (1)). It may then (II) be used in the bactericidal system of Klebanoff (1968) or may convert GSH to GSSG (III), which reoxidizes NADPH and thus activates the shunt (HMP). In some specie (e.g., guinea pig) NADPH may reduce pyruvate (IV), where the latter is in excess due to (I), also stimulating the HMP. The regular NAD^+-linked lactate dehydrogenase (LDH) is of course the main pathway for NADH (V). The dashed lines indicate transhydrogenation reactions (VI) via regular transhydrogenases or by lactate dehydrogenase-mediated exchange. Catalase also competes for H_2O_2 (VII).

D-amino-acid oxidase), and "Stale" H_2O_2 as added from a solution thereof. We may illustrate this with reference to two reactions characteristic of PMN and mentioned above i.e., catalatic oxidation of formate and oxidation of glutathione to the disulfide form. Thus, when H_2O_2 was added to a particle-free supernatant of guinea pig PMN in the presence of gluthione, NADPH and glucose-1-^{14}Cm the appearance of $^{14}CO_2$ was enhanced 49 ± 18% under optimal conditions. If the source of H_2O_2 was D-amino acid oxidase and tyrosine, the stimulation was 63 ± 33% (means and average deviations). In the case of ^{14}C-formate oxidation to $^{14}CO_2$, the relevant numbers are 0% and 1,690 ± 3%. Only nascent or fresh H_2O_2 might have optimal activity in the bacterialcidal system; excess might effectively be removed by the stimulation of the hexose monophosphate pathway via the GSG ↔ GSSG reaciton, discussed above. Figure 7.3 illustrated the generation and fates of H_2O_2, and summarizes the possible interaction of the metabolic and bactericidal pathways.

Chronic Granulomatous Disease of Childhood (CGD)

As so often happens, a pathological condition has helped to illumine a question of the origin, function, and fate of a metabolite. CGD of children has been studied in detail by a number of groups. The group in Minnesota has convincingly shown that the white cells of patient with this disease ingest bacteria normally but do not kill them. The combined data of the goups in Minnesota and Boston have shown that the PMN of patients with this disease fail to exhibit normal metabolic perturbations of respiration, hexose monophosphate shunt and peroxide formation (as reflected in catalatic formate oxidation) during phagocytosis (Holmes *et al* 1967; Baehner and Nathan 1967). The disease has been shown mainly to be an X-linked recessive trait, but recently some females have been described. A close examination of the cells of five patients compared with those of six control subjects in our laboratory yielded evidence that the NADH oxidase, described above, was present in the cells of the patients only to the extent of about 25% of normal (Baehner and Karnovsky 1968). This would lead to a deficiency in peroxide production and in turn cause a deficient stimulation of hexose monophosphate shunt during phagocytosis, a deficient increase in the catalatic oxidation of added formate, and a deficiency of the cells ability to kill bacteria by the Klebanoff mechanism. While it is true that not all investigators agree that the deficiency of this flavoprotein enzyme is the key to the disease, it seems to us that the evidence for its important role is rather strong. Certainly the disease manifests itself as a result, primarily, of hydrogen peroxide deficiency. Indeed the white cells of patients with CGD are able to kill those bacteria that are catalase-negative and produce their own hydrogen peroxide.

We have attempted to validate our hypothesis by introducing into leukocytes a hydrogen peroxide generating system. Thus we coated polystyrene latex spherules with glucose oxidase, and allowed the cells of normal individuals and patients with CGD to ingest uncoated and coated spherules in the presence of either glucose-1-^{14}C or formate-^{14}C. As shown in Tables 7.7 and 7.8, the generation of peroxide intracellularly due to the introduction of glucose oxidase into the cell on the spherules resulted in the significant restitution of stimulation of those metabolic concomitants of phagocytosis indicative of

Table 7.7
Formate-^{14}C and Glucose-1-^{11}C Oxidation by Control and Chronic Ghanulomatous Disease (CGD) Leukocytes*

	Formate-^{14}C		*Glucose-1-^{14}C*	
* Rest				
Control	0.30 ± 0.16	(4)†	5.71 ± 1.33	(4)
CGD	0.06 ± 0.05	(3)	1.65 ± 0.12	(4)
† Latex				
Control	2.69 ± 0.664	(4)	31.23 ± 2.30	(4)
CGD	0.23 ± 0.13	(3)	2.39 ± 0.12	(4)
† Coated Latex				
Control	1.05 ± 0.39	(4)	19.25 ± 2.61	(4)
CGD	0.83 ± 0.22	(3)	13.54 ± 1.74	(4)

* In nanomoles, mg^{-1} protein. hr^{-1} ($^{14}CO_2$ produced).

† Parenthess = number of studies.

Table 7.8
Effect of Intracellular H_2O_2 on Metabolism of Control and CGD Leukocytes*

Substrate	*Latex*	*Coated latex*
Glucose-1-^{14}C		
Control	5.6	3.4
CGD	1.5	8.2
Formate-^{14}C		
Control	9.0	3.5
CGD	3.8	13.8

* The data are given as ratios phagocytizing: resting, and are derived from Table 7.7. They refer to $^{14}CO_2$ produced.

peroxide production. Furthermore, our colleagues at Children's Hospital have demonstrated that the simultaneous ingestion of polystyrene spheres coated with glucose oxidase and bacteria, by cells of CGD patients, enhances the ability of the latter to kill the bacteria. These observations appear to us to indicate that, at least in the patients we have been studying, the lesion is in the NADH oxidase.

8

Lymphocytopoiesis

Traditionally, it has been a basic concept of hematology to recognize and to classify cells according to their morphology and to seek the relationship between them by considering transitional forms intermediate in morphology. Indeed, hematological diseases are recognized and classified by this very concept. Within this traditional way of thinking lie two dangers. The first is that of considering that all cells with the same name and morphology have the same life cycle, metabolic properties and function. The second hazard is assuming that the forms intermediate in morphology between any two distinct cell lines necessarily reflect a sequence of cellular transformation. A study of the quantitative aspects of lymphopoiesis as revealed by the research of the past ten years clearly shows that these aspects of the concept must be modified in order to permit the knowledge gained through basic research to be properly interpreted. From a practical point of view we must accept a morpholigical definition for lymphocytes although at the same time we must think of them as a heterogeneous category of cells. Differences in their kinetic properties and functional capacities may be used to subdivide them into groups that make up the entire category.

The problem with the morphological definition for the lymphocyte is that the lymphocyte must be identified by the absence of characteristics that other white cells possess rather than a by positive attributes of its own (Yoffey and Courtice 1956). A distinguishing feature of the small and medium cells is the high ratio of nucleus to cytoplasm and the clumped chromatin pattern of the smaller cells.

Some of the larger cells, however, have abundant cytoplasm while other show only a small basophilic rim of cytoplasm. Furthermore, a spectrum of cells intermediate in morphology lies between these cell types. The terms *large, lymphocyte, lymphoblast,* and *hemocytoblast* have been applied to these cells. For the sake of simplicity, we shall refer to them as blast cells. It must be realized, however, that cells of this morphology also represent a heterogeneous category of cells with widely different functional capacities.

In seeking to establish the developmental relationship between lymphocytes and other cell lines, classical hematology relied to a great extent on the presence of intermediate morphological forms. Within the past decade, new approaches to these problems have led to an increasing realization that stem cells for the lymphoid series are a migratory population of cells of myeloid origin. These stem cells are present in myeloid tissue in both the embryonic and adult states, and from myeloid tissue they feed into the remainder of the lymphoid complex in relatively limited numbers. In lymphoid tissue, they may undergo extensive proliferation, giving rise to many generations of cells. From radioautographic considerations of the kinetics of blast cells, it is evident that cellular tranformation and entry of any cell type into this category is less frequent than the occurrence of these intermediate transitional forms would suggest.

I. The Heterogeneity of the Small Lymphocyte Population

On the basis of life span, small lymphocytes may be divided into two main groups: long-lived and short-lived. Recent evidence indicates that long-lived cells may be considered as a single group according to life cycle, kinetics, and circulation. Shortlived small lymphocytes, however, are most likely not the same regarding these parameters and should not be thought of as a single group.

A. Long-Lived Lymphocytes

The long-lived lymphocytes comprise the majority of cells in what has been called the mobilizable lymphocyte pool or the recirculating lymphocyte pool. The experimental evidence indicates that they are the same as the thymic-dependent lymphocytes, the immunologically competent lymphocytes, and the antigen-reactive cells. All of these are new terms that have come into being in the last ten years. Thus, we will define each of them and summarize briefly the evidence that relates each to the long-lived small lymphocyte population.

The *mobilizable lymphocyte pool,* first defined by Caffrey *et al* (1962), refers to that group of small lymphocytes that may be drained from an animal via a chronic thoracic duct fistula before a low constant output is reached. The time usually required is two to

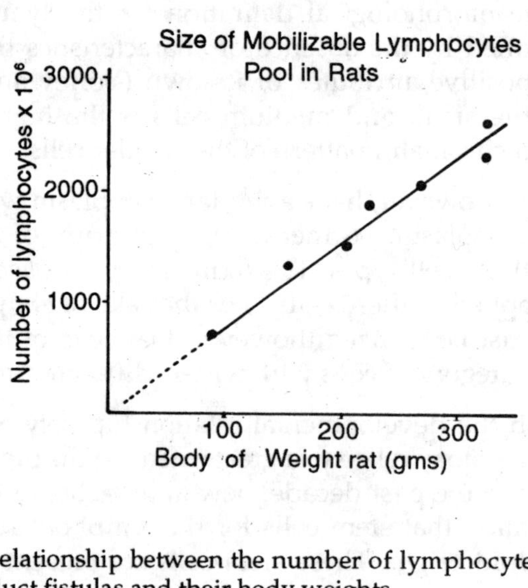

Fig. 8.1. Graph of the relationship between the number of lymphocytes that can be drained from rats with chronic thoracic duct fistulas and their body weights.

three days of drainage. It was found that the size of the mobilizable lymphocyte pool was proportional to the body weight of the animal and contained 7.8 × 10^6 lymphocytes per gram for the Sprague-Dawley rat. This number represents approximately half the total number of small lymphocytes in the animal (Everett *et al* 1964).

The *recirculating lymphocyte pool* was defined by Gowans and Knight (1964) as the population of small lymphocytes that is capable of migrating from blood to reach different lymph under normal conditions. They measured the size of the recirculating lymphocyte pool in rats by injecting labeled thoracic duct lymphocytes intravenously into syngeneic recipients and then determined the extent of their dilution by cannulating the thoracic ducts of the recipients 24 hours later. The pool of recipients' cells with which the labeled cells had mixed was estimated to contain between 1.5-2 × 10^9 small lymphocytes for male rats weighing 200 to 250 grams. This number is approximately the same as that obtained for the mobilizable lymphocyte pool in rats of this weight, although the two methods do not necessarily measure the same pool of cells.

Gowans (1966) has offered the criticism that the chronic drainage of lymph that measures the mobilizable lymphocyte pool may cuse a depletion of cells not normally a part of the recirculating pool. On the other hand, the measurements of the recirculaing lymphocyte pool may also be criticized in that 24 hours may not be an adequate time for a complete mixing of the pool if the entire pool is not in continuous recirculation. It is conceivable that a portion of the pool may be temporarily immobilized in the lymphoid tissue.

In order to avoid these conflicts, we shall speak here of the *long-lived lymphocyte pool* and define it as that group of small lymphocytes that has a life span of more than two weeks in the rat. We shall present evidence that long-lived small lymphocytes are a single group of cells measured by their kinetics, circulation, and life cycle, and that they comprise the majority of cells in both the mobilizable lymphocyte pool and recirculating lymphocyte pool.

The first evidence comes from experiments that showed that the rate of formation of long-lived small lymphocytes was proportional to the general body growth of the rat, and that this rate may be independently calculated using the rate of disappearance of labeled small lymphocytes from spleen, lymph nodes, thoracic duct lymph, or blood in rats previously labeled with ^{3}H-thymidine during the active phase of growth. Such an observation seems highly unlikely unless the long-lived cells were in equilibrium between these compartments.

Additional evidence comes from experiments in which local irradiation was given to the cervical lymph nodes of rats in which only cells of the long-lived population were lablled. The percentage of labeled lymphocytes in the locally irradiated nodes between two days and 14 days after irradiation was the same as that in the nonirradiated mesenteric nodes of the same animal and in the cervical lymph nodes of nonirradiated controls. Thus if the long-lived cells in any compartment are destroyed, that compartment is restored to normal by a migration of long-lived cells from the remainder of the pool.

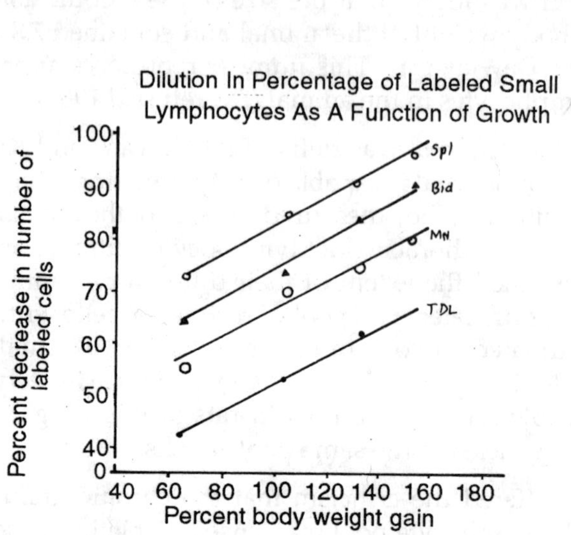

Fig. 8.2. Rats of this series received multiple injections of ^{3}H-thymidine for two weeks during their rapid growth phase in order to label a large percentage of the long-lived lymphocytes. The thymidine injections were then discontinued, and determinations were made for the decrease in percentage of labled small lymphocytes with the increase in body weight. (Bld, whole blood; Spl, spleen; MN, mesenteria lymph nodes; TDL, thoracic duct lymph). The common pattern of dilution as a function of growth for labeled cells within the respective compartments supports the concept of a single pool of long-lived lymphocytes.

Table 8.1
Percentage of Labeled Cells in Parabionts

Parabiotic Member	*Days of ^{3}HTH injection*	*Day of Sacri Post-^{3}HTH*	*Small Lymph*	*Lymph Blasts*	*Blood* *Small Lymph*	*Granulo-cyte*	*Mono-cyte*
1A	3	1	3.1	96	4.5	54	72
B		1	2.0	5	3.0	20	23
2A	5	1	3.0	97	9.5	76	76
B		1	2.3	4	4.8	26	19
3A	12	1	6.9	96	16.0	63	65
B		1	7.2	5	13.0	39	25
4A	12	14	12.5	0	14.0	0	0
B		14	11.3	0	15.0	0	0

Further evidence comes from experiments using rats joined in parabiosis. One member of each pair (A) was given ^{3}H-thymidine while occluding the cross circulation to the other rat (B). A variety of injection schedules was used (Table 8.1). All labeled cells seen in the noninjected members (B) were either immigrant cells formed in the injected members (A) or immediate progeny of immigrant cells. A comparison of the percentage of labeled monocytes or granulocytes of the injected versus the noninjected parabiont showed that these cells of blood had approximately a 25% chance of crossing from one rat to the other. However, the percentage of labeled small lymphocytes in the thoracic duct lymph was the same for both rats of all pairs irrespective of the number of ^{3}H-thymidine injections or the time of sacrifice postthymidine. This observation means that labeled cells of the recirculating lymphocyte pools were equilibrated in the two parabionts. In contrast, more than 95% of the blast cells in thoracic duct lymph of A rats were labeled, while in B rats less than 5% were labeled, showing that the blast cells do not recirculate to any great extent. Furthermore, in each pair of parabionts that was sacrificed at two weeks or more after the last ^{3}H-thymidine injection, the distribution of labeled small lymphocytes was comparable in all lymphopoietic compartments. These observations can only mean that the great majority of the long-lived lymphocytes of lymph nodes, spleen, and Peyer's patches had entered circulation during the two-week period and were part of a single pool equilibrated by recirculation from blood to lymph.

Gowans and Knight (1964) showed that the major route of recirculation is through the mesenteric lymph nodes and Peyer's patches via the postcapillary venules. Their studies showed that labeled thoracic duct lymphocytes transfused to recipients penetrated the deep cortex of the lymph nodes and entered the medullary lymph sinuses and efferent lymphatics. However, one should not think of the long-lived small lymphocytes as being confined to this route of recirculation. The results from the parabiotic rats showed that the long-lived cells were distributed throughout the nodes and spleens with the exception of the germinal centers. However, it is of particular interest that the corona of lymphocytes surrounding the germinal centers is composed primarily of these long-lived cells, since this is the region where they most likely contact an antigen. It has been shown by electron microscopic studies that following an injection of labeled antigen, the antigen is retained on the surface of long-branching processes of specialized reticular cells located in the cortical lymphoid follicle where it makes free contact with the surrounding lymphocytes.

Gowans and Knight (1964) did not observe labeled small lymphocytes in the corona during the first 24-36 hours after transfusion of labled thoracic duct cells. Thus, it is probable that these are the areas where the long-lived cells penetrate and remain for longer periods of time before again entering the circulation. They may home to these areas, and increased numbers may be retained at these sites during the active phase of an immune response.

Thymic dependent lymphocytes is a term originating from the work of Parrott *et al* (1966). It refers to those small lymphocytes that were found absent in specific areas of the spleen lymph nodes, and Peryer's patches in the adult animal subjected to neonatal thymectomy. The evidence indicates that these cells are the same as those of the long-lived lymphocyte pool. The areas of lymphocyte depletion in neonatally thymectomized animals are the same as those primarily occupied by the long-lived cells. Furthermore, neonatally thymectomized animals have a pronounced reduction in the number of small lymphocytes in thoracic duct lymph and in their mobilizable lymphocyte pool. Labeling studies have confirmed that the reduction in the total number of lymphocytes in the thoracic duct lymph is almost entirely due to the absence of long-lived cells and that short-lived lymphocytes and large lymphocytes appear in normal numbers. However, the neonatally thymectomized animals did not show a complete absence of long-lived cells. Additional evidence has also indicated that the entire pool is not formed under.

Neonatal thymectomy does not effect a change in lymphocyte content of the bone marrow, of the red pulp of the spleen, or of the germinal centers Ricke and Schwarz (1966) found that tissue and circulating short-lived cells were present in normal numbers after neonatal thymectomy and concluded that short-lived lymphocytes are derived from lymphopoietic centers other than the thymus and that the thymus is not necessary for their formation.

Thymectomy in young adult animals also reduces the output of cells in thoracic duct lymph, although the decrease is not as procounced as in the neonatally thymectomized animal. This evidence agrees with the concept that the long-lived pool is formed from birth to adulthood at a rate approximating that of body growth and that the formation of this pool is, mainly, thymic dependent.

The term *immunologically competent cell* was defined by Medawar (1963) as a cell fully qualified to undertake an immunological response; the term was coined by Medawar to distinguish immunological capacity from immunological performance. In contrast, an *immunologically active cell* is one already committed to and engaged in immunological activity. Three of the tests outlined for assessing immunological competence and directly related to the long-lived lymphocyte pool are:

1. the ability to restore immunological capacity to animals deprived of it,
2. the ability to produce splenomegaly, runt disease, or other manifestations of graft-versus-host reactions, and
3. the ability to produce a delayed type of inflammatory reaction by the intradermal injection of cells between animals of different antigenic makeup.

Still a fourth test that has come into being more recently is the mixed lymphocyte reaction.

An *immunologically incompetent animal* is one that does not show a normal capacity to mount a response to a large variety of antigens. In contrast, a tolerant animal is one tht cannot mount a response to a specific antigen although its response to unrelated antigens appears unimpaired. Methods shown to destroy a large percentage of the longlived pool also render the animal immunologically incompetent. Some of these are : administering high doses of total body irradiation, extracorporeal irradiation of blood, prolonged thoracic duct drainage, and treatment with antilymphocytic serum. Neonatal thymectomy, on the other hand, renders an animal incompetent by preventing the formation of a long-lived pool of normal size. With respect to Burnet's clonal selection theory tolerance arises from the deletion or inhibition of that small number of cells in the total pool that would otherwise respond to that specific antigen. Tolerant animals have a pool of normal size, but this indicates only that the number of cells within the pool that respond to any one antigen is extremely small. We shall discuss this point in more detail later on.

Radioautographic studies on the mechanism of action of antilymphocytic serum (ALS) have shown that a single injection of ALS may destroy a large percentage of the cells in the long-lived pool. In contrast, the number of short-lived cells is not reduced significantly by ALS treatment. Although the blood lymphocyte counts of ALS-treated rats may be higher than normal, lymphocyte counts of the thoracic duct lymph remain below normal for many months. Phagocytosis and destruction of the long-lived lymphocytes were evident in the liver, spleen, and lymph nodes within a few hours following an intraperitoneal injection of ALS to a rat. Macrophages laden with small lymphocytes were noted in the areas surrounding the postcapillary venules of mesenteric nodes as well as within the medullary sinuses. A single injection of ALS did not affect the lymphocyte content of thymus or of bone marrow. However, these results, it should be added, may not relate as much to specificity of ALS as they do to the life history of the long-lived pool. It might be expected, as suggested, that the long-lived cells would have more contact with ALS than the short-lived cells because of their extensive recirculation.

Immunological incompetence and tolerance should not be thought of as all-or-none phenomena: there are degrees of incompetence and tolerance. None of the methods used to render an animal incompetent completely obliterates the long-lived lymphocyte pool with the exception of lethal doses of irradiation. Also, in restoring an incompetent animal, it is not necessary to restore the entire long-lived pool. Transfusion of a relatively small number of cells obtained from the thoracic duct of normal donors can break tolerance to a long-standing homograft. Shielding a single Peyer's patch during lethal irradiation protects a sufficient number of cells to cause a rejection of a homologous or heterologous bone marrow graft. Still another aspect of quantitating competence is the antigenic disparity that separates the antigens from the recipient's own tissues. Animals capable of retaining a homograft may reject a heterograft. The degree of competence is considered in transplanting homografts by doing tissue typing prior to the transplantation. Such observations indicate that the number of cells in the long-lived pool capable of responding to a specific antigen increases as the antigenic disparity separating the donor and the recipient widens. At the same time, a long-lived cell may be capable of responding to a variety of antigens. A one cell-one antigen relationship is too limiting to provide an adequate system for the innumerable natural as well as artificial antigens that exist.

The term *antigen reactive cell* was defined by Mitchell and Miller in 1968. It is the same as the *antigen sensitive cell*, a term used by others prior to that time. These terms refer to the cells that first react to antigen by entering proliferation and then initiate the differentiation of *antibody precursor cells* into *antibody forming cells.* The evidence that Mitchell and Miller (1968) and others have presented from studies with mice is in conflict with the hypothesis that antigen reactive cells are the same as the antibody precursor cells. The antigen reactive cells appear to be equivalent to the long-lived small lymphocyte population. They have been shown to be thymic-dependent and present in the thymus in small numbers. They have been drained from normal animals by chronic thoracic duct fistula. Moreover, animals neonatally thymectomized showed a marked reduction in absolute numbers of antigen reactive cells in their mobilizable lymphocyte pools as compared to controls. Finally, antigen reactive cells were destroyed by treating animals with antilymphocytic serum. Antigen reactive cells were not found in the bone marrow, whereas antibody precursor cells were primarily of marrow origin. Thoracic duct lymph was found to contain a mixture of both antibody precursor cells and antigen reactive cells.

B. Short-lived Small Lymphocytes

Let us now summarize briefly what is known about short-lived lymphocytes of the different lymphopoietic compartments. Experiments measuring the rate of formation of small lymphocytes in the rat showed that the circulating life span of the short-lived cells is approximately 5 days, although for many of them it may be only a few hours. This rapid turnover rate must hold a significant meaning relating to the functions of these cells. Normally, lymphocyte destruction is most evident in the areas of tissues occupied primarily by short-lived cells (i.e., thymus, germinal centers, bone marrow) and these are also the cells most subject to the destructive action of cortical steroids.

Thoracic Duct Lymph

Approximately 7% to 10% of the small lymphocytes of the thoracic duct lymph are short lived. Unlike the long-lived cells, they continue to issue from a chronic fistula in normal numbers for at least several days after the mobilizable lymphocyte pool has been drained. Neonatally thymectomized animals show a normal number of short-lived cells per volume of lymph and thus they do not appear to be thymic dependent. Since thoracic duct lymph contains antibody precursor cells as well as antigen reactive cells, and since the evidence indicates that both belong to the small lymphocyte category, it is possible that the antibody precursor cells are found within the short-lived population.

Thymus

Lymphocyte turnover in the thymus has been measured by studying the rate at which small thymocytes become labeled in the rat and mouse during the course of giving repeated injections of ^{3}H-thymidine to label all cells entering DNA synthesis. 50% of the small thymocytes were labeled in both species by 36 hours of ^{3}H-thymidine treatment. The rate of appearance of labeled small thymocytes is not a linear function of time but a logarithmic one, which indicates that both labeled and nonlabeled cells disappear from the thymus (or die *in situ*) at random without respect to age. Thus it was calculated that the thymus of the rat forms a volume of cells equal to the thymic weight every 2½ days.

Thymus graft experiments, local thymic labeling experiments, and experiments involving thymectomized animals agree in showing that the majority of the cells formed in the thymus die *in situ*. A small percentage (less than 5%) of those formed appear to enter the blood and course to the spleen, Peyer's patches, and lymph nodes. Localized thymic labeling and experiments in which labeled thymocytes were transfused confirm that this small percentage is a part of the long-lived pool.

The relationship between the rapid production of the short-lived thymocytes and the continued formation of the small percentage of cells leaving the thymus and contributing to the long-lived pool remains one of the most intriguing problems of lymphopoiesis. The importance of understanding this relationship is emphasized by the evidence that links both tolerance and the development of certain autoimmune diseases with the proliferation in the thymus and its contribution of cells that serves in rendering an animal immunocompetent.

Bone Marrow

Bone marrow small lymphocytes of the rat have an even shorter turnover time than the thymocytes, as revealed by determining the respective rates of labeling with ^{3}H-thymidine. It was established that their average half-time renewal rate was 24 hours. As in thymus, the rate of increase in the percentage of labeled cells was not a linear function of time but a logarithmic one and approached 100% labeling at approximately 5 days.

Local marrow labeling experiments as well as the parabiotic experiments described above showed that more than 95% of the bone marrow small lymphocytes were formed in the marrow. It has been shown that many of these enter the blood. Bone marrow lymphocytes are not immunologically competent in that they do not confer graft-versus-host reaction nor do they restore immunological competence. As stated previously, the bone marrow has been shown to contain antibody precursor cells capable of coursing to the nodes and spleen and of giving rise to large blast cells that synthesize 19S antibody against sheep red cells. In view of the evidence implicating small lymphocytes as the precursors of antibody-forming cells, it is postulated that bone marrow small lymphocytes are the most likely candidates. Local marrow-labeling experiments lend further support for this postulate in that some labeled bone marrow small lymphocytes were found within the germinal centers and medullary cords of lymph nodes. Fluorescent antibody studies have established these areas as the primary sites of 19S antibody production in lymph nodes. A small number of the labeled cells of bone marrow have been reported to enter thoracic duct lymph (Brahim and Osmond in press), and these could account for the antibody precursor cells reported to be present in lymph. Direct evidence for this is still lacking, and it remains to be shown whether the labled bone marrow lymphocytes that have coursed to spleen and nodes can transform into blast cells and whether these same blasts are the precursors to the antibody-forming cells.

It is well established that in the bird the thymus controls the fomation of the long-lived pool as it does in the mammal Plasma cell production, however, appears to be dependent on another lymphoid organ, the bursa of Fabricius. The small lymphocytes of the bursa are also renewed at a rapid rate. If some of the bone marrow small lymphocytes are shown to be equivalent to the antibody precursor cells, then this population is most probably equivalent to those of the bursa.

This section of the chapter may be summarized by saying that the research of the past decade has emphasized the heterogeneity of the small lymphocyte category, and it points to the necessity of considering each group within the category as a separate popultion. The same research gives a strong indication that an interdependence between the various groups of small lymphocytes exists and that a traffic of cells between the hemopoietic organs is necessary to develop and maintain a normal immune system.

II. Stem Cells and the Interrelation of the Lymphopoietic Organs

The interrelationship of the various hemopoietic organs is further emphasized by chromosomal marker studies that have shown that stem cells for the thymocytes as well as for the long-lived lymphocytes lie within the myeloid tissue in both the embryo and adult. With respect to the thymocyte, Ford and associates (1956) identified donor type chromosomes in mitotic cells within thymuses of irradiated mice protected by bone marrow transfusion. They concluded that cells reconstituting the thymus were of donor origin. Evidence for a natural flow of stem cells into the thymus comes from experiments using parabiotic mice, one member of each pair bearing a chromosomal marker. The results demonstrated an appreciable movement of cells capable of undergoing mitosis from each animal into the thymus of its partner. Taylor (1965) reported that stem cells capable of lymphoid differentiation were present in embryonic liver before their appearance in the thymus rudiment. These studies wer subsequently confirmed by Owen and Ritter (1969) and by Auerbach and Globerson (1966). Their chromosomal marker studies clearly showed that the lymphoid elements of the thymus orignated in the embryonic liver.

The precursors of the immunologically competent cells have also been shown to be of myeloid origin and the formation of these cells was found dependent on an interaction of bone marrow and thymus. Tyan and Cole (1966) have used chromosomal marker studies to show that potentially immunologically competent cells derived from the mouse fetal liver migrate into the thymic tissue where they mature and/or proliferate prior to their appearance in peripheral lymphoid tissue. Using organ cultures, Auerbach (1966) reported that although cells within embryonic liver were not immunologically competent as measured by their ability to produce graft-versus-host reactions, competence was acquired when the liver explants were cultured for several days in combination with thymic tissue. Furthermore, when spleen rudiments were obtained from the embryo and cultured in a similar manner, no lymphoid development was observed. If a spleen graft was made in the anterior chamber of the adult mouse eye, lymphoid development was found and shown to be the result of cell migration. Auerbach concluded that the thymus, bone marrow, and spleen all participate in some interdependent way in the development of an immunologically competent animal McGregor (1968) has presented evidence that the immunologically competent cells of thoracic duct lymph develop from myeloid tissue. In adult rats inoculated at birth with parental strainbown marrow cell, the choracic duct lymph was shown to contain cells having the immunological capacity of the bone marrow donor.

These experiments are only a few that emphasize that the lymphoid stem cells are migrating population in both the embryonic and adult state, and that the development of a normal lymphoid complex depends on the interaction of cells from different organs. However, one must be aware that none of these experiments depends on a massive flow of cells from one organ to another. In a normal animal, labeled transfused cells of bone marrow, spleen, node or thymus origin do not home to the thymus in sufficient numbers to be recovered within the thymus of the recipient. Although there was a good exchange of labeled blood cells of all types in the studies employing normal parabiotic rats, less than one cell in ten thousand thymocytes was labeled in the noninjected member, whereas essentially all of the thymocytes were labeled in the members injected with ^{3}H-thymidine. The majority of the immigrant cells to the thymus had the morphology of a monocyte and more rarely a labeled small lymphocyte was encountered in the medullary areas. These observations simply mean that the absolute number of stem cells entering the thymus is small when compared to the number of large thymocytes present, and that the transformation of a stem cell into a blast is an event too rare to be observed in the normal thymus. The results of experiments in which a thymus bearing chromosomal markers was grafted to a normal recipient support this concept in that it takes from two to three weeks for the donor mitotic figures to be replaced by recipient cells. Thus the thymus has within it cells capable of giving rise to many generations of progeny, although the ability for self-renewal appears to be limited. The failure to recognize the possibility that stem cells may exist in such limited numbers that they may go undetected morphologically is perhaps the greatest criticism to most studies that in the past have relied on morphological criteria only for studying cellular derivation and differentiation. One of the greatest challenges for the future is to devise and employ new techniques that overcome this criticism.

The morphology of the stem cells for the thymus has been a subject of intensive interest in our laboratories in the last few years. Under conditions afforded by irradiation, in which the thymus was first depleted of the lymphoid population, it was possible to show a migration of labeled cells of marrow origin into the thymus. In parabiotic experiments employing irradiation and marrow shielding, and in experiments involving the transfusion of labeled marrow cells to irradiated rats, the only labeled cells migrating into the thymus were similar in morphology to blood monocytes. We have called these "monocytoid cells," since it is realized that all cells that look alike do not necessarily have the same functional capacities or metabolic properties.

Studies on the quantitative aspects of stem cells in peripheral blood and bone marrow clearly indicate that the stem cells capable of self renewal and the extensive proliferation necessary for reseeding a lethally irradiated animal are present in very limited numbers. Lewis and Trobaugh (1964), found five spleen colonies for every 10,000 injected marrow cells and five colonies for every 500,000 to one million injected blood leukocytes. Although the spleen-colony method does not assess the absolute number of stem cells in any transfusate, it should be obvious from such calculations that the changes of isolating a stem cell allowing for morphological characterization are remote. Nevertheless, the only cell type that entered the thymus had abundant pale staining cytoplasm a nucleus with many invaginations and folds and fine chromatin structure. The majority of these labeled cells entered the thymus of the irradiated rat via the blood vessels within the septa, and made their way through the connective tissue to the outer cortex. Labeled mitotic figures were seen and clusters of weakly labeled blasts were encountered at 24 to 48 hours posttransfusion.

In 1966 we presented radioautographic evidence in conflict with the classical concept of hematology, which advocates that cells of the fixed reticular network of the hemopoietic organs give rise to the free cells therein. The stromal cells of the spleen, thymus, lymph nodes and bone marrow were shown to be proliferating at a very slow rate. A small percentage were found to incorporate ^{3}H-thymidine and give rise to themselves. A larger percentage were labeled by multiple injections of ^{3}H-thymidine to growing animals, and a slow turnover time for reticular cells was confirmed by experiments measuring the disappearance rate for labled cells after long postthymidine intervals. Many reticular cells were still labeled in rats sacrificed at one year post-^{3}H-thymidine. It may be noted that stromal cells of the hemopoietic organs have long been recognized as being highly radioresistant. Thus, sublethal irradiation experiments were designed to stimulate blast cell formation and to test the capacity of the labeled reticular cells to transform. No evidence was obtained to support the view that reticular cells have stem cell capacity. The more recent evidence showing that the stem cells for both the short- and long-lived populations are of myeloid origin are a highly mobile population, and are radiosensitive further undermines this classical concept.

III. Small Lymphocyte Transformation

The results of radioautographic studies clearly show that the frequency with which a long-lived small lymphocyte transforms to blast cell *in vivo* is infrequent. Rats sacrificed at two weeks or more after multiple injections of ^{3}H-thymidine and which had as many as 50% of the long-lived lymphocytes labeled showed less than 1:10,000 blast cells to be labeled as calculated from radioautographs of tissue sections. Within the first 24 hours after antigenic stimulation with normal rabbit serum, this frequency was increased, in nodes and spleen, but it still represented less than 1:1,000 blast cells.

Miller *et al*(1967) determined the number of antigen reactive cells within the mobilizable lymphocyte pool of mice that responded to sheep erythrocytes. They reported that approximately 60 cells per million lymphocytes responded.

Studies employing radioautography as a means of estimating the number of small lymphocytes that transform in the *in vitro* culture systems also show that relatively small percentage of the lymphocytes respond. At least three independent studies have shown that less than 3% of the original small lymphocyte population respond in systems measuring immunological reactions. These approaches have included the monolayer culture sytem, analogous to the homograft reaction, the mixed lymphocye reaction, and the incubation of lymphocytes with antigens such as tuberculin.

More recently, Marshall *et al* (1969) have followed the proliferation of single blasts for three to five days of culture using time-lapse cinephotomicrography. They selected lymphoblasts derived from 48 hour cultures with tuberculin, pokeweed, or mixed lymphocyte cultures, and at that time the number of lymphoblast was approximately 2.3% of the initial small lymphocyte count. Examination of the film showed that the lymphoblasts divided and redivided to produce clones of 64 cells or more with an average generation time of eight to 13 hours.

The precursors to the antibody-forming cells also appear to respond in very small numbers to any one antigen as assayed by the plague-forming technique. Mitotic blocking agents such as colchicine or velban have been used in this system to inhibit the proliferation of antibody-forming cells in order to assess recruitment of antibody-forming cells. It was concluded that following antigeneic stimulation with sheep red cells, relatively few cells responded by synthesizing antibody and that these in turn entered a proliferative sequence. The magnitude of the antibody response was dependent primarily on the rate of division of antibody producing cells and not on new cell recruitment.

IV. Blast Cell Formation and Kinetics

If one accepts the evidence showing that stem cells comprise only a minute fraction of the cells in myeloid tissue and that the transformation of the small lymphocyte is a rare event in the nodes or spleen of the intact animal, then we are faced with the problem of what is the precursor to the relatively large number of blast cells that are readily observed. In order to answer this question, it is necessary to investigate the kinetics of blast cells.

Early hematologists realized that the cells that they referred to as *hemocytoblasts,* and were found in the lymph nodes, spleen, bone marrow, and thymus, had a short generation time as indicated by their mitotic index. Radioautographic studies have confirmed this concept. The average blast cells in lymph nodes and spleen have a generation time of 12 hours, and in thymus it is approximately 9½ hours.

Mesenteric lymph nodes from rats sacrificed within 15 minutes of a single injection of ^{3}H-thymidine had approximately 50% of the blasts cells labeled. Thus 50% of the blasts were in DNA synthesis at any one time. Rats sacrificed at 12, 24 and 36 hours after a single injection also had 50% of the blast cells labeled but the average grain count had decreased as a logarithmic function of time. The half time was 12 hours. These results show that the majority of the blast cells in the node are derived from themselves and that they represent successive generations of cells with the same morphological appearance. Although it is possible that the enlargement of a small lymphocyte or the transformation of a yet unidentified stem cell initiates differntiation, quantitatively speaking, cell reproduction by the blast cells themselves overwhelmingly outweigh the event of cell transformation.

This principal of differentiation is further illustrated by the bone marrow. Cells that have a morphology similar to the blast cells and lymph nodes and thymus are also present in bone marrow. The large and medium forms have been termed *transitional cells* by Yoffey (1962), who has considered them intermediate between the small lymphocytes of the bone marrow and the cells of the erythrocytic and granulocytic series. The local marrow-labeling experiments which showed that small lymphocytes are formed in the marrow, also gave evidence that at least some of the transitional cells gave rise to the marrow small lymhocytes. Recently, the transitional cells have been divided into two morphological type pale and basophilic. Studies of their kinetic behaviour show that the majority of the cells in each category give rise to themselves for many generations. Although some indirect evidence suggests that precursors to the proerythroblasts may be found in the transititonal cell category, this question must remain open.

Heterogemeoty of Lymphocytes

The lymphocytes constitute a family of cells of different origins, migration patterns, sizes, staining characteristics, ultrastructure, life span and function. The smaller lymphocytes have a small, dense nucleus in which nucleoli are rarely visible; the larger ones have a round or slightly indented nucleus with a loose chromatin structure, and nucleoli are always visible with proper staining techniques. Because the cytoplasm in lymphocytes of the smaller class is generally very pale, usually only, a small rim on one side of the nucleus is visible; electron microscopy shows that these cells have very few single ribosomes and no endoplasmic reticulum. However, some small lymphocytes presumably contain more ribosomes, since the cytoplasm is much more basophilic and stains intensely with pyronin. The larger lymphocytes have more numerous single ribosomes and in some instances, such as following the action of antigenic stimuli, one can observe polyribosomes with a faint endoplasmic reticulum in cells that may be in the process of transforming into plasma cells. Bovine thoracic duct lymphocytes have been shown to be of two overlapping size populations. The population of smaller cells has a median volume of 250 cubic microns with a 99 per cent confidence range from 142 to 425 cubic microns, while the population of larger cells has a median volume of 648 cubic microns with a 99 per cent confidence range of 370 to 1,150 cubic microns. The populations intersects at 312 cubic microns. For practical purposes, the cells with a volume of less than 312 cubic microns are considered to be the small lymphocytes, and those with a volume greater than 312 cubic microns the large.

The life span of lymphocytes has been reported to vary from a few hours to years. Little and associates (1962) have shown that the smaller class of rat lymphocytes is divided into those with relatively short life spans, and those with life spans greater than one year. The larger lymphocytes are also divided into two components; one with a life span of the order of one to two days, and the other with a maximum life span of about 60 days. Norman and associates (1965) have demonstrated that small lymphocytes have a mean life span of 530 ± 64 days in women.

On the basis of a study of mitotic indices and labeling with tritiated thymidine (^{3}HTdR), Osogoe (1963) concluded that there are two populations of lymphocytes; the first is produced rapidly, homes of the gastrointestinal tract and has a short life span; the other is smaller in size and has a very long life span. Everett *et al* (1964) also utilized single and multiple injections of ^{3}HTdR and analyzed the behaviour of lymphocytes in blood, thoracic duct lymph, and diverse organs. They concluded that 90 per cent of the cells in the thoracic duct lymph are long-lived. The long-lived cells are produced at a rate proportional to body growth and they recirculate from blood lymph. They also deduced that the thymus may be a source of the long-lived circulating lymphocytes. The small lymphocytes in the bone marrow, approximately 95 per cent of those in the thymus, and a major percentage of those in the spleen, are short lived (five days or less although it is nuclear whether these cells arise from the cortex, or the medulla, of the thymus.

Long-lived lymphocytes are immunologically committed and serve as a basis for immunologic memory.

Continuous intravenous administration of ^{3}HTdR in rats showed that the median survival time of small lymphocytes was about one month in animals that had received ^{3}HTdR for up to 271 days while 5% to 8% had a life span of more than nine months. Large lymphocytes constituted a homogeneous population in respect to labeling but small lymphocytes labeled nonuniformily, and appeared to comprise at least two populations differing in intensity of labeling and turnover rates with the more heavily labeled cells having the faster turnover.

The Generate Cycle of Lymphocytes and the Rate of Proliferation

Determining the time a cells spends in each phase of the generative cycle necessitates either direct observation or the introduction of a label at one of the subdivisions of the generative cycle; for example, by labeling all cells in the phase of DNA synthesis with ^{3}HTdR. Thereafter, one can observe changes in the fraction of cells that are labeled and in the flow of labeled cells through the premitotic rest periods and through mitosis. In the lymphatic nodules of the rat spleen, the autoradiographic data suggested a DNA synthesis time of about five hours and a minimum time for premitotic rest of 30 minutes, with a maximum between one and two hours. The diminution in intensity of label over interphase cells indicated a half-time of 13.4 hours but the grain count over mitotic figures showed a half-time of six to seven hours, which probably approximates the true generation time; this difference is probably an indication of the reutilization of tritium-labeled breakdown products of DNA. There is a great contrast in the rate of proliferation between the mantle-zone cells and the germinal-center cells. One to two per cent of mantle-zone cells surrounding the germinal center become labeled after a single ^{3}HTdR injection. The grain count data over these labeled cells are compatible with the idea that the cells undergo one division within the first twelve hours after injection of tritiated thymidine. Thereafter, further divisions may not occur for days and a half-time for the diminution in intensity of 260 hours or more may be calculated. This suggests that 98% of the mantle cells are in G_o or are resting with a long G_1.

Various phases in the generative cycle of thoracic duct cells in calves have been studied. These results showed that the generative time of the more basophilic cells is about 5½ to 6 hours, with a DNA synthesis time of 4 hours, while the populations of less basophilic cells had cycles about one to two hours longer. Mitotic time was found to be about 18 minutes, which is substantially shorter than the 40 minutes obtained by direct observation of an antibody producing cell in mitosis. Plasmablasts and hemohistioblasts in mesenteric lymph nodes of the rat have generative times of about 9 and 12 hours respectively. Mature plasma cells probably constitute a nondividing population, which is renewed in the lymph node in not more than five days.

Mouse spleen cells had a doubling time of 24 hours during the latent and log phases of primary antibody response, which decreased to 14 hours after antigenic stimulation. The doubling time can be assumed equal to the generation time only if all labeled cells divide and if there is no death of the progeny. There seems little doubt that antigens shorten the doubling time to a certain extent and stimulate immature plasma-like cells and lymphocytes to enter the cycle. The cell cycle of blast cells derived from spleens of primed donors in which a secondary response was initiated in diffusion chambers by the addition of antigen, showed a generation time of about 8 to 9 hours during the latent to log phase transition through the first mitosis, a mitotic time of 0.5 hours and a presynthesis rest of 0-1 hours. The short synthesis and generation times have been confirmed by Vincent *et al* (1969), using double labeling techniques.

Quantitative studies on lymphocyte production were begun by Yoffey (1936), but the initial measurements were high because of failure to consider the recirculation of lymphocytes from blood. Counts of mitotic figures throughout the lymph nodes, the thymus, and the spleen of the rat, assuming a one-hour mitotic time, show that approximately 67.6 x 10^6 lymphocytes are produced per day per 100 grams of body weight. If one reduces the mitotic time to the 18 minutes measured by Cunningham *et al* (1967), the production rate can be increased by a factor of about 3 or 4. About 0.5% to 2% of the DNA of rodent lymphoid tissue is renewed per hour in the lymph nodes and the thymus. Conversion of the DNA renewal rate into number of cells produced per unit of time has been done but is fraught with potential errors, such as the reutilization of labeled material from the death of cells and variations in size of metabolic pools. Therefore, by this method it is difficult to determine the total number of cells that are actually leaving the organs. Cronkite *et al* (1964) showed that the output in the thoracic duct of calves was about 2 × 10^8 per minute of which 10 per cent are newly produced and the others recycling. It was further estimated that four to 12 lymphocytes entered the blood from some other sources for every cell that entered the blood from some other source for every cell that entered through the thoracic duct. Single, normal, axillary lymph nodes produce about 0.5 × 10^6 cells per hour, but after antigenic stimulation by skin allograft this increase to 2.6 × 10^6, concluding that the increased production of cells is due to an increase in the number of cells replicating rather than to a decrease in the generation time. Their estimated generation time of nine hours is close to the value observed by Fliedner *et al* (1964) and Janeit *et al* (1966).

While it is simple to measure the number of cells coming out of the thoracic duct or an efferent lymphatic, it is still very difficult to get any realistic estimate of the absolute production rate of new lymphocytes in all the different morphologic categories. There are uncertainties in determining the migration pattern, the fraction of cells that are recycling from blood to lymph, the reutilization of DNA labeling materials, and the possible increased death of cells by antigenic or other stimuli; but it appears to be clearly established that antigens are effective in increasing the rate of proliferation.

Under normal conditions, the mass of the adult lymphoreticular system is relatively constant, implying a balance between the production and death of cells that may arise from a small constant input of antigens from the gastrointestinal tract or by absorption through the skin. One can determine the number of newly produced lymphocytes that leave a single lymph node by combining efferent duct cannulation with arterial ^{3}HTdR perfusion in order to label the DNA of all new cells. However, the absolute production can be determined from the replacement of unlabeled by labeled DNA per unit time divided by the average DNA per cell, plus the number of labeled cells leaving the node.

The replacement of unlabeled by labeled DNA in the steady state represents the intranodal cellular death rate of cells produced in the node. Imperfect knowledge of lymphopoiesis prevents accurate assessment of the absolute production rates at this time.

The lymphocytes are also heterogeneous in respect to their organ of origin—namely, the thymus, lymph nodes, spleen, gut-associated lymphoid tissue, or the bone marrow-and to their function. Various investigators have ascribed essential roles in primary immunity, secondary immunity, allograft rejection, delayed hypersensitivity, tolerance, transfer reaction such as graft *vs* host disease, as stem cells for hemopoiesis in general and in tropic functions. Finally, lymphocytes are heterogeneous in respect to their content of IgG, IgM, IgA, and antibodies; it is unusual, but not unknown, to find a cell with more than one Ig or antibody.

Migration Pathways

The migration pathways of the ubiquitous lymphocyte are shown in Figure 8.1. The flow of lymphocytes from the bone marrow to the blood and from blood to marrow has been studied over the years by many investigators. The concept that there is a major migration stream of small lymphocytes from the blood to the marrow accounting for the daily replacement factor, and that the migrant lymphocytes are transformed and serve as stem cells is not now accepted. In the dog, ^{3}HTdR-tagged small lymphocytes labeled at large in the body migrated to the bone marrow, but there was no evidence of transformation into erythroblasts. The evidence suggested that there are two populations of small lymphocytes, one that migrates to and one that is generated within the marrow.

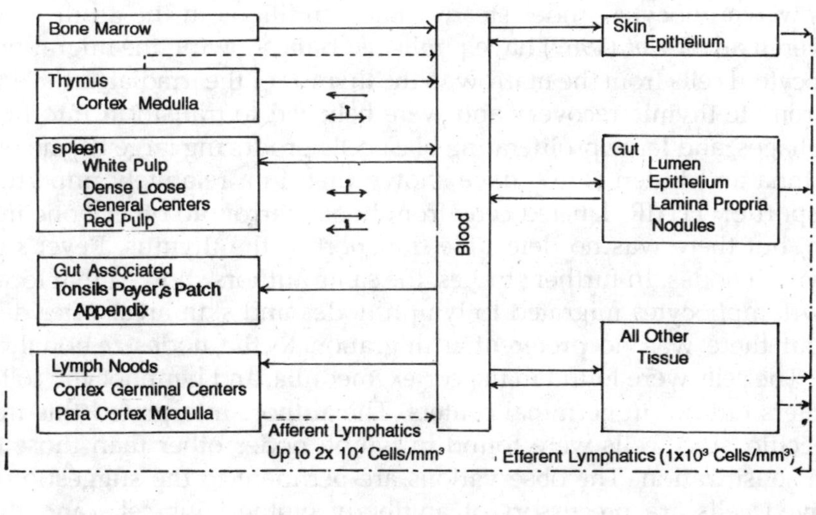

Fig. 8.3. The ubiquitous lymphocyte, its exchanges with blood and tissues.

There is strong evidence that some of the numerous small lymphocytes found in guinea pig bone marrow; are rapidly renewed by proliferation of precursor cells within the marrow. In these studies, Osmond and Everett used, in part, techniques of excluding circulation to marrow while ^{3}HTdR is administered, similar to those of Keiser *et al* (1964) in the dog. In addition, they studied the behaviour of marrow small lymphocytes in diffusion chambers where there can be no migration of lymphocytes into the chamber. They concluded that there is no large-scale migration of small lymphocytes into the marrow but some migration of large undifferentiated cells indicating intramedullary proliferation of precursor cells to form the marrow small lymphocytes. Rat studies also indicate that the marrow is a major site of proliferation of small lymphocytes. Although the evidence for proliferation of small lymphocytes in the marrow is secure, the nature of the precursor cell is not clear. It is conceivable that the small lymphocyte is in a long G_1 or G_0 phase that becomes the transitional cell of Yoffey (1958) after stimulation. The genetic relationship between the large and small-marrow lymphocytes remains to be determined. Further evidence for increased intramedullary production of lymphocytes by hypoxia confirms earlier comparable studies in guinea pig and mouse.

Since there is a large-scale intramedullary production of lymphocytes, as well as some migration of small lymphocytes into the marrow, steady state conditions demand a large-scale intramedullary death or migration out of the marrow. Hudson and Yoffey (1966) have demonstrated, by electron microscopy, that lymphocytes migrate between the sinusoidal endothelial cells of the marrow but not through them, and the direction of movement could not be determined. Syngeneic marrow transplantation using chromosome markers has shown that the marrow contains cells capable of repopulating the thymus, spleen lymph nodes, and bone marrow of otherwise fatally irradiated mice. The bone marrow to thymus to lymph node migration is slow, probably taking weeks although this has been established with certainty only in irradiated animals. The migration rate of marrow lymphocytes under steady state conditions in the adult is not known. However, Everett and Tyler (1969) have published data showing the migration of ^{3}HTdR labeled monocytoid cells from the marrow to the thymus of the irradiated rat. Presumably, these cells promote thymic recovery and were believed to transform into fibrocyte-like cells, macrophages, and large proliferating blast cells producing large thymocytes. Recent studies by Linna and Liden (1969) have shown that, in a relatively unperturbed state, there is transport of ^{3}HTdR labeled cells from bone marrow to other bone marrow and to the spleen, but there was no detectible transport to the thymus, Peyer's patches, or mesenteric lymph nodes. In further studies, the same authors showed that locally labeled bone marrow lymphocytes migrated to lymph nodes and skin areas after delayed type sensitivity, but there was no preferential migration to the nodes regional to the skin sensitization. The cells were found in the cortex, medulla, and lymphocytic collars around germinal centers but not in germinal centers. The authors interpreted this migration as being nonspecific, since cells were found in lymph nodes other than those regional to areas of skin sensitization. The observations are pertinent to the suggestion that bone-marrow-derived cells are precursors of anitibody-synthesizing-cells and that thymic-derived cells are antigenreactive-cells, which was supported by the observations that both 19S hemolysin-producing cells and immuno-competent cells in the graft-versus-host reactions (McGregor, 1968) were marrow derived.

In a recent study, cells in neonatal marrow were labeled by continuous. ^{3}HTdR infusion throughout pregnancy. The labeling of bone marrow lymphocytes dropped rapidly during the first week of life, as did the grain count overlying the cells, but both remained constant for 21 weeks thereafter. This suggests that there is a long-lived and short-lived marrow lymphocyte and may indicate migration out of the marrow, but does not provide information on the rate of migration.

Thymic Migration Routes

The apparent high production rate of cells in the thymus must be balanced by death or migration of cells or there will be progressive growth of the thymus. Dye exclusion studies indicated that 3% to 5% of mouse thymic cells were dying (stained) in the first three months while in from 3 to 12 months the dying cells increased to 15% to 20%. In foetal life, the death rate was higher on the sixteenth day of gestation than on the eighteenth. Logically, the lower death rates can be correlated with periods of higher migration rates. The question of migration versus *in situ* death of lymphocytes in the thymus in newborn mice has been studied by simultaneously measuring thymic growth and cell production in the thymus, and it was found that one-third of all cells present in the thymus were lost during the third day of life. In view of the low pyknotic index and Claesson's (1969) observation of low death rate discussed above, an extensive migration must have taken place during the third day. In view of the preceding, the earlier notion that 99% of thymic lymphocytes disintegrate within the thymus must be rejected for the time intervals studied. In young adult mice, it has been shown that cells migrate from the outer cortical zones into the perivascular lymphatic vessels near the corticomedullary junction; and that a large fraction of lymphocytes leave the thymus through lymphatics. There is also a series of papers suggesting that lymphocytes leave the thymus via the veins. Thus, the evidence for migration out of the thymus during fetal, neonatal and young adult life is unequivocal. The magnitude of the migration varies with the age of the animals, but its significance is not clear. Some insight into its possible importance can be gleaned from the following studies.

Neonatal thymectomy in mice leads to severe lymphocyte depletion from specific areas of the spleen and lymph node defined as *thymus-dependent areas*; somewhat similiar observation had been made earlier in the rat. Extracorporeal irradiation of the blood produces a depletion of lymphocytes in the paracortical areas of the lymph nodes, the cuff of small lymphocytes surrounding germinal centers in the spleen and lymph nodes, and the loose white pulp in the spleen. These areas of the spleen and lymph nodes are considered thymic-dependent. The proliferation of pyroninophilic blast cells, which accompanies cell-mediated immune reactions, has been shown to be confined to the "thymus-dependent" or paracortical areas of lymph nodes of guinea pigs and mice.

Syngeneic thymus cells, which have been labeled *in vitro* with tritiated adenosine, localize perferentially in the "thymus-dependent areas" after intravenous injection into mice. Mice with cogenital aplasia of the thymus show marked depletion of lymphocytes from the "thymic dependent areas" of the lymphoid organs. Goldschneider and McGregor (1968) labeled syngeneic rat thymocytes *in vitro* with ^{3}H-5-uridine and found similar pathways in normal and neonatal thymectomized rats and in rats depleted by thoratic dust drainage. Both large and small thymocytes filtered through lung more slowly than thoracic duct lymphocytes and accumulated in liver sinusoids. Large thymocytes entered splenic red pulp and the intestinal wall while small thymocytes entered splenic white pulp along the same route as small lymphocytes and penetrated into the diffuse lymphocytic fields of lymph nodes and Peyer's patches *via* post capillary venules. A few small thymocytes were found in the thymus and bone marrow. Large thymocytes were labeled by a single intravenous injection of ^{3}HTdR thymic lymphocyte suspensions were injected IV. The large thymocytes were not found in lymph nodes, thymus, or Peyer's patches, but were found in lung, liver, splenic red pulp, intestinal wall and, occasionally, in splenic white pulp. This approach, like all techniques involving the administration of thymic lymphocyte suspensions, is open to the criticism that some of the cells in such suspensions would not normally leave the thymus. Studies with thymus grafts or with chromosome markers have demonstrated the migration of thymic lymphocytes to the spleen and lymph nodes of mice, although whether this represents normal migration is still unresolved.

In situ labeling with ^{3}HTdR is preferable since it labels only cells in DNA synthesis using a single slow intraarterial injection via the thymic artery or direct injection in the thymic gland. Subcapsular injection may cause trauma to the thymus and its lymphatics while injection directly into the thymic artery may damage this vessel and cause interference to the normal flow of arterial blood into the injected thymus.

Sicne we were unsatisfied with the existing techniques, we developed a technique for long-term intraarterial ^{3}HTdR perfusion of the thymus of calf. In our studies, the perfused thymic weight is 20 to 83 grams or about 20% to 40% of the whole thymus. Studies on anatomic distribution of cells originating in the thymus of calves killed after two to eight days of infusion have shown that the majority of heavily labeled cells appeared in the "thymic-dependent areas" of the spleen and lymph nodes. The density was greater in the spleen, but few heavily labeled cells were seen in or near post capillary venules. Thymic cells were also found in the red pulp of the spleen, medulla, and the outer cortex of the lymph node. No heavily labeled cells were found in the bone marrow but large fraction of cells in Peyer's patches were lightly labeled. In other unpublished studies, it appeared that an occasional thymic lymphocyte found its way back to the contralateral thymus at a region of presumed exit (corticomedullary junction), suggesting that recycling may also occur in the thymus. Some heavily labeled cells are found in the thoracic duct, indicating that thymic cells enter the recycling pool. Howerver, the thymic cells appear to be short-lived or divide rapidly since none were found in the tissues 96 hours after termination of perfusion.

Our suggestion of migration of cells to the thymus is supported by observed changes in specific activity of DNA after administration of ^{3}HTdR , irradiation and chilling. The slow regeneration of bone marrow, thymus and spleen and lymph nodes after marrow transfusion in fatally irradiated mice is well-known and is shown schematically in Figure 8.4. The role of this route in restablishing immunocompetence has been generally accepted but the effect of the apparent large scale migration of cells to thymus in the studies of Field and Stanley (1966) is not clear, although it could represent migration from marrow to thymus to produce antigen-reactive cells.

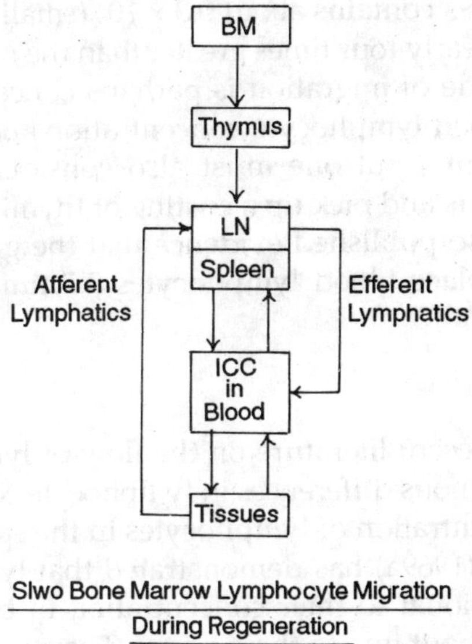

Fig. 8.4. Schematic presentation of the slow lymphocyte migration demonstarted during regeneration of hemopoietic tissues in otherwise fatally criadiated mice saved by syngeneic bone marrow transplantation.

Another approach that we have used to study thymic cell migration is the observation of cells with thymic specific antigen in the thymus, lymph, lymph nodes, spleen and blood. In these studies, it has been shown that the expression of surface, thymic-specific antigen (TSA) in the thymus, is inversely related to cell size and to expression of histocompatibility antigen. TSA-positive cells are found in thymic lymph, thymic vein, lymph nodes, spleen arterial blood, and thoracic duct lymph. The highest concentration of migrant TSA cells is found in the spleen, which is similar to the finding of more ^{3}HTdR labeled thymocytes in that organ (Iorio *et al* 1970). The 3% to 8% of cells in thymic vein blood with TSA pose a problem. The blood flow rate in bovine thymus is about 1 ml per gram per minute. If each cell in thymic vein blood with a coating of TSA were produced in the thymus, the number produced per day/kg. body weight would be:

$$A \times B \times C \times D \times E = (1.44 \times 10^3) \times (6 \times 10^6) \times (6 \times 10^{-2}) \times 1.97 \times 1 = 1.02 \times 10^9$$

A = minutes per day,

B = concentration of lymphocytes in thymic vein blood per ml,

C = fraction with thymus specific antigen in thymic vein blood minus fraction in arterial blood,

D = weight of thymus in grams per kg body weight = 1.97 (Chanana *et al* 1967),

E = blood flow (in ml) per gram per minute through thymus.

Since the blood of calves contains about 0.3 x 10^9 (small lymphocytes)/kg, the daily output from the thymus is nearly four times greater than the number of small lymphocytes in the blood. The magnitude of migration is perhaps conceivable and would certainly explain the reduction in blood lymphocyte concentration and the reduced thoracic duct output following thymectomy, but one must also consider the possibility that blood lymphocytes enter the thymus and pick up a coating of thymic specific antigen. Ernstrom and Larsson (1967) have also published evidence that the guinea pig thymus produces enough lymphocytes to replace blood lymphocytes 3.7 times per day, a number very close to our estimate in the calf.

Splenic Migration

There is considerable recent literature on the flow of lymphocytes into, and out of, the spleen based on arteriovenous differences in lymphocyte concentration, which indicate a substantially greater concentration of lymphocytes in the splenic vein, suggesting a net input into the blood. Ford (1969a) has demonstrated that lymphocytes recycle through the spleen at a rate proportional to their concentration in blood; the minimum transit time through the spleen is about two to three hours. The route of migration involves the

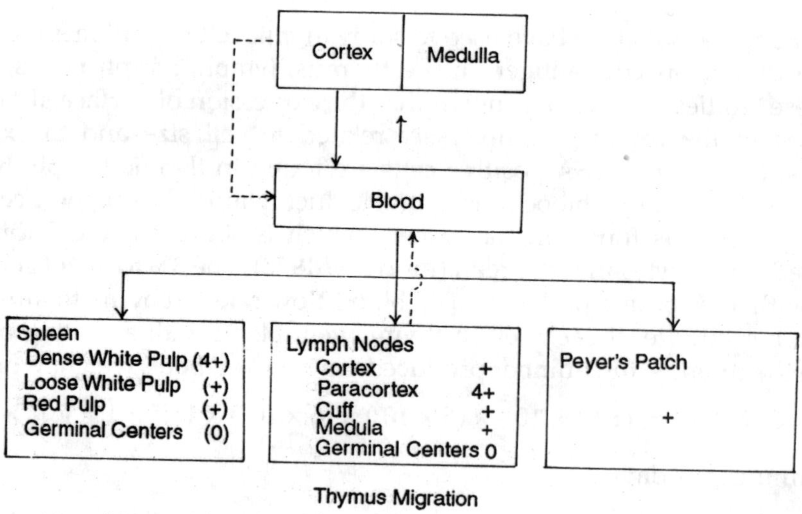

Fig. 8.5. Schematic routes of migration of thymic cells showing sites of relative concentrations.

trapping of lymphocytes in the periarteriolar sheath of the marginal zone and entering the white pulp, as previously suggested. The elegant morphological and ultrastructural studies of the spleen by Weiss (1962, 1963) show that tiny arterioles, which leave the central arteriole and terminate in the white pulp, rarely contain red cells but do contain lymphocytes. One presumes that plasma with lymphocytes is skimmed from the flowing column of blood and that lymphocytes are deposited in the marginal zone, thus providing a mechanism for the observed anatomic distribution, from which they make their way into the red pulp and presumably back into the blood. Ford (1969b) has also shown that cells recirculating through the thoracic duct can recycle through the lymph nodes; cells in both tissues have similar immunological properties.

Lymph Node Recycling

Recycling is so well-known now that discussion can be brief. The site of recycling is the postcapillary venule, known for years. The notion of recycling of lymphocytes from blood to lymph apparently was initiated by Renaut (1888) and again advanced by Sjovall (1936). In a series of elegant experiments Gowans (1959) and Gowans and Knight (1963) labeled syngeneic rat thoracic duct lymphocytes with tritiated adenosine, an RNA label, and conclusively demonstrated the recycling of lymphocytes from the thoracic duct to the blood and then through the postcapillary venules of the lymph nodes and back into the thoracic duct. Marchesi and Gowans (1964) showed by electron microscopy that lymphocytes pass through the endothelial cells rather than between them as granulocytes and monocytes do.

The outflow of lymphocytes from lymph nodes in efferent lymphatics indicates that there is a passive desquamation of cells apparently by population pressure pushing cells into the medullary sinuses. The output of cells, plus their type, remains unchanged for several days following cannulation and drainage of the efferent lymphatic of a lymph node, and the anatomic structure of the node remains the same. These results strongly suggest that the efferent small cells are recycling through the node from elsewhere in the body and that the large cells produced within the node continue to be produced at the same rate despite their loss from the body.

Information Obtained by Extracorporeal Irradiation of the Blood (ECIB) and Lymph (ECIL)

Although the notion of ECIB goes back to Gley and Heymans (1921), it was perfected as a tool for study of lymphopoiesis by Cronkite and his associates (1961, 1962; 1964; Jansen *et al* 1962; Sip *et al* 1965; Chanana *et al* 1966), who took advantage of the relative radioresistance of erythrocytes and the radiosensitivity of lymphocytes. Killing the blood lymphocytes should result in depletion of the lymphoreticular tissues in general since the blood lymphocytes exchange freely with some of the lymphocytes of lymphoreticular tissues. Irradiation of the blood and/or of the lymph has become a simple technique utilized in many laboratories. It has been useful in the induction of lymphopenia, depletion of small lymphocytes from lymphoreticular tissues, modifying allograft reactions and to some extent in the treatment of animal and human leukemia.

Depletion of the Lymphoreticular Tissues by ECIB

During ECIB, the thymic cortex is diminished in thickness, the corticomedullary ratio is decreased, and the splenic lymph follicles are markedly decreased in size, as a result of loss of small lymphocytes from the cuff surrounding the germinal centers. There is also a remarkable loss of lymphocoytes from the less densely populated areas of white pulp, as well as from the red pulp. The germinal centers in the spleen and lymph nodes are intact and have an incrase in mitotic activity. There is a striking diminution in the thickness of the cortical lymphocyte population in the lymph nodes, and in the relative density of lymphocytes in the medulla. Disintegrating cells are found in the intrafollicular zones of the cortex, or near the corticomedullary junction. The quantitative aspect of the depletion of lymphoreticular tissues with time have shown that all of them and the blood have a two-component depletion during 48 hours of ECIB. Approximately 50 per cent of the small lymphocytes in the cortex of the lymph nodes are tightly fixed and are mobilized very little, if at all, constituting a slowly mobilizable pool. Evidence for a mobilizable lymphocyte pool of 7.8×10^9 cells per kg body weight has been obtained from studies on thoracic duct drainage in the rat. The anatomic site of this was not determined as it was in the studies of Ruchti *et al* (1970).

Size of the Lymphocyte Pools Accessible by Thoracic Duct Drainage

The concentration of small lymphocytes in the peripheral blood and the output/kg/hr has been studied during 23 days of continuous ECIL. The output of thoracic duct lymphocytes decreasses in a way that can be expressed as 2 exponential components. The first component represents a pool of readily accessible lymphocytes that are mobilized with a half-time of about 11.2 days. The average size of this compartment in the 9 calves studied was estimated from the integral of the first 8 days to be 4.8×10^9 small lymphocytes/kg. This is about one half the size of the pool in rats reported by Caffrey *et al* (1962). The half depletion time of the less accessible lymphocyte pool cannot be determined with accuracy, but is of the order of 29.5 days. During this period, about 1.2×10^9 lymphocytes/kg were killed. The number of lymphocytes estimated in both the readily accessible and the slowly mobilizable compartments is an overestimate, since we have no good means of determining the absolute production rate of cells in either compartment during the depletion period.

Studies on restablishment of the pools following irradiation of the blood and lymph are incomplete at this time, but clearly follow a two-component process with an initial fast stage followed by a much slower stage. In some animals it has taken over a year for blood lymphocytes to attain pre-treatment levels. An analysis of the preceding data has been used to give a first approximation of the fluxes between blood and lymph nodes, the pool sizes and the time in pools. In blood the pool is about 0.3×10^9 cells/kg. The average time in the blood is 3.7 hours and about 27 per cent of the blood small lymphocytes are cleared per hour through the paracortical regions of the lymph nodes. In addition, an unknown flux of cells from blood into tissues is known to exist because of the return through the afferent lymphatics, but its magnitude cannot be measured. The pools of outer cortical lymphocytes and paracortical lymphocytes are both about the same size. The turnover rate of medullary and outer cortical lymphocytes is unknown.

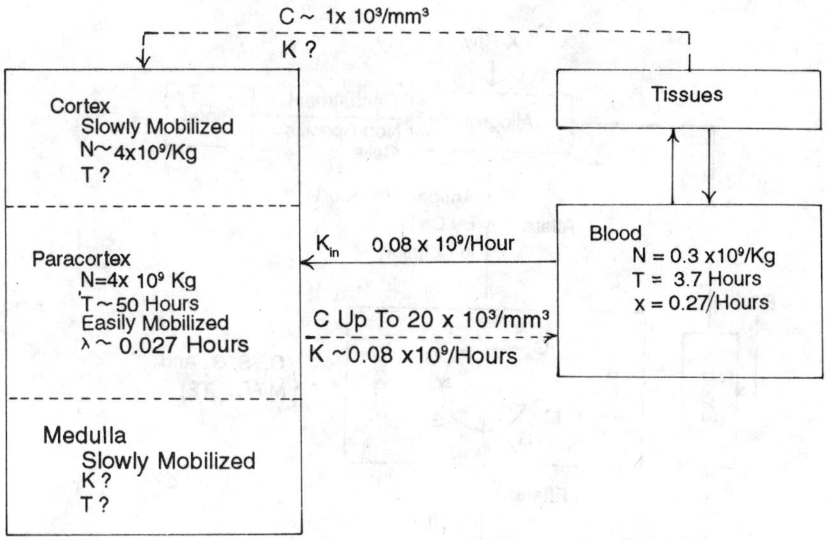

LYMPH NODE-BLOOD-TISSUES-CALF

Fig. 8.6. Schematic presentation of the flow of lymphocytes from blood to tissues, to lymph nodes with estmates of time, fluxes and sizes where possible.

N = number /kg body weight
T = average time in compartment
λ = fractional turnover per hour
K = flux (number per hour per kg)
C = concentration number per min.

Although much has been learned about the migration pathways and proliferation of lymphocytes, little is known about the factors that regulate the system. A schematic relationship of lymphocytes to allograft rejection is shown in Figure 8.7. The antigen is transported to the regional nodes either by cells or in solution. Within the nodes, there is transformation and proliferation and the chemotherapeutic agents active against the cell cycle can exert an immunosuppressive effect at this point. Activated cells migrate out in the efferent lymphatics where they can be attacked during ECIL or ECIB , thus reducing the flux of the activated cells through the allograft. At the allograft these cells can be killed by local irradiation and those that survive react with the antigen and kill graft cells either directly or indirectly. The inflammatory response results in recruitment of nonspsecific cells into the area. The rapidity of the ultimate rejection of the graft is a function of the number and strength of antigenic differences between host and donor, the flux of activated cells into the graft, and the intensity of the inflammatory response set up by nonspecific factors that result in necrosis following thrombosis and impairment of circulation.

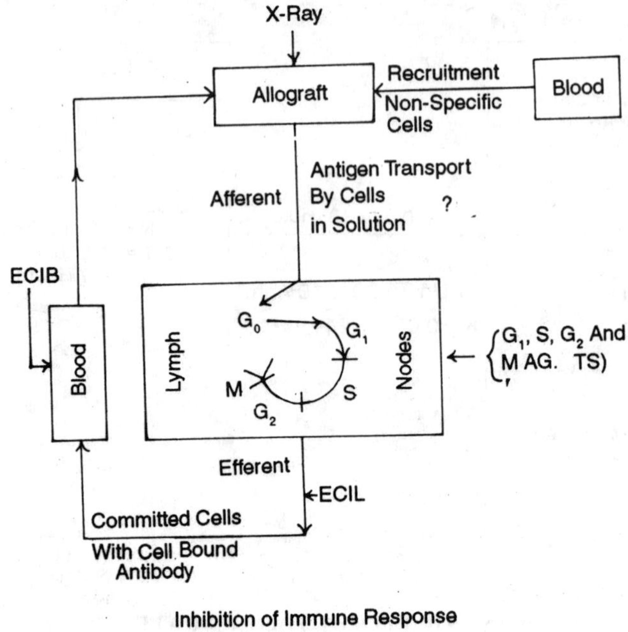

Fig. 8.7. Inhibition of Immune Response.

Hence, attack on the transplantation problem requires a knowledge of, and ability to control, lymphopoietic prolifertion and migration.

9

Formation of Monocytes and Macrophages

Monocytes and macrophages may be regarded as a continuum of cells of various degrees of differentiation or maturation. The circulating monocyte is only one stage of the cell line, which has its orgin in a cell in the bone marrow that has been called a *promonocyte*. The morphologic and metabolic characteristics of the promonocyte are virtually unknown, but there are reasons for believing that it shares a common ancestry with cells of the granulocytic series. Once it leaves the marrow cavity, the monocyte spends only a fraction of its life span within the bloodstream. Intravascular residence is measured in hours or, at most, days. The greater part of its life span is spent in the tissues, where it undergoes further differentiation into a macrophage. The total life span of this cell species from promonocyte to senescent tissue macrophage is not known. Studies of macrophages observed *in vivo* in ear chambers and of macrophages cultivated *in vitro* suggest that the life span may be at least several months.

Morphologic and Metabolic Characteristics

The concept of a continuum of cells from the blood monocyte to the larger tissue macrophage and multinucleate giant cell is important to the understanding of the function and metabolism of these cells. It is obvious that cells at different levels of differentiation have different metabolic and functional characteristics as well as distinctive morphologic features. The observations of Metchnik off early in the century (1905) and the later ones of Aschoff (1924) provided much of the basis for the concept of transitional forms between the blood monocyte and the tissue macrophage. In 1926, the Lewises demonstrated that circulating large mononuclear phagocytes of all classes of vertebrates were capable of maturing into "macrophages similar to those found in connective tissues, liver, spleen and lymph nodes and epithelioid cells and giant cells precisely like those found in tuberculous lesions."

Perphaps the most convincing evidence for the maturation of the blood monocyte in the tissues of the intact animal came from the work of Ebert and Florey in 1939. Using rabbit ear chambers, they observed that monocytes containing phagocytized particles migrate from small blood vessels into the surrounding connective tissue and there transform into large macrophages. As the cells mature, they increase in size and attain diameters of 50 to 200μ. They develop prominent cytoplasmic extensions that may extend impressive distances from the cell body. By cinemicroscopy, these cytoplasmic extensions can be observed to be in constant motion, sweeping about the cell until they contact a phagocytizable particle such as a microorganism.

As the cells age, multiple nuclei can often be seen within a single cytoplasm. The mechanism by which such multinucleate cells develop is not certain. Although many investigators believe that they arise from cell fusion, the evidence is not wholly convincing. Under some circumstances, macrophages in the process of maturation can be observed to incorporate radioactive thymidine into their nuclear material. Preliminary evidence suggests, however, that this thymidine is used largely for DNA repair rather than for DNA replication. Most studies have shown a very limited capacity for macrophage replication either *in vivo* or *in vitro*. Under unusual circumstances, such as intense antigenic stimulation *in vivo* or interaction with other proliferating cell types *in vitro*, macrophages show some proliferative capacity.

The most striking morphologic change that occurs with monocyte maturation is the accumulation of phase-dense granules that fill that cytoplasm. These are lysosomal structures, which are visible in the light and the electron microscope. Another morphologic feature of maturation is an increase in the numbers of mitochondrial elements in the cytoplasm.

Simultaneously with these morphologic alterations, a series of changes occurs in cell constituents and cell metabolism as the mononuclear phagocyte matures. With maturation, the cellular activity of a variety of lysosomal enzymes increases: acid phosphatase, β-glucuronidase, cathepsin, lysozyme and aryl-sulfatase. We have observed cellular acid phosphatase activity to increase 30-fold and lysozyme to increase 10-fold during a 14-day cultivation of human monocytes *in vitro*. This rich assortment of acid hydrolases seems appropriate for a cell whose major function includes phagocytosis, killing and digestion of microorganisms, and removal of damaged red cells.

The level of lysosomal enzymes, such as acid phosphatase and lysozyme, may be influenced by factors stimulating the reticuloendothelial system, such as tuberculosis. Mononuclear cells from rabbits resistant to tuberculosis are reported to have higher levels of acid phosphatase activity than cells from susceptible animals. The Golgi apparatus is small in monocytes and increases in both size and complexity with cell maturation. From available evidence, one can reasonably conclude that lysosomal enzymes are made in the endoplasmic reticulum and then packaged by the Golgi apparatus into primary lysosomes. These primary lysosomes may then fuse with phagocyte or pinocytic vacuoles, resulting in the production of combined structures called secondary lysosomes. These are rich in hydrolyte enzymes.

Pinocytosis, phagocytosis, high environmental concentrations of protein, and certain polyanions all appear to stimulate hydrolytic enzyme production *in vitro*. The mechanisms influencing maturation *in vivo* are largely unknown. Other metabolic concomitants of the differentiation from monocyte to macrophage are increases in the activity of mitochondrial enzymes such as cytochrome oxidase and increases in the rates of cellular

Table 9.1
Granule-Associated Enzymes of Monocytes and Macrophages

		Acid Phosphate		*Lysozyme*	
Cell type	*Time in culture*	*μgP/10⁶ Cells*	*μgP/μg Protein*	*μgP/10⁶ Cells*	*μgP/μg Protein*
Monocytes	4-6 hrs	0.7	12.5	4.0	50.0
Macrophages	14-16 hrs	21.1	14.4	37.6	72.4

respiration, glucose utilization, and lactase production. It appears, therefore, that the tissue macrophage is a larger, metabolically more active cell, and has a larger arsenal of hydrolytic enzymes than the antecedent monocyte. These metabolic differences are reflected in the greater functional capacity of the macrophage.

Functions

The monocyte-macrophage complex has three well-established physiologic functions: (1) the removal of damaged erythrocytes, (2) the interaction with lymphocytes at certain phases of the immune response, and (3) defense reactions against certain classes of microorganisms. These cells are probably also involved in wound repair and remodelling of embryonic tissues and bone; however, these functions are less well-characterized than the three cited above.

Erythrophagocytosis

The occurrence of hemosiderin-laden macrophages in diseases characterized by excessive red cell destruction (for example, hereditary spherocytosis) or extravasation of erythrocytes into tissues (for example, Goodpasture's syndrome or mitral stenosis with pulmonary hypertension) has been recognized by morphologists for years. Less well-known is that erythrophagocytosis is often a feature, of malignant diseases of the reticuloendothelial system in which morphologically mature mononuclear phagocytes abound; for example, monocytic leukemia and histiocytic medullary reticulosis.

The phagocytosis of erythrocytes by macrophages has been studied under a variety of conditions *in vitro* for several years. It was the studies of LoBuglio, Cotran, and Jandl (1967), however, that put the mechanism involved into sharp perspective. These investigators demonstrated that monocytes have surface receptors for IgG that interact with IgG-coated red cells. The attachment of coated erythrocytes can be blocked by intact IgG or by the Fab fragments, but not by the Fc portion of the molecule or by other proteins. Huber *et al* (1968) later demonstrated that monocytes also have receptor sites for the third component of complement.

Antibody-coated red cells form a rosette around the central monocyte. The red cells in this halo are more susceptible to osmotic lysis than free erythrocytes. Erythrophagocytosis by monocytes, like phagocytosis of other particles, depends on glycolytic energy production rather than on aerobic metabolism. Not surprisingly, a macrophage has a greater erythrophagocytic capacity than a monocyte.

At present, there is no direct evidence that mononuclear phagocytes are important in the destruction of IgM-coated erythrocytes. It has been inferred, but not proved, that the tissue macrophage complex is important in the destruction of senescent red cells. The mechanism by which the aged erythrocyte might be identified and destroyed is not known. Recently, Pimstone *et al* (1970) have identified heme oxygenase—an enzyme involved in heme catabolism—in animal peritoneal macrophages. The enzyme activity normally present at low levels increases greatly after the introduction of hemoglobin into the peritoneal cavity. It is likely that the macrophages equipped with this enzyme system are critical in the clearing of extravasated hemoglobin from the tissues.

Interaction of Macrophages and Lymphocytes

The interaction of mononuclear phagocytes with lymphocytes in certain phases of the immunologic response is supported by several observations: (1) Pure populations of lymphocytes containing no phagoccytes show a reduced "blastogenic" response to specific antigens *in vitro*; addition of phagocytes restores the response to normal levels; (2) RNA, containing trace amounts of antigen prepared from animal macrophages, can induce lymphocytes to produce the corresponding antibody; (3) Human monocytes and macrophages exposed to antigen *in vitro* and then washed free of extracellular antigen can induce transformation of autologous lymphocytes; (4) Normal, nonimmune lymphoid cells can induce antibody synthesis in X-irradiated recipient animals if living macrophages containing antigen are also transferred; (5) Close contact and cytoplasmic connections have been demonstrated between lymphocytes and macrophages *in vivo*; (6) After administration of a radioactive antigen to an intact animal, the label is found associated with medullary macrophages as well as with surface processes of dendritic reticular cells within the cortical areas of lymph nodes. The reticular cells are in intimate contact with the surfaces of surrounding lymphocytes.

The initial studies of the interaction of macrophages and lymphocytes in the early phases of the immune response suggested that the macrophage "processed" the antigen in some way and that the macrophage RNA "instructed" the lymphocyte or acted as in adjuvant enhancing the immunogenicity of minute amounts of antigen. The recent studies of Roelants and Goodman (1969) make the RNA-instruction hypothesis unlikely, although the adjuvant-hypothesis is still tenable. Small amounts of antigen are retained in immunogenic form within or on the surface of the macrophage for long periods of time, although the major portion is quickly degraded;. My own feeling is that macrophages probably act as sponges accumulating antigen and keeping a small amount available in a form capable of stimulating closely associated responsive lymphocytes.

Although the precise mechanism of macrophage-lymphocyte interaction in the immune response is not known, certain features of this interaction have been characterized. It seems clear that intimate contact between the surfaces of the mononuclear cell and the lymphocyte is necessary for maximal lymphocyte respons *in vitro*. Extracts of macrophages, conditioned medium from macrophage cultures, or macrophages separated from lymphocytes by a permeable Millipore membrane, are much less effective in inducing lymphocyte blastogenic transformation. *In vitro*, the central macrophage and surrounding lymphocyte form an "immunologic island"; the formation of such clusters is required for blastogenic transformation and continued division of antibody-forming cells. A metabolically intact monocyte or macrophage is necessary for this process.

Antigen-sensitized macrophages are more efficient than monocytes at inducing blastogenic transformation of lymphocytes *in vitro*. It appears likely that in the presence of sensitized macrophages, a higher proportion of the lymphocyte population enters the first detectable phase of DNA synthesis. Macrophages are more efficient than monocytes at making contact with autologous lymphocytes, and are capable of binding more antigen.

Early in the *in vitro* interaction of lymphocytes with mononuclear phagocytes, the invloved cells are always in close contact and are few in number. When blastogenic transformation is well-advanced, the cell clusters are large and contain many untransformed as well as transformed lymphocytes. The untransformed cells show no nuclear labeling and therefore are probably lymphocytes initially added to the cultures rather than those deriving from division of transformed lymphocytes. If these events observed *in vitro* reflect similar processes in the intact animal, they suggest that dispersion of immunologically stimulated lymphocytes and attachment of unstimulated lymphocytes to a cluster of reactive cells may be simultaneous phenomena.

A recent interesting observation in this exciting field of macrophage-lymphocyte interaction is that the presence of mononuclear phagocytes enhances the production of interferon by pure populations of lymphocytes stimulated with mitogen. This observation suggests that macrophages and lymphocytes may be coordinated in more than one type of host-defense reaction.

Bactericidal Activity

The neutrophil is generally regarded as the first line of defense against the common bacterial pathogens. The macrophage is thought to be the major cellular defense against facultative intracellulr parasites such as *Mycobacterium leprae, Mycobacterium tuberculosis, Listeria monocytogenes,* and Brucella species. Studies of genetic defects of neutrophil function, including chronic granulomatous disease (CGD) and absent neutrophil myeloperoxidase, suggest that a principal component of the neutrophil-bactericidal mechanism involves inctracellular hydrogen peroxide generation and interaction with myeloperoxidase. In some species, neutrophil cationic proteins may also play a role. Macrophages lack myeloperoxidase and probably lack cartionic proteins. What, then, are the bactericidal mechanisms of this cell?

The bactericidal activity of phagocytes may be thought of as having two components: as ingestion or phagocytic phase and a killing phase.

Phagocytosis

Particle ingestion by human monocytes has a broad pH optimum. The macrophage is in general a faster and more efficient phagocyte than the antecedent monocyte. Particle ingestion by human monocytes is accompanied by enhanced glucose oxidation and oxygen utilization similar to that in phagocytosis by neutrophils. Monocyte and macrophage phagocytosis occurs in the presence of inhibitors of oxidative metabolism and of RNA synthesis, but is inhibited by interference with glycolysis. In contrast,the pinocytotic activity of macrophages is markedly reduced by interference with aerobic mechanisms of energy production and of RNA and protein synthesis. In contrast to animal peritoneal macrophages or the human macrophage grown *in vitro* from blood monocytes, the human alveolar macrophage appears to require both aerobic and anaerobic mechanisms of energy production for phagocytosis of microorganisms.

Killing

The mechanisms by which macrophages kill an organism once phagocytized have been little studied. We have recently begun to investigate this problem, using cultivated human macrophages and *Listeria monocytogenes* as the test system. Certain facts have emerged. The first is that bacterial killing is at least in part dependent on availabel oxygen; i.e., the fraction of organisms killed is greatly reduced at partial pressures of oxygen below 16 mm of mercury.

While studying drugs used in the treatment of intracellular parasitosis, we observed that Clofazimine (B663), a compound used in the treatment of leprosy, enhanced macrophage killing ability without impairing the viability of the organisms in short-term cultures. This observation opens up the possibility of exploring the mechanism by which macrophages kill. B663 is a phenazine derivative. Like other phenazines, it acts as a redox agent and is able to stimulate cellular oxygen consumption and hydrogen peroxide generation. These two observations—dependence on molecular oxygen and stimulation by B663—suggest that macrophage-killing mechanisms may in part depend on intracellular hydrogen peroxide formation.

Table 9.2
Phagocytosis by Human Macrophages, Monocytes and Neutrophils

Particle	Time for Phagocytosis (min)	Cells with Ingested Particles (%)		
		Macrophage	Monocyte	Neutrophil
Candida albicans	15	98 ± 2	90 ± 7	97 ± 3
	60	98 ± 2	94 ± 5	99 ± 1
Staphylococcus aureus	15	90 ± 8	58 ± 10	74 ± 3
	60	98 ± 2	97 ± 2	99 ± 1
Listeria monocytogenes	90	95 ± 2	49 ± 3	NT

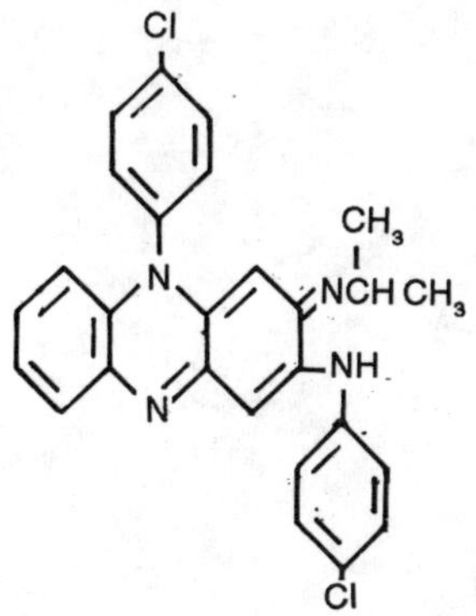

Fig. 9.1. Structural formula of Clofazimine.

We have considerably more to learn about the ability of macrophages to kill microorganisms. Mackaness and his colleagues, as well as other investigators, observed that macrophages from mice immunized with living tubercle bacilli are better able to control these organisms than cells from nonimmunized animals. The enhanced resistance seems to be nonspecific in that it is directed against Brucella, Listeria, and certain other intracellular parasites, as well as the immunizing organism. Nonlethal infection with any of these facultative intracellular bacteria is characterized by the development of delayed hypersensitivity, by a form of acquired resistance that cannot be passively transferred with serum, and by enhanced antibacterial activity of the macrophages of the host. The mechanisms of this enhanced resistance are still completely unknown.

10

Thrombocytopoiesis

Blood Platelets are produced by megakaryocytes, and the numbers of platelets produced appear to be influenced by a homestatic control mechanism. Perturbation of the thrombocytopoietic system by depletion of circulating platelets is followed by changes in the megakaryocytes that, in turn, seem to lead to production of increased numbers of platelets. However, these changes are initiated, in large measure, at the level of megakaryocyte precursors rather than by a direct effect of the feedback mechanism on the recognizable megakaryocytes. Since cellular division does not occur in the compartment of recognizable megakaryocytes, and only a portion of the most immature forms retain the capacity for nuclear replication, proliferative potential and the consequent implied responsiveness to stimulation should be properties of precursor cells that cannot be identified as being committed to megakaryocytopoiesis by morphological criteria. Responses of the thrombocytopoietic system to the stimulation of platelet depletion have suggested, in fact, what some of the characteristics of these precursor cells might be.

Thrombocytopoiesis After Acute Platelet Depletion

Acute depletion of circulating platelets by thrombocytopheresis in rats is followed by a gradual increase of the platelet count to supranormal values. This reactive thrombocytosis suggests that there is stimulation of platelet production as a result of thrombocytopenia. Platelet production does not increase immediatley; rather, there is an initial period of two days during which the numbers of platelets that are produced remain about normal. Thereafter, production rate increases, and thrombocytosis develops. During the two-day lag period, several changes in megakaryocytopoiesis have been described. For the first nine hours, megakaryocytes remain normal in size. The macromegakaryocytosis that occurs in response to the stimulus of thrombocytopenia is apparent in the immatur recognizable megakaryocytes 24 hours after onset of thrombocytopenia. Macrocytic cells pass in a wave-like manner through the compartment of recognizable megakaryocytes, appearing and disappearing first in the most immature, or stage 1, cells. The maximum degree of macrocytosis occurs in stage III (mature, granular megakaryocytes) two days after platelet depletion. The sequential appearance and disappearance of macrocytes suggests that the stimulus or production of large cells is effective at the level of stage I megakaryocytes or unrecognizable precursors rather than at the level of more mature differentiated megakaryocytes. The delay in appearance of macromegakaryocytosis after initiation of the thrombocytopenic stimulus may be due to the time required for affected precursors to differentiate, but it may also be a reflection of the time required for elaboration or accumulation of a critical concentration of a thrombopoietin. The fact that the three maturation stages of recognizable megakaryocytes achieve comparable degrees of macrocytosis further suggests that macrocytosis is due not simply to stimulation of cytoplasmic growth of differentiated cells. In response to thrombocytopenia, it appears that cells are macrocytic when they differentiate from the precursor compartments and that their subsequent growth is normal.

During the first postthrombocytopenic day, differentiation into and maturation through the compartment of recognizable megakaryocytes occur at normal rates. Acceleration is apparent during the second postthrombocytopenic day. The megakaryocytes that differentiate under the influence of the thrombocytopenic state mature more rapidly than normal, but the rate of replacement of unlabeled by labeled megakaryocytes after an injection of tritiated thymidine (^{3}HTdR) suggests that the prexistent megakaryocytes, which were differentiated before induction of thrombocytopenia, may also be stimulated to mature and produce platelets during the second postthrombocytopenic day.

Table 10.1
Thrombocytopoiesis after Acute Thrombocytopenia in Rats

A. 48 Hours: Normal numbers of platelets produced

1. 9 hours: Recognizable megakaryocytes normal
2. 24 hours: Macrocytosis of stages I and II megakaryocytes
3. 24-48 hours: Acceleration of megakaryocyte turnover

   Increasing numbers of megakaryocytes.
4. 48 hours: Maximum macrocytosis of stage III megakaryocytes

B. After 48 hours: Increased numbers of platelets produced

After a single, short-lived episode of thrombocytopenia, we observed no shift in the differential count of megakaryocytes of the three maturation stages in conjunction with accelerated maturation. Therefore it appeared that accelerated influx balanced accelerated maturation so that little, if any, increase in numbers of megakaryocytes would occur. When thrombocytopenia was maintained by repeated injections of antiplatelet serum, Odell *et al* (1969) found that megakaryocyte number just began to increase 24 hours after the onset of thrombocytopenia. Thus sustained thrombocytopenia may be necessary to produce a demonstrable increase in megakaryocyte numbers.

Thrombocytopoiesis with Sustained Platelet Depletion

When thrombocytopenia is maintained for four to six days, the pattern of labeling of megakaryocytes by ^{3}HTdR indicates that acceleration of their turnover rate persists. Thus there are increased numbers of megakaryocytes being produced and, in turn, producing platelets in any given period of time. For this reason, quantification of megakaryocytopoiesis from a static determination of cell numbers without consideration of turnover rate would tend to underestimate total megakaryocytopoiesis.

The capacity of the megakaryocytic system to expand in terms of numbers of cells is not completely clear. Harker (1968a) found that megakaryocyte numbers were only moderately increased in rats after four daily thrombocytophereses, but that after ten days, they had increased to more than three times normal. Odell *et al* (1969) found that

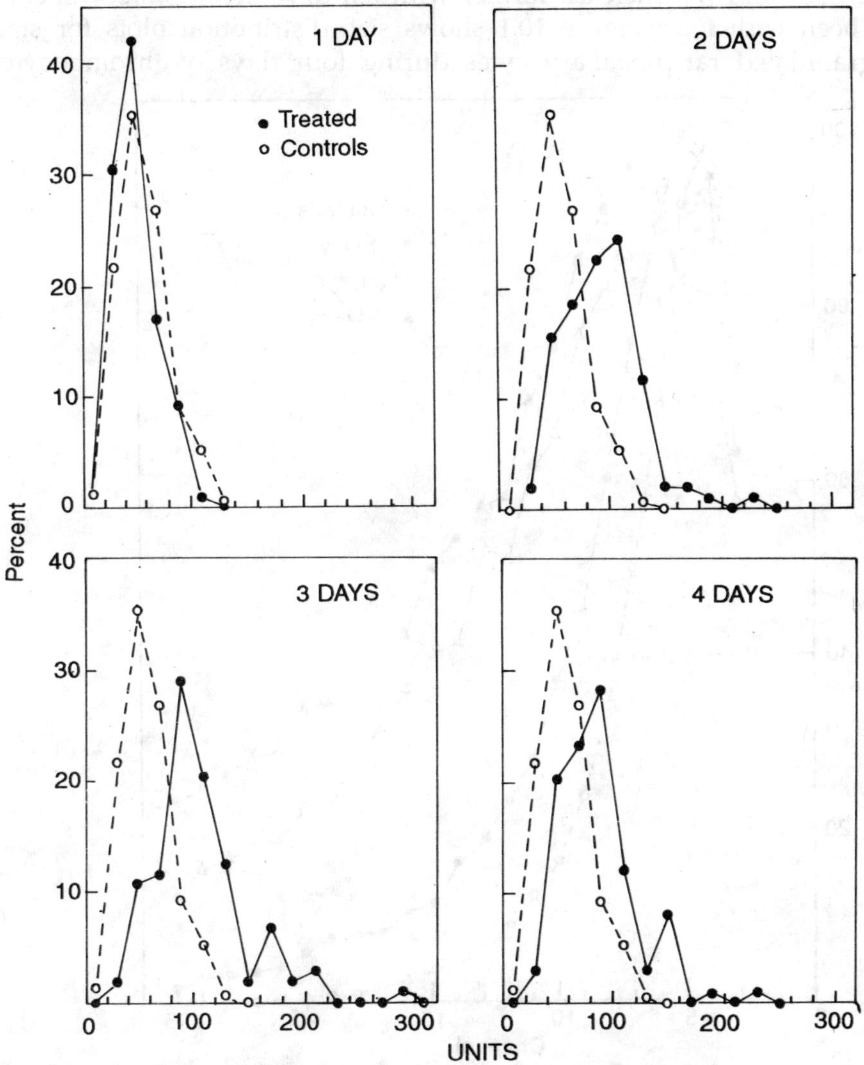

Fig. 10.1. Size distribution plots of stage III rat megakaryocytes during sustained thrombocytopenia produced by daily injection of rabbit antirat platelet serum on days 0, 1, 2 and 3. Cell size is expressed in arbitrary units. Each curve for treated rats represents 99 to 112 megakaryocytes from 3 rats. The control curve represents 153 megakaryocytes from 4 rats.

daily injections of antiplatelet serum (APS) resulted in megakaryocyte numbers of more than two times normal in 2.5 days after initiation of the stimulus with no further increase during the next 1.5 days.

While numerical expansion is not clear, available data indicate that megakaryocytes have only a limited potential to become macrocytic and that they achieve maximum macrocytosis early in the response to thrombocytopenia. The degree of macrocytosis may be partly dependent on the severity of the thrombocytopenia, but Harker (1968a) found that cell size did not increase further with ten days of thrombocytopenia over what it had been with four. Figure 10.1 shows size distribution plots for stage III, completely granulated rat megakaryocytes during four days of thrombocytopenia

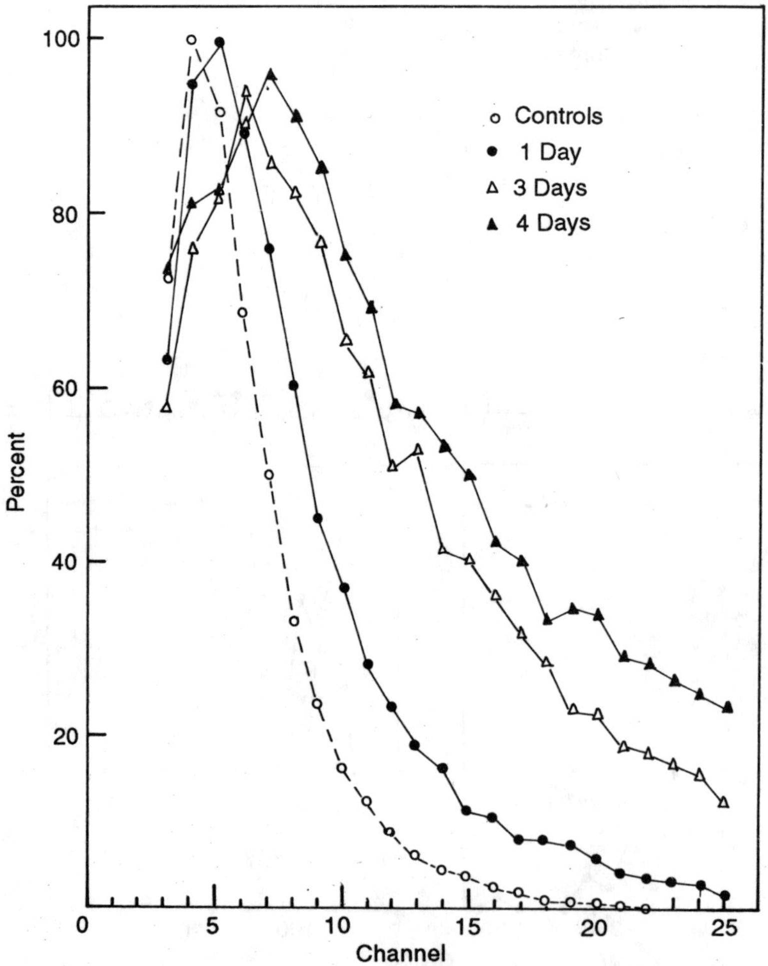

Fig. 10.2. Size distribution plots for the platelets from the same rats shown in fig. 10.1. The abscissa shows channel number of the plotter, and the ordinate is expressed as percentage of the modal value. For each rat, 2 plots were done and averaged; each curve shown is the average of 3 treated rats or 4 controls. The plotter was calibrated with suspensions of rat and human red blood cells, and the control modal value at channel 4 for rat platelets corresponds to an average volume of 3.3 cubic microns. Values included in channels 3 through 25 ranged from 1.9 to 23.5 cubic microns.

maintained by daily injection of rabbit antirat platelet serum. Size estimations were made from bone marrow smears as previously described. The units of size differ from those previously reported because a different microscopic magnification was used. As in the experiments with a single episode of platelet depletion, macrocytosis became prominent in stage III megakaryocytes two days after onset of thrombocytopenia. Sustained thrombocytopenia did not result in a further increase in megakaryocyte size.

In the same animals, relative platelet volumes were also determined, and these are shown in Figure 10.2. Platelet rich plasma (PRP) was separated from cardiac blood (collected under ether anesthesia), anticoagulated with ACD-A, by centrifugation at 140 × g for 15 minutes at room temperature. Before and after centrifugation, the blood and PRP were kept in a constant temperature room at 37°C. PRP was diluted in Isoton also at 37°C, and platelet size distribution was plotted immediately on a Coulter model J plotter with a 50-micron aperture tube. The Coulter counter was kept at regular room temperature. Plots obtained of platelets separated by this method of centrifugation were identical to those of platelets separated by sedimentation of red cells at 37 °C.

Platelets circulating one day after initiation of APS injections were somewhat larger than normal. These platelets were formed from normocytic megakaryocytes, and their size may be typical of normal, newly formed platelets, which have been reported by others to be larger than platelets that have aged in the circulation. No two-day curve is presented in Figure 10.2 because platelet counts were too low at that time to permit separation and plotting. On days three and four of sustained thrombocytopenia, platelet sizes were considerably increased, and a substantial proportion of the population appeared to be larger than any produced normally. These large platelets were presumably produced by macromegakaryocytes, and this suggests that large megakaryocytes may produce platelets of large size rather than simply producing large numbers of platelets. Dilution of normal rat platelets *in vitro* with normal rat plasma or plasma from a rat after four daily injections of APS did not result in a change in size of the normal platelets, so neither low platelet numbers nor a plasma factor could be implicated as producing a factitious macrothrombocytosis.

During recovery from thrombocytopenia, macromegakaryocytosis was prominent for two days after the final thrombocytopenic stimulus. Thereafter, the size of stage III megakaryocytes gradually returned to normal. In these animals, macrothrombocytosis became progressively less prominent also. Correlation of platelet and megakaryocyte size is more tenuous under these circumstances than in those rats shown in Figures 10.1 and 10.2 where circulating platelets were destroyed daily by APS and, hence, pltaelets did not age in the circulation. The animals represented in Figures 10.3 and 10.4 were recovering from thrombocytopenia, and their platelet counts gradually increased from about $0.25 \times 10^6/mm^3$ on day one to about $2 \times 10^6/mm^3$ on day five. Consequently, the decrease in platelet size may have been due, in part, to aging of the cells in the circulation as well as to production of smaller platelets.

The magnitude of the thrombocytopoietic response to thrombocytopenia has been judged in part by the number of platelets produced, and these observations indicate that

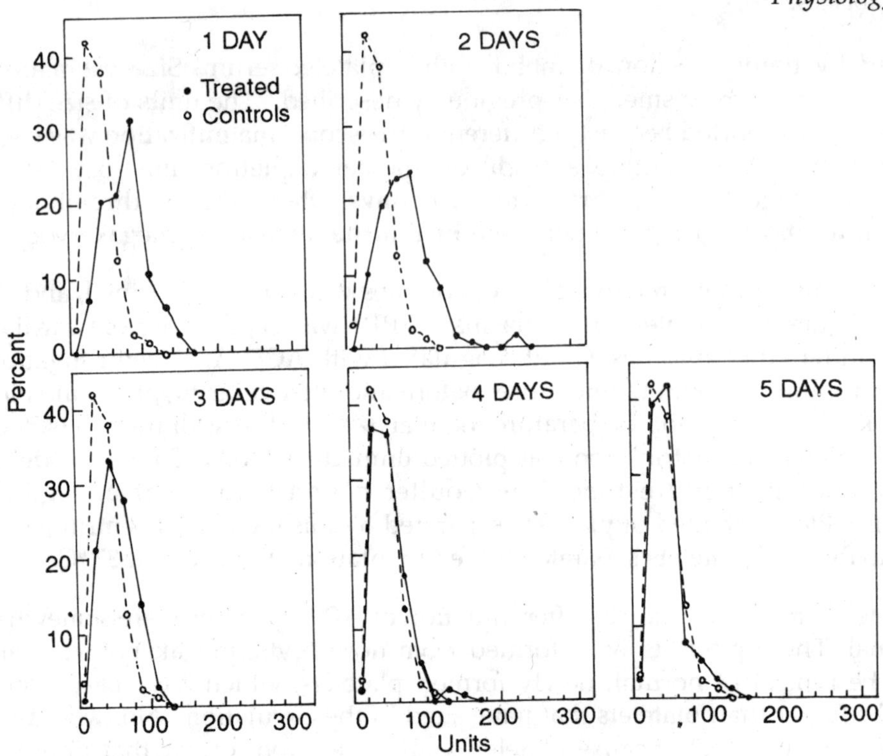

Fig. 10.3. Size distribution plots of stage III rat megakaryocytes during recovery from thrombocytopenia. Antiplatelet serum was given to induce thrombocytopenia on days -2 and 0. Cell size is expressed in arbitrary units. Each curve for treated rats on days 1 to 4 represents 108 to 112 megakaryocytes from 3 rats; on day 5, 79 megakaryocytes from 2 rats; the control curve represents 190 megakaryocytes from 5 rats.

increased numbers are produced. The results of the studies reported here do not permit an accurate correlation between size of megakaryocytes and the size of the platelets they produce. However, they do indicate further that states of stimulated thrombocytopoiesis may be associated with alteration in platelet size as well as platelet number.

It could be suggested that production of macrothrombocytes may be a mechanism to compensate partially for the hemostatic defect of thrombocytopenia. Cronkite *et al* (1955) reported that newly formed platelets in the blood of dogs during recovery from irradiation were more active in accelerating prothrombin conversion than the aging platelets present in the blood during the degenerative phase. The new platelets also appeared larger than the aging ones. More recent studies have tended to confirm the greater hemostatic effectiveness of newly formed platelets. However, with regard to specific platelet functions such as adherence to collagen or glass beads, discrepant results have been reported. In view of the rapid turnover of megakaryocytes in response to thrombocytopenia, macrothrombocytes may represent platelets that are released from megakaryocytes that are more immature than those that would normally release platelets. Rapid maturation may also interfere with complete formation of platelet demarcation membranes within the megakaryocyte cytoplasm.

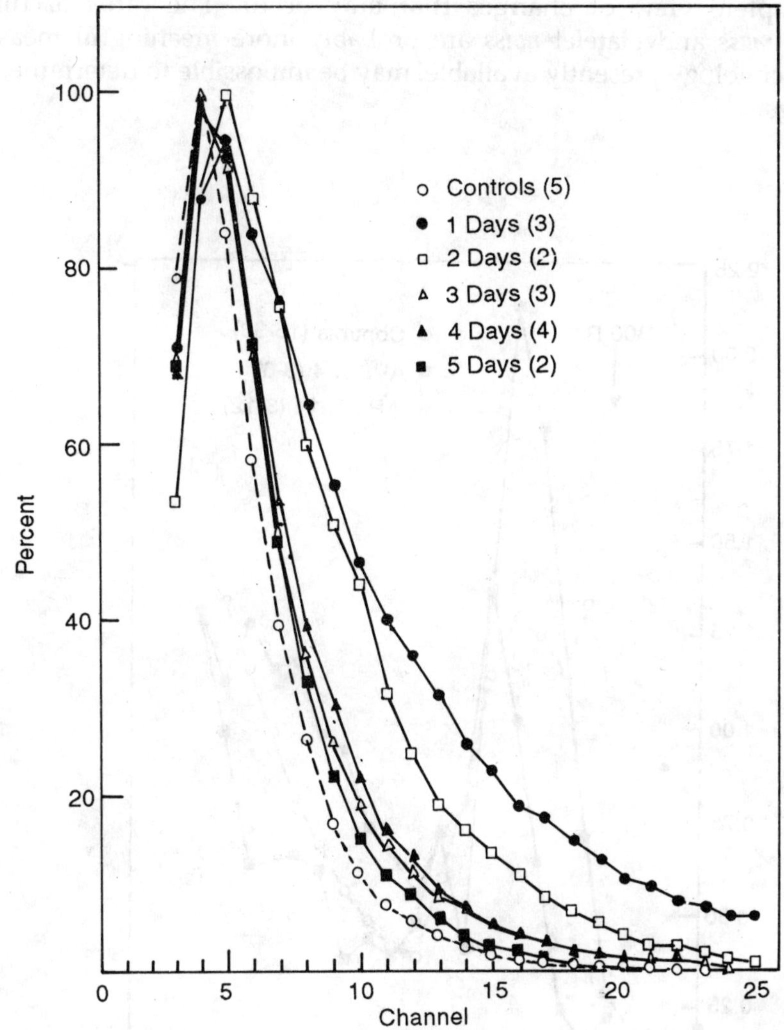

Fig. 10.4. Size distribution plots for the platelts from the rats shown in fig. 10.3. The number of rats represented by each curve is shown in parenthesis. See legend of fig. 10.2 for further explanation.

The turnover rate of newly formed platelets during recovery from thrombocytopenia is not clear. When a population of rat platelets, all two days old or less, was labeled with tritiated diisopropylfluorophosphate (^{3}H-DFP) and transfused to normal rats, they were destroyed at a normal rate (Ebbe *et al* 1970). Adelson *et al* (1963) reported similar findings with dog platelets labeled with ^{32}P-orthophosphate. Estimation of platelet turnover *in situ* during recovery from thrombocytopenia has been hampered by the apparent labeling of megakaryocytes by ^{3}H-DFP.

From the observations summarized so far, it seems clear that many of the measurements previously used to quantify platelet production and turnover probably give an incomplete view of changes that may occur. The rates of turnover of megakaryocyte *mass* and platelet *mass* are probably more meaningful measurements, but, with the technology presently available, may be impossible to determine, especially in human beings.

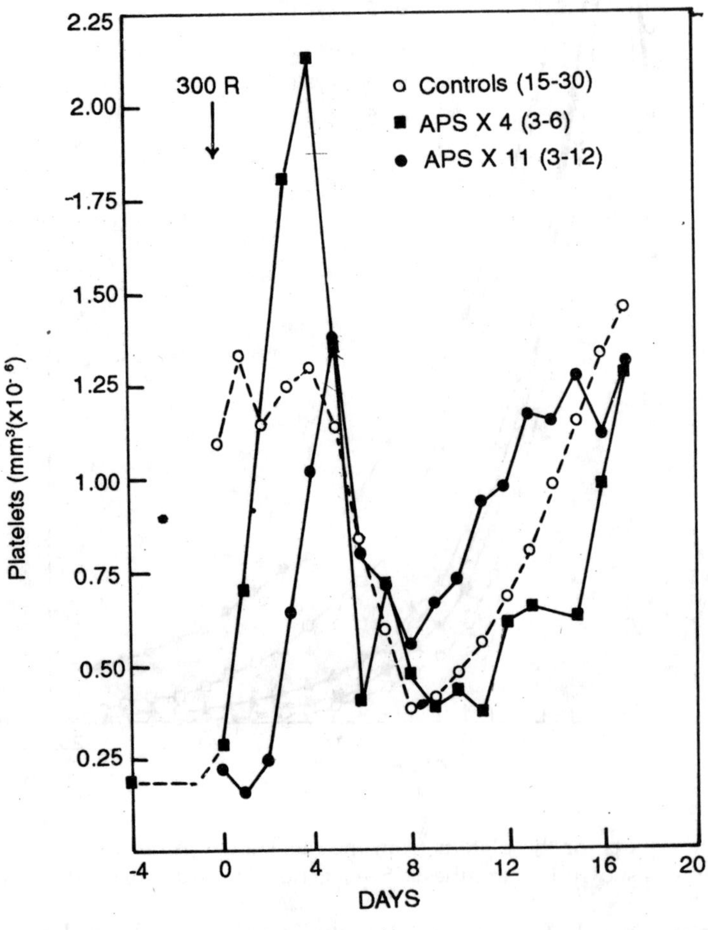

Fig. 10.5. Average platelet counts of mice given 300 R total body x-irradiation on day 0. Number of mice represented by each point is shown in parenthesis. "APS × 4" means that the mice received antiplatelet serum on days -3, -2 and -1 before irradiation; platelet counts were checked by tail vein puncture ~3 hours after the initial injection. "APS × 1" means that the mice received a single injection immediately before or after irradiation.

Effect of Radiation on the Response to Thrombocytopenia

When normal mice are exposed to sublethal doses of X-radiation (200-400 R), their platelet counts show a characteristic response. For the first four days after irradiation, there is no substantial decrease. This means that there are cells resistant to these doses of radiation and capable of maintaining platelet production for about four days.

Discontinuance of heterologous antiplatelet seum (APS) injections after four daily injections to maintain thrombocytopenia in mice is followed by a prompt increase in levels of circulating platelets to thrombocytotic levels before they gradually retun to normal (Ebbe and Stohlman 1970). Sublethal irradiation, given after the four days of thrombocytopenic stimulation, does not prevent the development of postthrombocytopenic thrombocytosis during the first few days after irradiation. Platelet counts go as high in the chronically stimulated mice exposed to radiation as in nonirradiated controls. This finding indicates that changes established in a radioresistant compartment, such as increase in cell number, size, and maturtion rate, are the determinants of the degree of reactive thrombocytosis. However, treatment of mice with 300 R immediately before or after a single injection of APS prevents the thrombocytotic response to acute immunothrombocytopenia. Therefore, the early, initial response to thrombocytopenia appears to depend on stimulation of a radiosensitive cell population.

Effect of Thrombocytopenia on the Response to Radiation

Sublethal irradiation of mice produces thrombocytopenia, and the platelet counts begin to fall after the lag period of four days described above. Lowest platelet levels occur on the eighth or ninth postirradiation day as expected if production ceased on the fourth day and the platelets had a life span of four to five days. With an X-ray dose of 300 R, platelet counts return to the normal range on the thirteenth or fourteenth postirradiation day. When mice were irradiated after four days of stimulation to the thrombocytopoietic system by repeated injections of APS, recovery from radiation-induced thrombocytopenia appeared to be somewhat delayed even though the degree of thrombocytopenia was not changed. This finding implies an increased radiosensitivity that, in turn, suggests that chronic stimulation may result in an increased proportion of the megakaryocytic precursors being in active cell cycle and, hence, susceptible to damage by radiation.

Acute stimulation, produced by a single injection of APS and shortlived platelet depletion during the period immediately before or after exposure to sublethal doses of radiation, had a different effect. The radiation-induced thrombocytopenia was neither as severe nor as prolonged as it was in control irradiated mice. This modification suggests that the feedback stimulant (thrombopoietin) acts on a cell population that is in part radioresistant. The effect of acute platelet depletion on the course of radiation-induced thrombocytopenia was apparent from the peripheral platelet counts eight and more days after the stimulus was applied. At that time, the animals that had been treated with APS immediately before or after irradiation were making more platelets. Thus, stimulation of radioresistant cells by thrombocytopenia appears to result in expansion of the compartment of mature megakaryocytes eight days later. In normal, nonirradiated mice, the response to the paltelet depletion induced by a single injection of APS consists of a gradual development of a transient postthrombocytopenic thrombocytosis which had subsided by the eighth day with return of platelet levels to normal. Persistence of the stimulatory effect in irradiated mice may have been due to the failure to develop postthrombocytopenic thrombocytosis and consequent inhibition of megakyocytopoiesis, or it may have been related to changes in the cellular environment due to bone marrow depopulation by radiation. Acute stimulation at the time of irradiation may simply have resulted in expansion of the cell population, which was capable of responding to the decrease in concentration of circulating platelets that first began about five days postirradiation.

Conclusions

Figure 10.6 summarizes our current hypothesis about the constitution of the

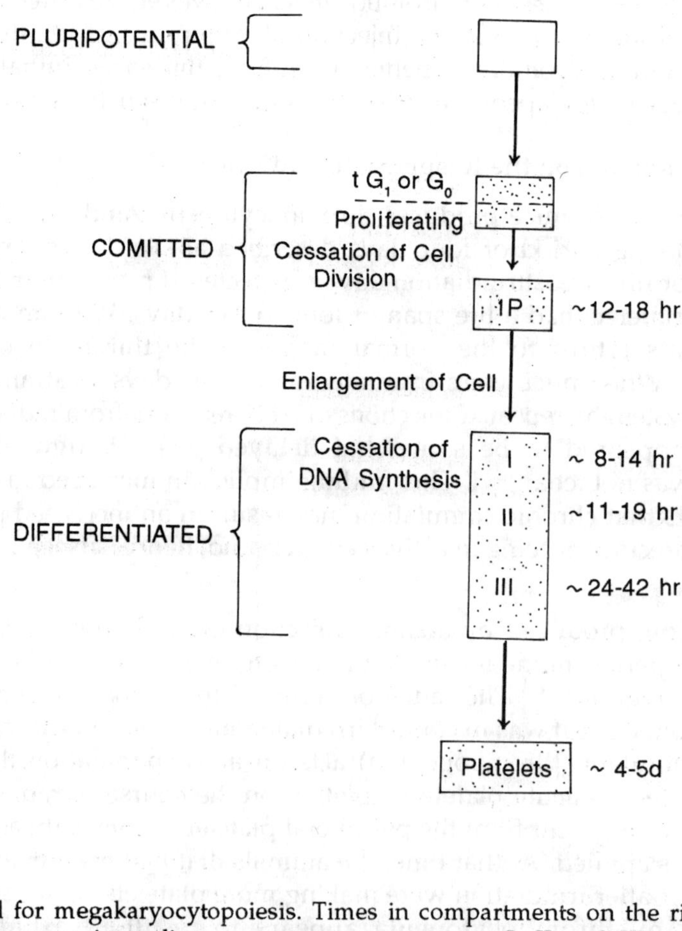

Fig. 10.6. Model for megakaryocytopoiesis. Times in compartments on the right are estimates for normal rats. IP means immediate precursor compartment. I, II and III refer to morphological subdivisions of the compartment of recognizable megakaryocytes.

thrombocytopoietic cell system. The times in compartments are estimates for the normal rat. The role of the pluripotential stem cell in maintaining normal megakaryocytopoiesis and in adjusting to states of perturbed thrombocytopoiesis has not been defined. The evidence that megakaryocytes originate from the same common precursor as red cells and granulocytes has been reviewed, as have the reasons for postulating an intermediate committed stem cell compartment in which cell proliferation is followed by DNA synthesis without cell division and consequent polyploidy in the immediate precursor compartment (IP) before differentiation into recognizable megakaryocytes.

The earlier committed stem cell is thought to be the 2N megakaryocyte previously assigned mainly a proliferative role. However, if one assumes that thrombopoietin does not directly affect the pluripotential stem cell, then the studies in irradiated mice indicate that there is a cell population, in the thrombocytopoietic system that is both partially radioresistant and responsive to thrombopoietin. For this reason, the earlier 2N megakaryocytes have been proposed to be in a state of prolonged cell cycle, with prolonged G_1. or no cell cycle (G_0). If this postulate proves to be correct, then comparisons between megakaryocytopoiesis and erythropoiesis could be drawn. In the sublethally irradiated dog, erythropoiesis is responsive to stimulation by acute anemia during the immediate postirradiation period, and the erythropoietin-responsive stem cell has been demonstrated to differ from the pluripotential stem cell and to be in a state of prolonged G_1 in the normal steady state.

After irradiation, normal thrombocytopoiesis may be temporarily maintained (for about four days in mice) by radioresistant differentiated and immediate precursor compartments. After that, platelet production would drop, owing to radiation-induced damage to the proliferating precursor compartment, and the rate of subsequent recovery would depend on rate of replacement from precursors that had not been damaged by radiation. Acute stimulation shortly before or after irradiation may hasten recovery by stimulating proliferation of quiescent precursors and making more cells available to respond to the stimulus of the radiation-induced depletion of bone marrow megakaryocytes or peripheral platelets. Alternatively, it may simply provide an early stimulus or proliferation, which is automatically followed by an orderly maturation and differentiation of megakaryocytic cells. With more chronic stimulation, a new steady state may be established in which the precursor cells are at least as radiosensitive as normal ones and perhaps, slightly more so if more than a normal proportion enter active cell cycle.

It has been proposed that there is a correlation between ploidy and cell size and that macromegakaryocytosis is due to an increased content of DNA in megakaryocytes. This effect could be achieved by stimulation of nuclear replication in the immediate precursor compartment or in those early stage I megakaryocytes that retain the ability to synthesize DNA. With prolonged thrombocytopenia, it might be suggested that the thrombopoietic stimulus would be more intense than with a single, short-lived episode of thrombocytopenia. The fact that megakaryocytes do not become progressively larger when thrombocytopenia is prolonged suggests that thrombopoietin does not directly stimulate DNA synthesis in these compartments. Alternatively, maximum stimulation may be achieved with a brief period of thrombocytopenia, but this seems somewhat unlikely in view of the report of a progressive increase in megakaryocyte numbers with prolongation of the thrombocytopenia and the differences between the effects of acute and chronic stimulation on the response to radiation.

An alternative explanation for increased ploidy and macromegakaryocytosis would be the influx of cells into the nondividing compartment at higher than normal ploidy values in response to stimulation. Maturation of the later stages of megakaryocytopoiesis is accelerated in the thrombocytopenic animal and, by analogy to erythropoiesis, it could be proposed that stimulation of the proliferating committed stem cells causes them to mature rapidly, skip final division, and enter the nondividing immediate precursor compartment with twice the normal complement of megakaryocyte volume as the maximum increase that has been reported in rats and man responding to peripheral platelet depletion.

HUMORAL CONTROL OF THROMBOPOIESIS

Much evidence exists that production of platelets by megakaryocytes reflects the level of circulating platelets. Thrombocytopenia whether produced by exchange transfusion or administration of platelet antiserum is followed by increased production of platelets, and platelet levels rise to greater than normal ("rebound thrombocytosis"). This is associated with an increase in the number and size of megakaryocytes, an increase in their rate of maturation; and an increase in the influx of precursor cells into the pool of identifiable megakaryocytes. Conversely, thrombocytosis produced by hypertransfusion of platelets is followed by rebound thrombocytopenia, which has been interpreted as secondary to suppression of platelet production.

Various isotopic labels have been used to study thrombopoiesis following transfusion-induced thrombocytosis. In studies of acute thrombocytosis, produced by a single infusion of platelet, Ebbe *et al* were not able to demonstrate alterations in platelet production in rats in which platelet levels had been raised to 2½ times normal, using either platelets that had been labeled with tritiated diisopropylfluorophosphate (^{3}HDFP), or by studying labeling indices or differential counts of megakaryocytes following the *in vitro* administration of tritiated thymidine (^{3}HTdR). Some animals in which platelet levels were acutely raised to six times normal showed a slight decrease in immature (Stage I) megakaryocytes, suggestive of suppression of thrombopoiesis. However, there was no significant change in the labeling indices or mean grain counts, and there was no reciprocal increase in more mature (Stage III) megakryocytes. The authors concluded that neither rate of maturation nor influx of precursor cells into the compartment of megakaryocytes had been affected by thrombocytosis. In these experiments, ^{3}HTdR was administered before induction of thrombocytosis, and it is possible that changes would have been detected if the isotope had been administered after elevation of platelet counts. Sustained thrombocytosis (levels 3 times normal for 5 days) decreased the proportion of Stage I megakaryocytes, and increased the proportion of Stage III megakryocytes in the bone marrow of rats, 4-5 days after initiation of thrombocytosis; but labeling indices remained normal.

Table 10.2
Effect of Transfusion-Induced Thrombocytosis on Incorporation of Isotopes into Platelets, In Vivo

		Thrombocytosis			
Isotope	*Recipient*	*No. Days of Transfusion*	*Platelet Count (X normal)*	*% Decrease of Incorporation of Isotope*	*Reference*
$Na_2{}^{35}SO_4$	Rat	3	9 X	52%	Odell *et al* (1967)
$NA_2{}^{35}SO_4$	Rat	4	4 X	62%	Harker (1968)
^{75}SeM*	Rabbit	5	4 X	41%	Shreiner and Levin (1969)

* Selenomethionine-^{75}Se.

Measurements of the rate of appearance of radioactively labeled platelets in the circulation, after administration of isotopes that are incorporated into megakaryocytes, has provided evidence that thrombocytosis suppresses platelet production, as summarized in Table 10.2. Incorporation of $Na_2{}^{35}SO_4$ and selenomethionine-^{75}Se (^{75}SeM) in platelets was significantly reduced by sustained elevation of platelet levels at 4-9 times normal, in rats and rabbits. Reduction of numbers of megakaryocytes three to four days following induction of thrombocytosis and a decrease in megakaryocyte number and size after four to ten days of thrombocytosis also suggest decreased thrombopoiesis. Harker demonstrated a correlation between megakaryocyte mass and incorporation of $Na_2{}^{35}SO_4$ in circulating platelets.

These data suggest that sustained thrombocytosis is a more potent suppressor of thrombopoiesis than acute thrombocytosis. Furthermore, the duration of thrombocytosis appeared to influence the level of suppression of thrombopoiesis (Fig. 10.7). Elevation of platelet levels to greater than 2-3 times normal may be necessary to demonstrate these changes. Therefore, it appears that thrombopoiesis is not totally suppressed by sustained thrombocytosis, just as erythropoiesis is not uniformly suppressed by polycythemia.

Both stimulation and suppression of thrombopoiesis, after production of thrombocytopenia or thrombocytosis, respectively, are detectable only after a delay of approximately 24 hours. An increase in the duration of thrombocytopenia or thrombocytosis results in more marked alterations in the rate of thrombopoiesis. The studies of Ebbe *et al*, Harker, and Odell *et al* have indicated that adjustments in the rate of thrombopoiesis occur at the level of megakaryocytic precursors or Stage I megakaryocytes; and that following such changes, a population of megakaryocytes that has been altered in number, size, and rate of maturation can be identified in the bone marrow. Maximum rebound thrombocytosis and rebound thrombocytopenia, following

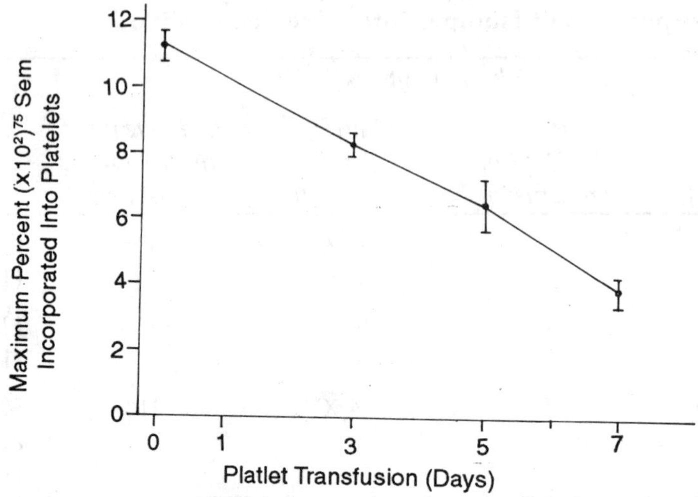

Fig. 10.7. Effect of duration of thrombocytosis on maximum levels of ^{75}SeM in circulating platelets. Platelet transfusions were administered daily for the number of days indicated. Plateler levels were maintained 2 to 4 times normal in each group. The Mean ± 1 SE is shown. Increased duration of thrombocytosis was associated with a decrease in levels of ^{75}SeM in platelets.

induction of thrombocytopenia or thrombocytosis, occur approximately six days after alteration of the platelet levels of rabbits and rats. This period of time is that required for two consecutive populations (cohorts) of megakaryocytes to enter the marrow pool, mature and release platelets. These observations suggest that there is an effective feedback mechanism by which the rate of thrombopoiesis is affected but the level of the circulating platelet mass. Odell *et al* (1969) and Ebbe *et al* (1968c) have suggested that the time lag between alteration of platelet levels and detection of altered megakaryocytopoiesis reflects either mechanisms effective at the level of precursor cells, or a delay in the production of a humoral susbtance that is responsible for altered thrombopoiesis.

Evidence for Humoral Control of Thrombopoiesis

In many studies, elevations in platelet counts have been interpreted as indicative of the presence of thrombopoietic stimulating factor (s), and these have been summarized in two recent reviews. Dependence on alteration of platelet levels may not be a reliable measure of thrombopoietic activity, since circulating platelet levels do not necessarily reflect only alterations in rate of production. Variations in platelet counts may occur due to a variety of factors. Elevation of platelet counts in animals following administration of test plasma has not always been reproducible. Nevertheless, these studies have suggested the presence of thrombopoietic stimulating factor (s) in normal plasma; plasma from thrombocytopenic donors; and plasma from patients with myeloproliferative disorders and idiopathic thrombocytopenic purpura. Two families have been reported in which some members apparently had a deficiency of a plasma component necessary for normal thrombopoiesis. Sullivan (1969) recently reported one patient in whom plasma, obtained during a period of alcohol-induced thrombocytopenia produced elevation of platelet levels when administered subsequently.

More recently, the isotopes $Na_2{}^{35}SO_4$ and ^{75}SeM have been used to detect thrombopoietic stimulating factor(s). Both isotopes are incorporated into megakaryocyte cytoplasm and subsequently appear in circulating platelets when they are released from

Table 10.2
Detection of Thrombopoietic Stimulating Activity by Measurement of Incorporation of Isotopes into Platelets, in Vivo

Isotope	*Recipient*	*Test Plasma*	*Alteration of Incorporation of Isotope*	*Reference*
$Na_2{}^{33}SO_4$	Hypertranfused Rat	Normal rat	Increased 100%	Harker (1969)
		Thrombocyto-penic rat	Increased 400%	
		Thrombocyto-tic rat	No change	
^{75}SeM*	Hypertransfused Rabbit	Normal rabbit†	Increased 52%	Shreiner and Levin (1969)
		Thrombocyto-penic rabbit †	Increased 78%	
		Thrombocyto-tic rabbit†	No change	
	Normal Rabbit	Normal rabbit†	No change	Evatt and Levin (1969)
		Thrombocyto-penic rabbit†	Increased 36%	
Na_2	Normal Rat	Normal rat	No change	Cooper *et al* (1970b)
		Thrombocyto-penic rat	Increased 49%	
	Normal Mouse	Normal mouse	No change	
		Thrombocyto-penic mouse	Increased 58%	

* Selenomethionine-^{75}Se.
† The dose of test plasma was 40 ml/Kg.

labeled megakaryocytes. These isotopes are not directly incorporated into circulating platelets.

Evatt and Levin (1969) were not able to demonstrate thrombopoietic stimulating activity in the plasma of normal rabbits when such plasma was given to normal recipients. This confirmed previous observations that normal plasma did not elevate platelet counts of normal recipients when donor and recipient were of the same species. However, plasma from thrombocytopenic donors produced a significant increase in the levels of ^{75}SeM in the platelets of normal recipients, suggesting that plasma from thrombocytopenic donors contained a substance that increased the rate of thrombopoiesis. Cooper (1970a) recently reported similar findings in rats and mice, using $Na_2{}^{35}SO_4$.

Animals with suppressed thrombopoiesis, secondary to platelet hypertransfusion, provide a more sensitive assay for the detection of thrombopoietic activity. Harker (1969) and Shreiner and Levin (1969) have demonstrated thrombopoietic stimulating activity in the plasma of both normal and thrombocytopenic animals following the administration of such plasma to rabbits or rats with transfusion-induced thrombocytosis. This resulted in increased levels of incorporation of ^{75}SeM or $Na_2{}^{35}SO_4$ into platelets (Table 10.3). Plasma from thrombocytopenic donors produced a greater increase than plasma from normal donors. Plasma from donors with transfusion-induced thrombocytosis did not contain detectable thrombopoietic stimulating activity. Furthermore, Shreiner and Levin (1969) were able to demonstrate a dose-response relationship between the volume of test plasma administered and the level of isotope that subsequently appeared in the circulating platelets. Penington (1970) recently reported detection of thrombopoietic activity in plasma from patients with idiopathic thrombocytopenic purpura. Assays were performed by measuring levels of ^{75}SeM in platelets of mice given test plasma during the period of reactive thrombocytosis that followed the administration of platelet antiserum to these animals.

Discussion

Thrombopoiesis is responsive to the level of circulating platelets. The apparent difficulty in totally suppresssing thrombopoiesis following transfusion-induced thrombocytosis may reflect a degree of regulation independent of humoral factors contained in blood, or relative insensitivity to elevations of platelet counts. Platelet mass also may play a role in the regulation of thrombopoiesis, as evidenced by the persistence of thrombocytopenia in patients in whom there is sequestration of platelets within an enlarged spleen.

The definite delay between alteration of platelet levels and demonstrable changes in megakaryocytopoiesis is compatible with a feedback mechanism that operates via a humoral substance or substances. This mechanism (or series of mechanisms) eventually alters influx of precursors into the compartment of megakaryocytes, megakaryocyte size and number and rate of maturation. However, the site of action of thrombopoietic stimulating factors (thrombopoietin) remains unknown. Furthermore, since in some studies alterations in levels of isotope following stimulation of thrombopoiesis were not associated with detectable alterations in platelet counts, it is possible that, in part, thrombopoietin acts by increasing platelet size. It has been reported that young platelets are larger and more dense than old platelets. In addition, thrombopoietin (s) may alter the number of platelets produced per megakaryocyte, as suggested by the studies of Harker (1968), Harker and Finch (1969), and Ebbe *et al* (1968b). It is likely that such factors act on megakaryocytic precursors and immature megakaryocytes, affecting both ploidy and cytoplasmic volume. Large megakaryocytes may produce either large or increased numbers of platelets.

The site of production and chemical nature of thrombopoietin(s) are unknown. The development of more sensitive and simpler assay procedures hopefully will lead to characterization of thrombopoietin(s), along with detection of the location and insight into the nature of the mechanism that senses platelet levels or platelet mass.

11

Blood Groups

Blood group substances are produced in the erythroblast, which is a nucleated cell, and are detected on the surface of the mature erythrocytic membrane. They are genetically induced and independent membrane alloantigens.

They are genetic products that express gene activity either directly or through an enzyme intermediate, such as ABO-group glycosyl transferases. These products differ between subjects and are categorized into group systems that correspond to different genetic units.

The genetic units are transmitted independently of each other during meiosis, in conformity with Mendel's second law. Two given genetic units are located on different chromosomes or are separated very far from each other or the same chromosome.

These substances are antigens and are thus immunogenic, that is, capable of stimulating antibody formation. This property is the basis for interhuman alloimmunization following pregnancy or transfusion.

THE ABO AND ASSOCIATED SYSTEMS

Two main cell lines produce ABO substances: the erythroblast, in which synthesis of erythrocytic blood group antigens occurs, and mucous cells of the digestive tract, which, in 80% of humans, the so-called secretors, are the site of synthesis of an ABH-group substances in hydrosoluble form. A and B antigens are the end product of a long series

Table 11.1
Discovery of the Main Blood Groups

ABO	1990	Lewis	1946
MN	1927	Duffy	1950
R	1927	Kidd	1951
Rh	1939	Yt	1956
Lutheran	1945	Xg	1962
Kell	1946		

of metabolic transformations in which several independent genetic systems collaborate. These systems are not neccessarily identical in a given subject's erythroblast and salivary cell.

There are three antigen systems in the erythroblast and two others in the mucous cell, which show numerous interactions. The three erythroblast systems are the classic Landsteiner ABO *systems,* which controls the presence of A and B antigens on the erythrocyte, the Hh *system* distinct from the ABO system, which was discovered after recognition of the Bombay phenotype, which determines the presence of the H substance (the H substance of O-group erythrocytes is an acceptor necessary for elaboration of A or B specificities; it is produced by the Hh system, not the ABO system), and the recently discovered I *antigen.* The role of the latter is discussed here because of the existence of complex HI, AI and BI antignes. I specificity is probably in part an acceptor of H, A and B substances.

The two systems unique to mucous cells are the ABH *secretion system.* Sese, which controls the presence of A, B, or H antigen in saliva (the Se gene appears to be a regulator of H-gene activity), and the *Lewis system,* which controls the presnce of Le^a substance in saliva (according to present theories, Lewis antigens on erythrocytic surfaces are not produced by erythroblasts but come from the plasma and secondarily adhere to erythrocytes).

ERYTHROBLASTS

ABO system

A and B Antigens and Anti-A and Anti-B Antibodies of ABO Blood Groups

In 1900, Landsteiner discovered that the serum of certain subjects agglutinated red blood cells from other subjects. He thus identified two antigens, A and B, and labeled "O" any erythrocytes not agglutinated by either of these antibodies. Subjects whose erythrocytes bear the A antigen have an anti-B agglutinin in their serum. Conversely, subjects with B antigen-bearing erythrocytes possess serum anti-A agglutinin. Subjects whose erythrocytes have no A or B antigen possess anti-A and anti-B agglutinins in their serum. Two years later, a fourth group was discovered, subjects whose erythrocytes

Table 11.2
Four Classic ABO Groups

	Antigen	*Antibody*	*Frequency in equation (%)*
A group	A	Anti-B	15
B group	B	Anti-A	9
AB group	A and B	None	3
O group	Neither A nor B	Anti-A and Anti-B	43

contained both A and B antigens and whose serum contained no anti-A and anti-B agglutinin. The scheme of "natural" anti-A and anti-B human agglutinins was thus already perfectly clear; by convention, the four classic blood groups are defined in terms of erythrocytic antigen(s): A,B,AB, and O. In fact, the O group is recognized by negative reactions to anti-A and anti-B antibodies and not by direct identification of the specific antigen.

By 1910, Von Dungern and Hirzfeld demonstrated that A and B characters were genetically controlled; Bernstein showed in 1924 that transmission was mendelian, with erythrocytic blood groups depending on the presence of two out of three A,B or O alleles (or R according to Bernstein) on two loci of the corresponding erythroblast chromosome.

Phenotype and Genotype

Serologically defined groups characterize phenotypes. The phenotype may differ from the genotype for the A and B groups. Indeed, if erythrocytes from an individual are agglutinated only by anti-A antibodies, they are said to belong to the A group, but this classification does not indicate whether the corresponding chromosome of their erythroblast nucleus contains two A genes or only one A gene associated with one O gene. Thus, the individual genotype of A phenotype may be AA or AO. Only family study permits in some cases differentiation of these two possibilities.

This distinction does not apply to AB and O groups, for which serologic study permits identification of not only the phenotype but also the genotype. In fact, both alleles are here recognized either directly (AB group) or indirectly (O group). In the latter case, the absence of A and B antigens implicated O-gene homozygosity.

Table 11.3
Frequency of ABO Groups in Various Ethnic Groups

	Phenotype (%)			
Population	*O*	*A*	*B*	*AB*
France	44	45	8	3
Scotland	50	32	15	3
Sweden	37	48	10	6
Switzerland	40	47	9	4
Pakistan	25	33	36	5
India	32	29	28	11
American Indians	88	12	0	0
Eskimos	54	43	1.5	1.5

A Variant

Serum from B subjects contains an anti-A antibody absorbed by certain types of A (A_2) erythrocytes that agglutinated red blood cells of 80% of groups-A subjects that are called A_1. Serum from B subjects, in fact, contains two distinct anti-A antibodies: anti-A_1 is active only against A_1 erythrocytes, while anti-A reacts with both A_1 and A_2 red blood cells. The same applies to serum anti-A anitbodies in O subjects, in whom anti-B antibody is also present. Thus, a specific anti-A_1, antibody can be obtained by absorbing B subject serum onto A_2 red blood cells.

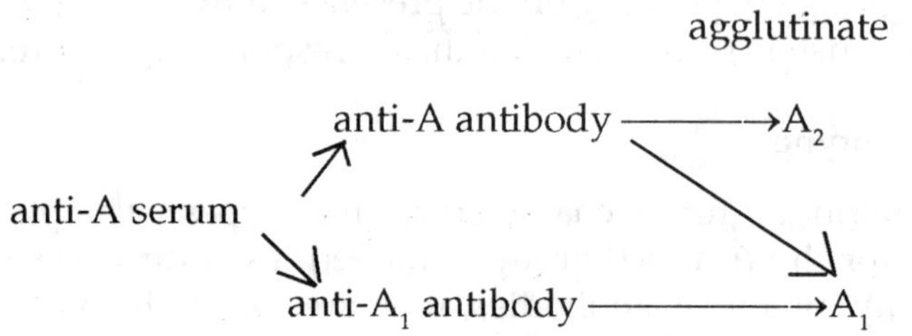

There are still other A and B group variants, the weak A and B antigens.

Enzymes

ABO blood group antigens are glycolipids. For each group, the immunodominant sugar that is responsible or immunologic specificity has been identified. This sugar is *N-acetylgalactosamine* for the A group and galactose for the B group. It is obvious that these blood group sugars are not primary ABO gene products. A and B gene products are, in fact, specific transferases, respectively, N-acetylgalactosaminye transferase and galactosyl transferase, that transfer *N*-acetylgalactosamine or galalctose to an "acceptor", the H substance. The latter substance (with fucose as the dominant sugar) is itself coded for by an H gene located in the Hh genetic unit independent of ABO genes.

The System

Erythrocytes from O-group subjects, which possess neither A nor B antigen, contain an antigen related to the ABO system, the H antigen. This antigen is, in fact, the precursor of A and B antigens, in other words the basic material on which A and B gene products act. The H antigen is recognized by a specific antibody present in some A_1 or A_1B subjects. O subjects who have neither the A nor B gene cannot transform the H precursor substance into A or B substance. Thus, all individuals, irrespective of ABO group, contain H gene, which enables them to produce H substance. There is, however, one exception to this rule. It was discovered in Bombay, in the 1950s, that rare individuals, apparently of the O group, had no H substance on their erythrocytes and produced not only anti-A and anti-B antibodies (like the usual O indididual) but also anti-H antibody. Their serum aggluminated all red blood cells, except their own. Family studies of these subjects have shown that the Bombay phenotype in the homozygous state represents a non functional gene at the H locus. These subjects have normal genes of the ABO system, because they are able to transmit those genes to their children. In the example shown, the Bombay proposita transmitted to her first daughter a B gene obviously

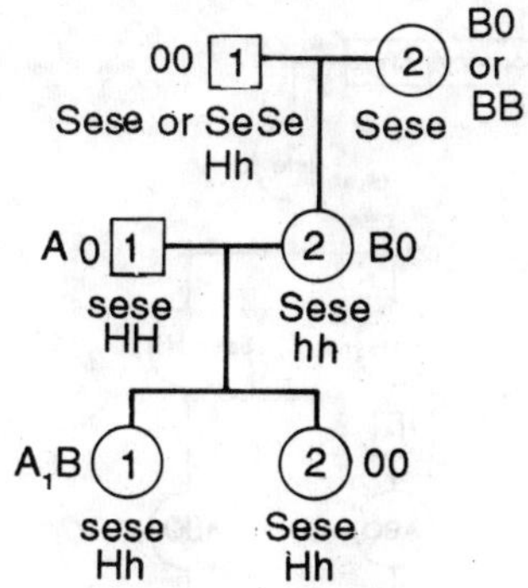

Fig. 11.1. Family pedigree of a subject who carries the Bombay genotype. The Bombay proposita (no. 2 of the second generation) transmits the B gene to her daughter, although she is apparently of the O group.

obtained from her mother. This interpretation was corroborated by demonstrating the presence of the corresponding galactosyl transferase enzyme. This enzyme has no H substrate to transform, and the B antigen is therefore not produced. Study of the Bombay phenotype is additional proof that the H substance is, indeed, the acceptor for A and B substances. It also shows that the H substrate is produced by a locus independent of ABO loci; the Bombay proposita whose family is represented in Fig. 11.1 had consanguinous parents and thus the hh genotype. At the same time, genetic analysis demonstrated that she was BO, that is heterozygous at the ABO locus. This discordance between heterozygosity in one system and homozygosity in the other proves the genetic independence of the two systems. Indeed, in a subject homozygous for a rare gene, born of consanguinous parents, the chromosomal pair that carries the rare gene is a copy of the original chromosomal segment that originated in the common ancestor. The same reasoning demonstrated the independence of Hh and Sese loci (the latter is responsible for ABH secretion). For the sake of completeness, let us mention also that the enzyme that carries the specific fucose for the H substance is a fucosyl transferase.

Erythroblast I Antigen

The H substrate probably overlays the I antigen, which is also produced by an ABO-independent locus. At variance with H, I specificity is, however, not absolutely necessary or A and B antigen formation, because rare subjects without I antigen express H and ABO specificities. Interestingly, I reactivity of Bomaby subjects and of H-deficient subjects is much greater than that of normal subjects.

Other Systems

The analysis of reactive structures on the erythrocyte surface is not yet complete.

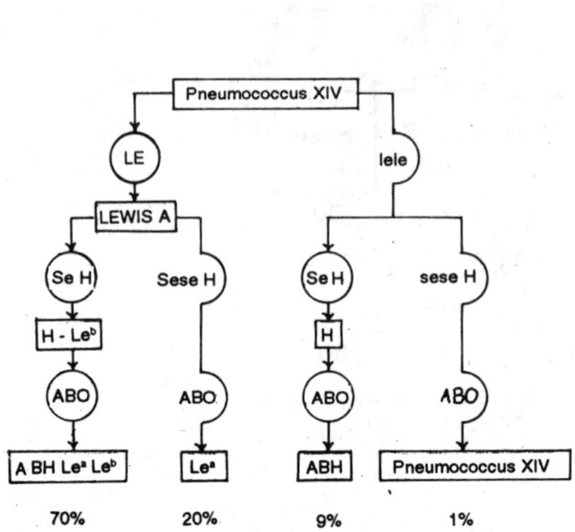

Fig. 11.2. ABO system substances.

Several genetic observations suggest that other systems, independent of ABO, H, and I, may also exist (Y, Z).

MUCOUS CELLS

Mucous cells, especially those of salivary glands, are capable of extracting and then secreting in hydrosoluble form certain blood group antigens. Here again, three genetic systems are involved: Lewis, secretion, and Hh, which has already been described.

Genetic Aspects

Only subjects with the Le gene produce the Lewis susbtance. Genetic analysis shows that this substance is a mendelian system that is independent of the systems mentioned earlier. The same is true for the Sese secretor system, whose genes control secretion of ABH substances. We have already discussed an argument that favours independence of these systems from ABO and Hh. The Hh system is present in salivary cells. Subjects who carry Se and H genes secrete H substance in their saliva, whereas subjects without Se gene, for example, sese homozygotes, cannot secrete it. In ddition, it is obvious that the newly formed H substance is immediately converted into an A or B substance by the ABO system enzymes coded for by the genes present in the genome.

The salivary secretions may appear as four different phenotypes, shown in Table 11.4. It is interesting to note that the quantity of Lewis substance is much greater in type-2 subjects than in type-1 subjects and that only type-2 subjects have the Lewis substance on their erythrocytes, because the Lewis soluble substance circulating in great quantity in the plasma may absorb onto red blood cell surface. As in the case of the erythroblast, new genetic systems are appearing. Thus, in some subjects called OH_m, the H substance is present in the saliva but not on the erythroblast.

Table 11.4
Genes and Substances of Salivary Mucous Cells

Gene		*Substance*
LeSe	Le[a]	H
Le sese	Le[a]	—
Lele Se	—	H
sese lele	—	—

Table 11.5
Hydrolysis of A and B Substances

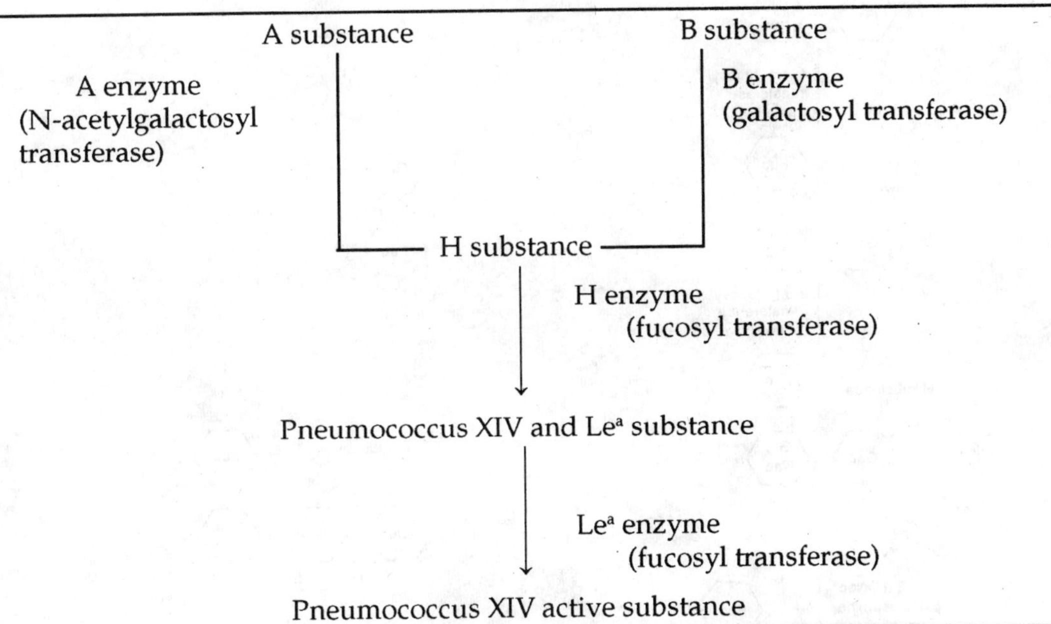

Biochemical Aspects

Biochemical studies have permitted definition of the relationships among the Lewis H, and ABO systems. Unexpectedly, group-specific substances, when purified and isolated, reveal multiple specificities. For example, A and B specificities are found on the same molecule in AB subjects. Salivary blood group-specific substances are glycoproteins that contain a central protein backbone on which oligosaccharide chains are attached laterally. Their immunologic specificity has been verified by enzymatic hydrolysis; proteolytic enzymes do not destroy immunologic specificity, whereas glucidolytic enzymes, which detach terminal sugars from lateral oligosacharide chains, cause disappearance of specificity. It thus appears that group antigens relate to lateral chain sugars, and not to proteins, which indicates that the antigens are not primary gene products but result from activity of specific (gene-produced) enzymes.

If one adds to the soluble susbtance from an A-group subject (who secretes ABH and Le[a] substances encoded by AH, Le and Se genes), the N-acetylgalactosaminidase enzyme N-acetylgalactosamine is removed and, at the same time, A specificity disappears. H specificity is then observed. Similarly, if fucosidase is added, only Lewis specificity remains. This specificity may, in turn, be removed by addition of another fucosidase, which splits fucose from C-4 in *N*-acetylglucosamine; a residual specificity of pneumococcus XIV now appears. This disaccharide, present in all subjects either in the

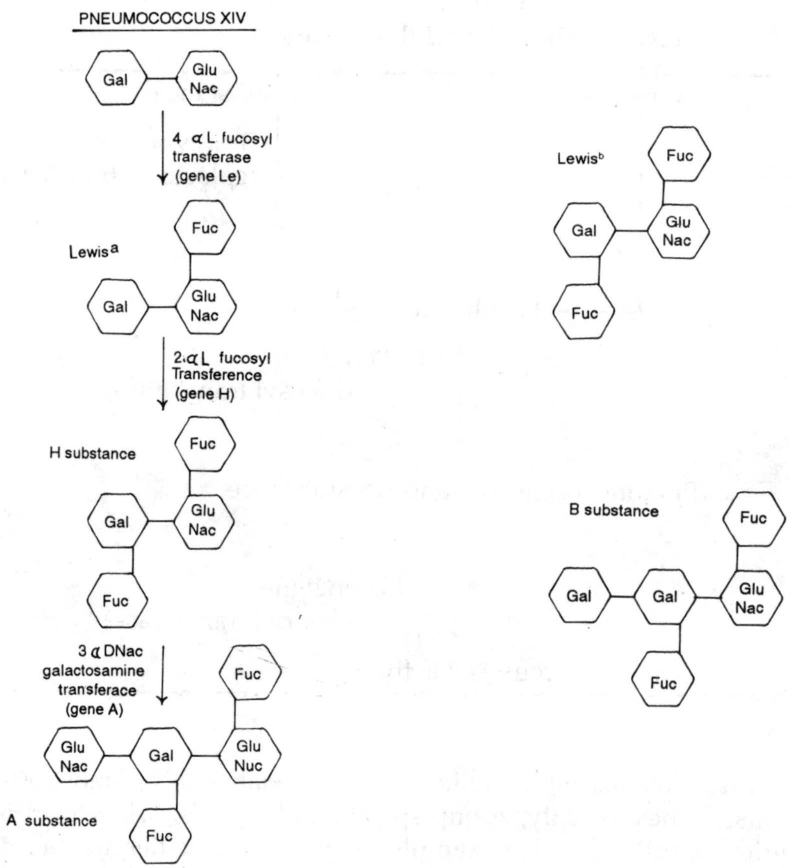

Fig. 11.3. Biosynthesis of A, B, H, and Le specificities.

form of 1,3-glucosamine, or 1,4-glucosamine, could be called an isotype. If the order of antigen construction in living cells is the reverse of that seen *in vitro* destruction of antigens, one deduces the existence of a basic galactose-glucosamine disaccharide on which a Lewis gene binds a fucose to C-4 of glucosamine; at the same time, an H gene binds another fucose to C-2 of galactose, if the Se gene is present. Finally, an A or B gene binds either an N-acetylgalactose mine or a galactose to the C-3 of the terminal galactose.

This hypothesis implies that there are specific enzymes for each gene: 4α-L-fucosyl transferase for Lewis, 2α-L-fucosyl transferase for H, 3α-D-*N*-acetylgalactosminyl transferase for A, and 3α-D-galactose transferase for B. This hypothesis has been entirely confirmed in recent years by direct demonstration of these enzymes. The principle of this demonstration is the following : N-acetylgalactosamine, labeled with ^{14}C, is incubated with the serum in which the enzyme is being searched for. The acceptor onto which the enzyme is capable of transferring the sugar is then added. This substrate may be found in O erythrocytes or in extracts of a human breast milk in the form of fucosyl-lactose. If the enzymes are present, the erythrocytes acquire A antigenicity or a radioactive tetrasaccharide is formed, depending on whether the substrate is a red blood cell or fucosyl-lactose.

Similarly, by incubating mucous gland extract from subjects with Lewis genes or, simply, serum of these subjects with the galactose-1, 3-*N*-acetylglucosamine acceptor, α-L-fucose is transferred onto C-4 of glucosamine, indicating that subjects who possess the Lewis gene do have a 4α-L-fucosyl transferase that allows in vitro conversion of the basis XIV substance into Le^a specificity substance. It is also possible to obtain in vitro (by use of extracts or serum from O-secretors) conversion of the base XIV disaccharide into H substance whether the disaccharide is formed by either 1,3 or 1,4 binding, which demonstrates that the H gene codes for another fucosyl transferase, a 2α-L-fucosyltransferase. When using an extract or serum from a subject with both H and Le genes, transfer of both 1, 4-fucose and 1,2-fucose is obtained at least for the disaccharide substrate with 1,3 binding. Here, both H and Le^a transformations occur.

An extract or serum from an A subject converts the H substrate into A substance; an extract or serum from a B subject transforms H substance into B substance. In the first case, the presence of 3α-D-*N*-acetylgalactosamine transferase is demonstrated; in the second case, 3α-D-galactose transferase is detected. Thus, one finds, A enzyme in A subjects and B enzyme in B subjects, A and B enzymes in AB subjects, and no enzyme in O subjects. Nonsecreting subjects have enzymes of their ABO genes but do not contain (in their mucous cells) the fucosyl transferase that is present in their serum. Bombay subjects have no fucosyl transferase but have the enzymes that correspond to their ABO genome. Thus, the existence of a logical masterplan of synergistic functioning of independent genetic units is shown, as is a precise description of biochemical mechanisms associated with cell differentiation. Se and Le genes contribute within mucous cells to the production of H and Lewis immunologic specificities but do not participate in production of these antigens within the erythroblast. For the same final product for example, the A group, two different genetic pathways may be used by two differntiated somatic cells.

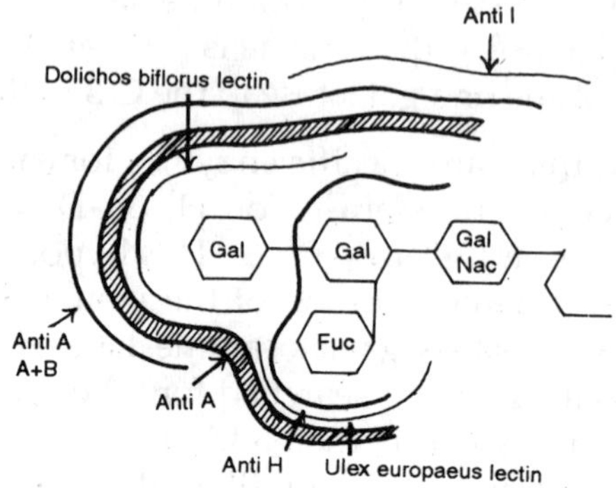

Fig. 11.4. Antigenic sites of AB red blood cells and lectin receptors.

ANTI-ABH ANTIBODIES

We have seen that in the ABO system, a given subject always possesses antibodies that correspond to the antigen(s) not present in his erythrocytes. This rule has no exception. These antibodies are normally consistently found in all individuals. They are called"natural" because they seem to be present prior to any known stimulation. If a new A or B specific antigen is introduced into an organism that does not carry it, specific anti-A or -B antibodies appear, as if the angtigen had determined the appearance of new molecules with an apparent identical specificity but different behaviour. These antibodies, superimposed on the already present natural antibodies, are observed only after stimulation and are called "immune" antibodiess.

The distinction between natural and immune antibodies is of great theoretical importance and has generated considerable thought. However, this differentiation is not absolute. Sera from subjects without any known prior stimulation may sometimes contain antibodies with some immune antibody properties, such as hemolytic ability. In addition, the determinism of the formation of the two types of antibody is not necessarily different. Detailed study of these two antibody categories is important due to their unique serologic and physiochemical differences.

Natural Antibodies

Natural (or normal) antibodies include anti-A in B subjects, anti-B in A subjects, anti-A and anti-B in O subjects, and anti-H in the Bombay phenotype. These antibodies are always observed in subjects who lack the corresponding antigen. Less commonly occurring antibodies that do not follow any known stimulation, include anti-A_1, anti-A of "weak A" subjects, and anti-H in some A_1 or A_1B subjects (aside from the Bombay phenotype).

Natural anti-A and -B antibodies have some characteristics different from those of immune anti-A and -B: permanence, spontaneous agglutination, no hemolyzing ability, maximum activity at 4 °C, neutralization by soluble substances, thermolability at 70°C, relatively homogeneous association constant for the homologous antigen (Wurmser). They are mostly IgM, which never cross the placenta.

Immune Antibodies

Immune antibodies are only found after stimulation. Even if the environment is the soruce of unknown stimuli responsible for natural antibody formation, these antibodies (IgM class) are called "primary-response" antibodies, whereas immune antibodies (IgM class) are "secondary-response" antibodies. The role of the environment in natural and immune antibody production is well-established (soluble blood group substances are found in animals and in vegetables) but is not exclusive.

Anti-A and -B immune antibodies differ from natural antibodies by the following criteria: their appearance is inconstant, they do not agglutinate spontaneously: they can hemolyze: their activity is maximal at 37°C they are difficult to neutralize with solubel substances; they are thermostable at 70°C; their affinity for homologous antigen is very heterogeneous (Wurmser); and they are mostly IgG antibodies, which cross the placenta.

Anti-A immunization may appear under numerous and not always known circumstances:

Vaccination by diphtheria or tetanus toxoids: the toxoid antigen city relates to the presence in the culture medium of hog stomach extracts rich in A substance.

Antitetanus or antidiphtheria serotherapy: until recently, most antisera were purified by pepsin enzymatic digestion. Sera thus treated are very rich in A substance.

Table 11.6
Average Concentration of Anti-B Allohemagglutinins in Various Pathologic Situations

Alcoholic cirrhosis	12	$N_4^* \times 10^6$
Autoimmune "complement-type" hemolytic anemia	6.5	$N_4 \times 10^6$
Autoimmune "IgG-type" hemolytic anemia	3.5	$N_4 \times 10^6$
Acute leukemia	2.5	$N_4 \times 10^6$
Healthy subjects	2.5	$N_4 \times 10^6$
Chronic lymphocytic leukemia	0.5	$N_4 \times 10^6$

* N_4 the maximal number of exythrocytes agglutinated at 4°C by a given serum. This number is proportional to the concentration of specific ABO antibodies.

Injection of certain pharmacologic preparations of animal origin that contain the A substance; examples are dealbuminated hog stomach extracts used in the treatment of gastroduodenal ulcers or pernicious anemias.

Injection of antigenic substances related to A antigen: an example is the Forssman antigen, which is present in paratyphic B bacilli (TAB vaccine).

Pregnancy: when the fetus is A or B and the mother is O.

Immunization duration is highly variable. Regular follow-up of donors known to be immunized against the A antigen have shown the disappearance of the immune antibody within a few weeks to a few months, occasionally as long as 20 months after immunization. Note that the ability to artificially induce immune antibody formation in high titer enables to obtain anti-A or -B test sera by injection of small amounts of A- or B-soluble substances.

ANTI-I AND ANTI-LEWIS ANTIBODIES

I-system Antibodies

Antibodies that correspond to the I system are IgM autoantibodies. These generally exothermic antibodies are responsible for cold agglutinin disease.

Lewis-system Antibodies

Anti-Lewis antibodies (anti-Le^a, anti-Le^b, anti-Le^*) are not infrequent and may be considered natural antibodies in man. Their appearance in relation to the erythrocytic and salivary phenotypes of the subjects who produce them is not completely understood. The classic anti-Le^a antibody appears in all Le (a-b-) subjects of the A,B, or AB group who secrete ABH substance (Se, Lele); anti-Le^b appears in Le(a-b-) subjects who do not secrete ABH substances (sese, lele).

Anit-Lewis antibodies are generally agglutinating but may also be detected by Coombs' test in the presence of complement. In certain cases, they may show hemolyzing ability, especially if test erythrocytes have been treated with trypsin. Anti-Lewis antibodies are IgM and do not cross the placenta. Because of this property and the fact that fetal erythrocytic phenotypes are usually Le(a-b-), they have no role in immunologic fetomaternal disease. Their existence must, however, be considered in cases of transfusion, because anti-Le^a or -Le^b hemolyzing antibodies may cause hemolytic accidents.

III RH SYSTEM

The classic Rh system had to be modified in 1961 when the differences between Rh and LW groups were clarified. There are in fact two genetically independent systems, although they are phenotypically associated.

In the serum of most women having had a new born with hemolytic disease, an alloantibody is present that recognizes 85% of the erythrocytes of white subjects (Rh positive). This alloantibody is anti-Rh. This type of antibody was first identified by

Levine in 1939. Conversely, if a rabbit or guinea pig is immunized with human or *Macacus rhesus*, monkey red blood cells the animal elaborates heteroantibodies that agglutinate not only *M.Rhesus* red blood cells but also all human red blood cells, with very few exceptions. This antibody is anti-LW antibody, first detected by Landsteiner and Wiener in 1940. After adequate dilution and absorption of species-specific satellite heteroantibodies, anti-LW heteroantibodies recognize the red blood cells of only 85% of white subjects, those defined above as Rh^+. Rh^+ subjects have, in fact, larger amounts of LW antigens than do Rh^- subjects, and it is this fact that caused the confusion between Rh and LW^-. The very rare subjects who are not recognized by the nondiluted reagent are called LW^-. They may produce an anti-LW alloantibody.

The clinically important antigen is the antigen recognized by the immune alloantibody in fetomaternal alloimmunization. The use of the term "Rhesus" is therefore improper, but because of long precedence, Levine has proposed that the antigen common to the M. *rhesus* monkey and man, indentified by the bcteroantibody or by the exceptional human alloantibody, be labeled LW antigen in honor of Landsteiner and Wiener. The name, anti-Rh, has been retained for the alloantibody responsible for the hemolytic disease of the newborn.

IMMUNOLOGIC ASPECTS

Subjects whose erythrocytes are agglutinated by anti-Rh alloantibody (85%) are said to have the Rh^+ or D^+ phenotype. The 15% of subjects who are negative are Rh^- or D^-. Techniques that permit artificial agglutination, developed between 1940 and 1945, especially Coomb's test, allow recognition of other antigens of the Rh system. These antigens include C, present in 70 % of white subjects, E(30%), c(80%), and e antigens (98%). Rhesus-negative subjects who possess the C antigen are termed rh', and those with E antigen are known as rh". It has been noted that these antibodies form couples and give antithetic reactions. Because anti-C and anti-c and anti-E and anti-e are antithetic, their specific antigens are presumed to be produced by alleles.

Phenogroups with Three Variation Units

The recognition of these antithetic reactions led Fisher to postulate the existence of three closely linked locus pairs, or pseudoalleles (D(d), Cc, Ee). Block transmission of various haplotypes has been really observed. Major common haplotypes are shown in Table 11.7.

However, each series of antigens produced by the three genetic units shows many variations. The D standard Rh antigen itself is concerned and there are numerous varieties of weak antigens (D^u) that have considerable practical importance. Thus, D reactivity presents a quantitative variability with a gaussian distribution; the tail of the curve represents a population of very weak reactivity. Weak D antigens are the classic D^u, only detected by certain techniques and reagents. Thus, for standard Rh, as for many other blood group antigens, there are weak variants that are genetically transmitted.

Weakly reactive D antigens are seen in two other situations; some partial Rh antigens, which are genetically transmitted, and depressed Rh antigen, due to a positional

Table 11.7
Definintion of the Main Haplotypes of the Rhesus System

Three-unit haplotypes (Fisher)	*Current names (Wiener)*	*Approximate frequency*
Haplotypes that possess the standard Rh gene (D)		
DCe	R_1	0.40
DcE	R_2	0.15
Dce	R_0	0.02
DCE	Rr	0.00
DC^we	$R^w{}_1$	0.01
Haplotypes that do not possess the standard Rh gene (D)		
dce	r	0.39
dCe	r′	0.01
dcE	r″	0.01
dCE	r_y	0.00

abnormality caused by allelic interaction. D^u antigens are of clinical importance, because they may cause immunization in a Rh^- subject. Sensitive techniques are used to detect them to avoid alloimmunization of an Rh^- recipient who would othrwise be transfused with "weak" D blood. Conversely, it is wise to avoid needless injections of anti-D immunoglobulins into D^u women.

Phenogroups with Five Variation Units

It was soon discovered that these three variation units did not explain all reactivities. The phenogroup produced by various Rh haplotypes also included two other antigenic types: compound antigens and G antigen.

Compound antigens are produced only by haplotypes that possess two contiguous genetic markers. For example, Ce, ce, cE, and ce^s antigens are produced only when the corresponding variants of Cc or Ee are in the *cis* position in the same haplotype.

The G antigen is defined by a reactivity present in all subjects who have either C antigen, D antigen, or both C and D and only very rarely in subjects who lack C and D antigens. Phenogroups thus include five variation units : C or c, G or non-G, D or non-D, compound antigens, and E or e.

Polarized Antigen Production

Depressed Antigens

Certain phenogroups have only weakly expressed Ee reactivities or, usually, weak expression of both Cc and Ee, To date, any such phenogroup, including weak C or c and normal E or e reactivities has not been observed. The main haplotypes known presently, which are transmitted as a block, are the D (C) (e), D (c) (E), -(c)(e) complexes.

Silent Antigens: "Dash" Phenogroup

The "dash" phenogroup is a silent phenotype, either for the Ee antigens (Dc-) or for the Cc and Ee antigen s(D—). Antigenic D reactivity is then in excess. These individuals are very readily immunized, because they produce antibodies to naturally absent antigens, which appear as antigens produced by the Cc or Ee zone, the incidence of which is very high. They also are targets for autoantibodies of the IgG type, especially Hr, nl, Ee, or Rh 18.

Rh-Null Phenotype

The Rh-null phenotype defines subjects who lack all of the known Rh antigens. Two types are known: one is extremely are (silent type) and results from the existence of two entirely silent haplotypes. The other phenotype (regulator type) is less exceptional. It seems to result from interactions with another genetic system by substrate inhibiton or defect. In fact, within the ABO group, the O gene at the ABO locus is also silent; it resembles the first mentioned Rh^{-} null phenotype. The second is reminiscent of the Bombay phenotype, in which A and B genes cannot express themselves due to lack of a substrate, although the corresponding enzymes are synthesized.

Associated LW Antigen

The anti-LW antibody produced by guinea pigs immunized with M.*rhesus* erythrocytes or by the very rare LW-human erythrocytes reacts weakly with D-red blood cells and more strongly with Rh+ red blood cells. This difference caused the early confusion between the Rh and LW systems. Rh-null erythrocytes, which possess no DCE antigens, do not contain either the LW antigen, and this is prorbably not a coincidence.

Rh Antigens and the Membrane

Rh antigens are most likely a part of lipoprotein structures responsible for integrity of the erythrocytic membrane. D-reactive sites are much less numerous than those of the ABO system. Their number varies from 10,000 to 30,000 for normal phenotypes, with a maximum of 100,000 for the exceptional D— phenotypes. The larger site number of D— erythrocytes explains why they are readily agglutinated by anti-D antibodies (which are normally nonagglutinating). In addition, both with the regulator and the silent-type Rh-null, there is nearly constantly an abnormal fragility of Rh-null red blood cells in vivo. Levine has postulated that lipoprotein Rh antigens are functional membrane components, unlike glycolipid ABH antigens. Fragile Rh-null red blood cells and intact Bomaby erythrocytes are thus explained, according to Levine, by the fact that ABH sites are more superficial and less imbedded within that membrane than are Ra sites.

Rosenfield's Nomenclature

In view of the complexity of Rh-reactive structures and the difficulty involved in their genetic interpretation, Rosenfield has proposed a practical nomenclature that attempts to more precisely classify the antigens studied. Each defined test serum is given a number that corresponds to the Rh determinant that it recognizes. Thus, factors 1,2,3,4 and 5 correspond to D,C,E, c and e. A given phenotype is expressed by the test serum utilized for its characterization; a number is preceded by a minus sign if the raction is negative. For example, a Rh negative phenotype may be written: -1, -2,-3, 4, 5 (ddccee). Such a nomenclature has obvious advantages for computer use but may be difficult to introduce into clinical practice.

Table 11.8
Rosenfield's Numerical Nomenclature and Wiener's Classificaiton

DCE	*Numerical*	*Rh-Hr*	*DCE*	*Numercial*	*Rh-Hr*
D	Rh 1	Rh_0	—	Rh 17	Hr_0
C	Rh 2	rh'	—	Rh 18	Hr
E	Rh 3	rh"	—	Rh 19	$^0hr^s$
c	Rh 4	hr'	vs or e	Rh 20	—
e	Rh 5	hr"	c^G	Rh 21	—
ce	Rh 6	hr	CE	Rh 22	—
Ce	Rh 7	rh_1	D^w	Rh 23	—
C^w	Rh 8	rh^w	E^t	Rh 24	—
C^x	Rh 9	rh^x	LW	Rh 25	—
V or ce^s	Rh 10	hr^v	(c-like)	Rh 26	—
E^w	Rh 11	rh^{w2}	cE	Rh 27	—
G	Rh 12	rh^G	—	Rh 28	hr^H
-	Rh 13	Rh^A	—	Rh 29	—
-	Rh 14	Rh^B	D^c_{or}	Rh 30	—
-	Rh 15	Rh^c	—	Rh 31	hr^B
-	Rh 16	Rh^D	—	Rh 32	—
				Rh 34	—
				Rh 35	—

GENETIC ASPECTS

Fisher and Race's classic scheme introduced the concept of pseudoalleles. The existence of three pairs of genes is considered: Dd, Cc and Ee. The antigen that corresponds to d has not yet been found. In addition, there are probably more than three antigenic variations and the analysis of compound antigen leads us to consider that C and E belong to the same cistron and do not complement in the *trans* position. Two genetic units are proposed: the D zone, which produces the D antigen or not, and the Cc Ee zone, which produces a large series of proper antigens. Any overview of the genetic nature of the Rh system must also explain three more phenomena:

That formation of specificities of the Rh gene complex is polarized. None of the composed antigens so far discovered associates D to E, but, conversely, all of them associate C with E. In addition, the fact that the D— — haplotype shows D excess suggests a failure of a basic substance conversion, as if there were polarity from D to C and then to E. But so far, no complex of — — E or — — e has been detected. Such polarity might be explained by sequential action of one or several operons.

That several independent genetic systems are involved in manifestations of a coordinated genetic activity. It has been demonstrated by segregation analysis that Rh and LW are independent. In addition, a Rh-null subject (of regulatory type) may transmit a normal Rh gene, just as a Bombay subject may transmit a nórmal A or B gene. However, the imaginary basic substance cannot be LW, because some LW subjects have normal Rh antigens. Nevertheless, all Rh-null subjects are LW-. Therefore, the initiating substance must be a substrate for both Rh and LW.

That silent-type Rh-null subjects are also LW-. These subjects do not lack a priori the substrate produced by the X_1r gene. Jouvenceaux and Gibblett imaginatively proposed a sequential activity, involving, alternatively, Rh, the LW, and, again, Rh. The first cistron involved is D, the second is LW, and the third is CE. If one notes that LW suppression is observed only when the Rh complex is totally silent but not when the complex is partially silent (D- or De-, one must agree with Jouvenceaux that LW expression requires an active Dd segment. The antigenic relationship between D and LW would then be explained by the fact that D type permits formation of a greater quantity of LW than does d type. The Dd segment would therefore transform the substance produced by X_1r into substance 2 (Rh 29), onto which independent LW and CE units would then act.

Rosenfield's Hypothesis

Rosenfield, Allen, and Rubinstein have recently proposed a genetic basis for Rh antigen production that takes into account the polarization mentioned above. The operator R^{29} gene first permits elaboration of the Rh 29 basic substance and then acts on operator genes R^1, R^{17} and R^{18}. This genetic model explains a certain number of complex findings, but it must be admitted that the genetic function that leads to formation of Rh and LW antigens is still uncertain.

RH-SYSTEM ANTIBODIES

These antibodies are the most important of the immune antibodies in immunohematology. The D antigen itself is the most immunogenic antigen of all blood group systems. It is the main antigen responsible for fetomaternal alloimmunization. However, anti-E and -c antibodies are also frequently observed in polytransfused subjects and in women immunized by pregnancy, unlike anti-e, which is very rare. Thus, the Rh sytem is the second most important red blood cell group system, after ABO. Even in primary responses, anti-Rh antibodies are IgG antibodies. They usually do not agglutinate Rh+ red cells, and one must resort to artificial techniques of agglutination in searching for them in serum and in Rh grouping. Note also that some high-frequency antigens, (Rh17 and Rh18 in Rosenfield's nomenclature), are particularly common targets of IgG autoantibodies in autoimmune hemolytic anemias.

OTHER BLOOD GROUP SYSTEMS

The erythrocytic membrane has numerous other antigenic markers that express genetic "allotypic" variations within our species. It is possible to distinguish highly immunogenic antigens, such as the Rhesus system, which are responsible for most alloimmunizations in our species (Kell, Duffy, Kidd, and Bg systems), and those that are conversely poorly immunogenic but may, in certain cases, lead to the formation of irregular natural antibodies (MNS, P, and Lutheran systems). Finally, the Xg^a antigen merits particular attention, because it is produced by a genetic unit localized on the X chromosome, hence the interest it has in human genetics.

About 15 genetically independent blood groups systems have been identified. They are not, as is sometimes claimed, "subgroups," because each expresses the activity of an autonomous genetic unit. Some of them are highly polymorphic and equilibrated, for example, the MNS system. Others have great hemotypologic value. They include Di^a antigen of the Diego system, which has been found only in mongoloids, and the Js^a antigen of the Kell system, which is peculiar to blacks.

More and more complex relationships between reactive structures of the erythrocytic membrane which appear as various blood group systems are being uncovered. Indpendent of the classic relations between A and B or between H, I or i antigens, there is coupling between Rh and Duffy, Lutheran and Auberger, and i and P_1. The significance of these relationships may either be genetic or phenotypic and is presently under study.

IMMUNOGENIC SYSTEMS

Kell System

The Kell antigen is present in about 8% of white subjects and is one of the most immunogenic antigens, frequently responsible for antibody formation in polytransfused subjects.

The Kell system is relatively complex. It includes a series of haplotypes, the most current of which produces the Cellano, Kp^b, and Js^b antigens, with several variants.

Mutant haplotypes may produce the Kell antigen more common in whites than in blacks), the Kp^a antigen in whites, and the Js^a antigen in blacks. In fact, here again, synergistic activity is suggested between the basic system Kx, which may be produced by an X-linked gene, and the Kell gene complex itself. The Kx antigen may be present on normal leukocytes. It would be lacking in children with aX-linked disease called septic granulomatosis, in which polymorphs are unable to destroy previously phagocytosed bacteria. Anti-Kell antibody is an example of immune antibodies that may appear after transfusion or fetomaternal stimulation. It is usually revealed by Coombs' test (IgG type) but may also be detected directly when red blood cells are suspended in human serum. Its clinical importance has already been mentioned.

Duffy System

The Fy^a antigen of the Duffy system, present in 65% of white subjects, is more immunogenic than the Fy^b antigen. Both antigens represent the product of two Fy^a and Fy^b alleles, but in black populations, subjects are not infrequently deprived of one or the other and thus exhibit the Fy (a-b-) phenotype. The anti-Fy^a antibody is the most commonly occurring antibody. It may be responsible for transfusional hemolytic accidents. It has also been incriminated in fetomaternal alloimmunization accidents. It is generally detectable by the indirect Coombs' test by use of anti-IgG antibodies.

Kidd System

This system has tow alleles (Jk^a and Jk^b). Here again, the Jk^a antigen, present in 80% of white subjects, is the most immunogenic. Very rare subjects have neither Jk^a nor Jk^b and may produce an anti-Jk^a Jk^b antibody. Recently, it was demonstrated that this antibody recognizes all leukocytes from Jk(a+) or Jk(b+) subjects but not leukocytes from Jk(a-b-) subjects. Paradoxically, neither isolated anti-Jk^a nor anti-Jk^b reacts with normal leukocytes. It has been suggested that the antigen recognized by anti-Jk^a Jk^b antibody may be a Jk^a and Jk^b precursor present on leukocytes, similar to the Kx antigen of the Kell system.

The anti-Jk^a antibody is relatively common in polytransfused subjects, and its identification is technically difficult. Nonetheless, it may cause hemolytic blood accidents and hemolytic disease of the newborn if it is an IgG antibody. The best technique for detection is a Coomb's test that employs trypsin-treated red blood cells in the presence of complement and of anticomplement serum. The anti-Jk^b antibody is rarer but may also cause transfusion accidents and hemolytic disease of the newborn.

Bg Antigens

There are on human erythrocytes antigens that correspond to selected HLA antigens (SD) of leukocytes and platelets. The Bg^a antigen is identical to HLA-B7, Bg^b to HLA-BW17, and Bg^c to HLA-A28. Antibodies that correspond to these antigens are frequently observed in polytransfused subjects, especially in subjects who possess complex mixtures of immune alloantibodies, which greatly increases the difficulty of analyzing the specificities of antibodies present in these sera.

Conclusion

Anit-Rh, D, C, E, e anti-Kell, anti-Fy[a], and anti-Jk[a] represent more thatn 98% of the antibodies found in transfusional immunization. They always appear first. The corresponding systems (Rh, Kell, Duffy and Kidd) must therefore be considered first when transfusion is indicated.

WEAKLY IMMUNOGENIC SYSTEMS

MNS System

This system includes two series of pseudoalleles, M and N and S and s, organized in four haplotypes of decreasing frequency, Ns, Ms, MS and NS. The fact that the frequencies are well equilibrated account for the polymorphism of the MNS system and for its contribution to segregation analysis. In fact, this system is further complicated by the existence of rare alleles in which the antigen is defined by a specific antibody (e.g.), Mg antigen) and by the presence of alleles whose antigens are revealed by discrepancies that depend on which reagent is used, whether of human or animal origin. Their link with the MNS system is demonstrated by segregation analysis, e.g., for the Mi[a] antigen.

Considerable biochemical breakthroughs have been made in recent years. M and N specificities are linked to the presence of sialic acid [*N*-acetylneuraminic acid (NANA)]. They are carried by complex glycoprotein molecules, where oligosaccharidic lateral chains are linked to the amino acids, of the protien chain (Pro, Lys, Arg) by O-glycosidic bonds. M and N specificities might result from specific sialyl transferase activities, which transfer two NANA units to different points of a basic disaccharide that bears T and Tn specificities that characterize hidden antigens. This hypothesis explains the polyagglutinability of neuraminidase-treated red blood cells.

P System

The P system is a relatively complex one that has two main phenotypes: P_1, which carries P_1 and P specificities, P_2, which has only P specificity, and very rare phenotypes, which apparently represent nonconcerted substrated [P^k, which lacks P, and Tj(a-), which lacks P_1, P, and P^k]. P_2 subjects sometimes produce an irregular natural anti-P_1 antibody; Tj(a) sera contain anti-P+P_1+P^k antibody, for example. These sera recognize antigens of all other subjects, except the Tj(a-) ones. P^k subjects produce an anti-P antibody that recognizes antigens of all other subjects, except P^k and Tj(a-).

At variance with M and N specificities (T and Tn, Pr_1 and Pr_2), which are glycoprotein in nature, P^k, P, and P_1 specificities are glycolipid in nature, just like ABH specificities of the erythrocyte. Lactosyl ceramide is the basic disaccharide structure onto which specific α-galactosaminyl transferases successively bind P^k and P specificities. So formed, lacto-*N*-neotetraose ceramide is the basic tetrasaccharide structure, very similar to ABH specificities, onto which and α-galactosyl transferase adds the P_1 specificity. The P_2 phenotype, that is, the noncoverted P, could be due to the absence of the transferase.

Lutheran System

This sysem is characterized by the existence of two alleles, Lu^a and Lu^b, which give phenotypes Lu(a+b-) (0.2%), Lu(a+b+) (5.8%), and Lu(a-b+) (94%) in whites. Here again, there is a very rare silent phenotype, Lu(a-b-), of two types, one recessive and the other dominant.

SERUM PROTEIN GROUPS

Immunoglobulins present a genetic polymorphism, called allotypy, to be compared in many respects to those mentioned on the preeceding pages for erythrocytes. Numerous other serum proteins present a similiar polymorphism, and some authors have decided to designate them also under the term "allotypy." We will briefly review the major human serum protein allotypes.

IMMUNOGLOBULIN ALLOTYPES

Four Ig allotype systems are recognized in man: Inv, Gm, ISf, and Am systems. The first one distinguishes the light chains of every Ig, the second and the third (Gm and (Isf) determine heavy chains of certain IgG, and the Am sytem determines heavy chains of certain IgA subclasses.

Methodology

The allotypic character of human Ig is recognized by hemagglutination inhibition techniques. A specific antibody recognizes the allotype borne by 1g that is bound to erythrocytes, and this recognition induces red blood cell agglutination. For example, an anti-Rh specific antibody that bears a Gm (1) marker on its Fe fragment may bind to Rh+ erythrocytes. When the sensitized erythrocytes are incubated together with specific anti-Gm (1) antibody, the marker on the heavy chains of the bound antibody is recognized and causes agglutination of red blood cells. Some human sera inhibit such agglutination. One may deduce that these sera possess Gm (1) specificity on their own immunoglobulins.

The initial source of anti-Gm sera was subjects with rheumatoid arthritis [rheumatoid arthritis γ-globulin (Ragg)], and, in fact, in this setting, Grubb first discovered anti-Gm antibody. Unfortunately, these sera are often polyspecific and thus difficult to use despite their generally high titer. Recognition of an iallotypes of low titer but of restricted specificity in normal subjects [sera normal agglutinators (SNagg)] represented significant technical progress, which led to the discovery of the Inv system. The immune nature of SNagg has been demonstrated in certain situations, such as fetomaternal immunization and injection of blood or blood derivatives. However, anti-Gm post-transfusion immunization is fairly rare.

INV System

This system includes three specificities, Inv(1), Inv(2), and Inv(3), with five phenotypes, Inv(1,2-3), Inv (-1,-2,3), Inv (1,-2,-3), Inv(1,2,3) and Inv(1,-2,3). In this nomenclature, the specificity is indicated by the number, and the absence of any specificity is denoted by a minus sign. The three all types are formed by a series of polyallelic genes: $INv^{1,2}$, Inv^{1}, Inv^{3} and Inv^{-}. The latter is a silent gene, which explains the sixth silent phenotype, Inv (-1,-2,-3), when it exists in a double dose. The biochemical basis of the Inv system is described elsewhere.

GM System

Allotypic specificities within the Gm system are now very numerous. Gm (1) to Gm(25) by the international nomenclature most generally used. Each specificity is transmitted like a mendelian character, but segregation analysis has shown that some allotypes are transmitted as a block. Studies that involve formal genetics combined with population analysis have permitted recognition of the most frequent haplotypes within the human races:

White race: Gm 1,17,21; Gm 1,2,17,21; Gm 3,5,8,10,13,14

Black race: Gm 1,5,13,14,17; Gm 1,5,14,17; Gm 1,5,6,14,17

Mongoloid race: Gm 1,17,21; Gm 1,2,17,12; Gm 1,13,17; Gm 1,3,5,13,14

It should be noticed that Gm (1) and (5) allotypes are never present in the same haplotype in whites, whereas coexistence is always the case in blacks, which means that black individuals are always of the Gm (1,5) phenotype. Similarly, all mongoloid people are Gm (1), because all haplotypes of mongoloid races include the Gm1 gene. Conversely, Gm (6) specificity is found only in black people. This specific polymorphism has made the Gm system particularly important in studying cross-breeding and evolution in primates. It has thus permitted dating the appearance of certain mutations during evolution. The mechanism by which such polymorphism is maintained is, however, unknown.

The various Gm specificities are borne by different molecules within each individual's serum. They represent the subject's phenotype. By use of methods similar to those previously described for Inv, it was recognized that Gm specificities are borne by IgG and that most markers are located on the Fc of the heavy chains. Only Gm (4) and Gm (17) specificities are located on the Fd fragment and need for their expression the quaternary structure of the IgG molecule. Interestingly, each marker is borne by a different IgG molecule.

Relationships between Allotypy and Isotypy

The Gm system provides an example of the very close relationship between allotypy and isotypy. Table 11.9 demonstrates by use of four antisera [anti-Gm(1), anti-Gm(4), anti-Gm(5), and anti-Gm(21) along with anti-non-a and anti-non-g sera], how it is possible to define the isotypic class of a myelomatous protein or a purified antibody.

As can be seen, IgG1 does not bear the same markers as IgG3: the first contains Gm (1,17) or Gm (3,4), and the second contains Gm(5) or Gm(21). This means that in subjects whose genome bears the haplotype "1,17,21," 1 and 17 markers are present in differentiated cells that synthesize IgG1, whereas the 21 marker is found in differentiating cells that synthesize IgG3. It must be admitted, then, that the two contiguous zones are not activated within the same differentiated cell.

Such an analysis has been profitably put to use in studying modifications of genetic markers that occur during certain myeloproliferative diseases. By this means, it has been shown that in some cases, the changes bear on the characteristics of only one of two haplotypes, which argues in favour of genetic determinism of the abnormality. Note that when one determines the Gm phenotype of a subject, one is, in fact, grouping the precursor stem cells form which Ig-forming lymphocytes are made.

Table 11.9
Relationships between Allotypy and Isotypy of Human Immunoglobulins

	Allotypy				*Isotypy*	
Isotypy	*Anti-Gm (1)*	*Anti-Gm (4)*	*Anti-Gm (5)*	*Anti-Gm (21)*	*Anti-"non-a"*	*Anti-"non-g"*
IgG1	+	—	—	—	—	—
	—	+	+	—	+	—
IgG3	—	—	+	—	+	+
	—	—	—	+	+	—
IgG2	—	—	—	—	+	+
IgG4	—	—	—	—	—	—

Biochemical Basis of Specificities

The biochemical basis for Gm specificities of IgG heavy chains has already been discussed. Note that the Fe fragment of Gm (1) IgGI differs from that of Gm(-1) IgGl by two noncontiguous amino acids of a pentapeptide located toward the middle of the Fc fragment. IgG2 and IgG3 chains, but not IgG4, have a peptide analogous to the Gm(-1) peptide of IgGl chains. This peptide explains "non-a" specificity. In other words, the "non-a" peptide represents an immunologic specificity defined by an antibody that recognizes (9G.n(-1) IgG1, IgG2, and IgG3, as though it were an allotypic specificity for IgG1 and an isotypic one for the other two. Such specificities are presently called isoallotypic.

Applications to the Study of Genetic Funcitons

Functional Haploidy

In the heterozygous state, no molecule is marked simultaneously by both alleles. For example, in a 1, 5 subject, no single protein has both markers.

Either Gm (1) or Gm(5) is present but not Gm (1, 5). An analogous phenomenon has never been observed in AB subjects, in whom all erythrocytes are both A and B. This means that only one of the chromosomes is involved in antibody synthesis.

Allotype Production in Lymphocyte Cultures

It has been shown by Ropartz that homozygous Gm (4,5) lymphocytes placed in culture can produce Ig of Gm(1) and Gm(17) allotypes. Analogous results have been obtained after phytohemagglutinin stimulation or in mixed-lymphocyte cultures.

This finding has suggested that all subjects have a genetic potential that enables them to synthesize any Ig that carries the various allotypes. Gm system genes could therefore be regulatory genes transmitted by mendelian inheritance that repress structural genes. Artificial culture condition would then modify the action of the regulatory genes and derepress structural genes.

ISF System

The third system of Ig allotypic markers is the ISf system, presently represented by only one allotype, ISf(1), whose specificity is borne by the Fc fragment of IgG1 molecules. It is interesting to note that in several myelomatous protein, a Gm and an Isf factor have been found to occur simultaneously, which indicates that the heavy chains relate to at least two independent genetic systems. Another unexpected finding was the discovery that frequency of the ISf(I) marker increases with age.

Am System

This marker is specific for certain IgA2 immunoglobulins. It is borne by α_2 heavy chains. The character identified in serum is also present in saliva. Two Am specificities are presently known, Am(1) and Am(2), but their relationships have not yet been clearly determined. Familial studies indicate that there is a relationship between the Am(2) and the Gm locus.

α_2-GLOBULIN ALLOTYPES (GC GLOBULINS)

The Gc polymorphism ("group-specific component") relates to α_2-globulins. In animals, antisera have been described that react with certain types of α_2-globulins that differ between individuals. On immunoelectrophoresis, there may be one precipitation arc, either a rapidly migrating on a slow migrating protein, or two arcs that react with two protein types. A genetic system is thus defined, in which two alleles, Gc_1 and Gc_2, determine three phenotypes. In additon, there exists a silent allele of very rare frequency and numerous rare variants of Gc_1 and Gc_2.

β-LIPOPROTEIN GROUPS

Two "allotypic" genetic β-lipoprotein systems have been identified, Ag ("Antigen"') and Lp ("lipoprotein").

Ag system

In performing simple gel immunodiffusion with antibodies against human serum in polytransfused subjects, Allison and Blumberg (in 1961) observed that one of the sera was capable of precipitating 50% of normal human sera and that this trait was a dominant mendelian genetic character with autosomal transmission. They called this substance Ag^a antigen. Other factors were soon recognized: Ag^x, Ag^y, Ag^z and Ag^1. Genetic analyses showed that the Ag^x and Ag^y systems are probably alle'es and that the Ag system is at least as complex as Rh, Kell, and Gm. Ag^x and Ag^y characters are observed in heterozygotes; there is no functional haploidy, as in the Gm system.

Lp System

This allotype is transmitted as a dominant and autosomal mendelian character. Two antigens are known, Lp^a and Lp^x, associated with three phenotypes, a+x-, a+1+, a-x-. This genetic system is independent of the Ag system and of most other marker systems. Berg, who discovered this system, has shown that only part of the circulating β-lipoproteins of Lp(a+) sera have the character and that antigens of the Lp and Ag systems are borne by entirely separate lipoprotein molecules. Thus, when an Lp(a+) or an Ag(a+) serum is treated with an anti-Lp^a antibody to remove (by precipitation) all Lp(a+) molecules, the supernatant still reacts with anti-Ag^a serum.

APPENDIX: ERYTHROCYTE GROUPING

Erythrocyte grouping is a prerequisite to any transfusion. The routine is to study the standard ABO and Rh groups. We will only discuss the main methods of grouping in detail but stress that in some circumstances, especially multiple transfusion, it is necessary to determine the entire Rh group (C,c, E, e) along with the Kell, Duffy, Kidd and Lewis groups.

ABO Grouping and Its Difficulties

ABO grouping is performed by two complementary tests on both erythrocytes and serum.

The red cell test incubates known anti-B, anti-A and anti-A plus anti-B sera with the erythrocytes to be tested. The erythrocytic antigen(s) defines(s) blood group A,B, AB, or O.

The serum test consists of incubating the serum to be tested with known A_1, A_2 and B erythrocytes. Every individual has in his serum the antibody(ies) that corresponds to the absent erythrocytic antigen (s).

If red blood cells are agglutinated by anti-A and anti-A plus anti-B but not by anti-B, they bear only the A antigen. The subject may be tentatively considered to belong to the A group. His serum does not agglutinate A red blood cells (A_1 and A_2) but does agglutinate B red blood cells. He therefore possesses an anti-B antibody, which confirms the fact that he belongs to the A group. Concordance of findings in red blood cell and serum tests is rquired. If there is a discripancy, no ABO group conclusion can be reached. The order of reagent examinations (anti-B, anti-A, anti-A+B) is unimportant but, once chosen, must not be chanaged.

The two most widely used techniques of agglutination are performed in Kahn tubes or on opalin slides. Although currently studied in certain laboratories, A_1, and A_2 subgroup determination is of no consequence in intransfusion. Note that A_1 red blood cells are agglutinated by anti-A_1 reagents but not by anti-H reagents, while the reverse is tru for A_2 red blood cells.

ABO group determination is generally uncomplicated. Any discrepancy between red blood cell and serum tests requires three additional controls, following preliminary washing of test erythrocytes:

"Auto control" involves patient's serum plus patient's own red blood cells. If the results are negative, this control eliminates spontaneous erythrocytic agglutination.

"AB control" involves AB serum plus erythrocytes to be tested. When negative, this control excludes erythrocytic polyagglutination and verifies the red cell test.

"Allo control" involves the patient's serum plus compatible O erythrocytes. This is, in fact, a simple agglutinin detection. This control, when negative, verifies the serum test.

Table 11.10
Red Cell and Serum Tests of ABO Grouping

Anti-B	*Anti-A*	*Anti-A+B*	*A_1*	*A_2*	*B*	*Groups and frequency in Frame (%)*
—	+++	+++	—	—	+++	A, 45
—	—	—	+++	+++	+++	O, 44
+++	—	+++	+++	+++	—	B, 8
+++	+++	+++	—	—	—	AB, 3

If there is a discrepancy between erythrocyte and serum tests, with negative control, the cause is usually a rare but normal group less often, hypogammaglobulinemia is responsible for negative serum tests. If one of the controls is positive, one must think of an associated immunologic disease.

Discrepancies with Negative Controls

O Subjects with Hemolysin

The tested serum may react less with A than with B erythrocytes. This occurs rarely in O-group subjects and must never be accepted without further study. It may represent anti-A hemolysin in the O subjects's serum. Serum inactivation (20 min at 56°C), which destroys complement, suffices to normalize the serum test. Less commonly there is an unknown A_x, but in this case, A_2 erythrocytes are not agglutinated in the serum test.

Weak A Groups

There are three main weak A groups (all very rare): A_3, A_x and A_m.

A_3 is detected by anti-A and anti-A+B. It gives a dual population pattern on slide grouping. A_3 is sometimes associated with serum anti-A_1. A_x is detected by anti-A+B and sometimes also by anti-A. Agglutination is weak, and there is no dual-population pattern. A serum anti-A is always present. A_m gives no agglutination with test sera. The fixation elution test, employing anti-A, is required to detect the antigen. Similar B-group varieties (B_3,B_x,B_m) are even rarer.

Dual Population

Double populations are recognized on opalin slides. Whereas agglutinates are normally seen on the white background of opalin, dual population agglutinates appear on a pink background made of nonagglutinated red blood cells. A dual population may be due to an A_3 leukemia or malignant hemopathy of the myeloproliferative type, previous transfusions with O blood, or a chimera or mosaic (very rare).

A_2B Subjects with Anti-A_1

This phenotype presents the only real difficulty in ABO typing, because the A antigen may be considerably weakened, independent of any relevant clinical disorder. Its presence can therefore not be recognized, and because there is an anti-A_1 in serum, one may erroneously conclude that it is a B group. This pitfall justifies the use of A_2 erythrocytes in the serum test. Similarly, it is wise to check the red blood cell test results of all B subjects by use of a strongly positive anti-A reagent.

Leukemic Modifications

Certain malignant hemopathies may induce a very important alteration in A or B-antigen expression, either on a fraction of red blood cells (giving then a dual-population pattern and simulating A_3), or on all erythrocytes (thus simulating A_x or A_m). But, there are no anti-A antibodies in the serum. The abnormality represents an acquired modification of blood group. It may normalize during clinical remissions.

Absence of an Expected Antibody in the Serum Test

The natural antibody expected in the serum test in relation to data obtained in the red blood cell test, may be absent when the subject is unable to produce antibodies, either due to new born immune immaturity (antibodies present being of maternal origin) or to congenital or acquired agammaglobulinemia, myeloma or chronic lymphocytic leukemia.

Discrpancies with Positive Controls

There exist three possibilities: the auto control is positive (presence of cold agglutinins or rouleau formation), only the AB control is positive (polyagglutinability), or the allo control alone is positive (because of an irregular agglutinin).

Cola Agglutinins

This is a most difficult situation in which all three controls are strongly positive (agglutination is already seen in the tube in which blood is collected). Agglutination is most often due to autoantibodies bound to the patient's erythrocytes and less commonly to free antibodies in the serum. The bound autoantibodies may be eluted by washing red blood cells at 37, 40, or 45°C; the free antibodies can be absorbed onto O-group erythrocytes (the grouping may also be performed at 37°C).

Rouleau

In macroglobulinemia, myeloma, and hyperfibrinemia, abnormal red blood cell sedimentation may simulate agglutination. However, the AB control performed prior to erythrocyte washing is positive, while mere red blood cell washing is followed by a normal red blood cell test. The serum test is performed by slightly diluting serum in saline (1/2, 1/3). The protein responsible for the effect is then insufficiently concentrated, and the rouleaux disappear. One should note, however, that anti-A and anti-B hemagglutinins have also been diluted and may sometimes be difficult to detect.

Polyagglutinability

The polyagglutinability phenomenon (recognized by an AB positive control) may be due to contamination of the blood sample (it then suffices to obtain another blood sample) or to certain infectious diseases. There are several types of polyagglutinability: T, Tn and acquired B. Diagnosis is difficult and requires the experience of a specialized blood center.

Contribution of ABO Grouping to Pathology

We have named several diseases whose diagnosis may be recognized by irregularity in ABO typing. Let us briefly review them.

An ABO dual population (or, possibly, Rh) may be due to acute leukemia, refractory anemia, or myeloproliferative diseases.

A double population in several group systems, for example, ABO, MNS, Rh, and Kidd, may represent a mosaic or chimera with possible hermaphroditism (XX-XY).

Large quantities of A or B substance in the plasma suggest the presence of a gastrointestinal carcinoma (e.g., stomach or pancreas). These substances inhibit agglutination in the red blood cell test.

The presence of an anti-P_1 antibody may indicate the existence of a hydatic cyst.

The absence of detectable antibody on serum testing should lead to a search for a primary or secondary immunodeficiency (e.g., chronic lymphocyotic leukemia).

Massive autoagglutination usually denotes cold aggluytinin hemolytic anemia.

The rouleau phenomenon suggests Waldenstrom's macroglobulinemia or myeloma.

Rh Grouping

Determination of the standard (D) Rh phenotype is always performed along with ABO typing and is, of course, recorded on the usual blood group card. Rh+ refers to any subject whose red blood cells contain the standard Rh antigen (85% in the white race), and Rh-denotes any subject who lacks this antigen. Unlike the ABO group, there is no possible serum test, because Rh—subjects do not normally have anti-Rh antibody. Standard Rh grouping must be performed not only for all subjects to be transfused but also for pregnant women with possible fetomaternal alloimmunization.

Technique Description

The anti-Rh reagent is a mixture of bovine serum albumin and selected antisera obtained either from pregnancy-immunized women or from male volunteers previously immunized. The anti-Rh antibody is not capable alone of causing agglutination of Rh+ red blood cells. The addition of bovine serum albumin modifies the dielectric constant of the medium and leads to agglutination of sensitized erythrocytes.

The technical conditions of Rh grouping are different from those of ABO grouping. The reaction is performed at 40°C on a slide or at 37°C in microtubes. The utilization of proteolytic enzymes, such as papain, bromelin, or trypsin, considerably increases sensitivity and permits immediate recognition of weak Rh (D^u) antigens. Automatic techniques (Autoanalyzer or Groupamatic) generally include use of bromelin or Polybrene (a bicationic molecule).

The albumin control must always be performed. Erythrocytes sensitized by any IgG antibody generally agglutinate in bovine serum albumin, which explains why red blood cells from patients with hemolytic anemia due to IgG-type autoantibodies, already

Table 11.11
Results of Rhesus Grouping

Anti-D (1)	*Anti-D(2)*	*Anti-G*	*Anti-E*	
+	+			Rh+
—	—			Rh-
+	—			D^u (weak Rh+)
—	—	+	—	rh′
—	—	—	+	rh″
—	—	+	+	rh′rh″

coated with antibody before contact with anti-Rh reagent, agglutinate in the presence of albumin even when they are Rh-. Rh grouping of these patients is dificult. Elution of autoantibodies by heating to 56°C is not possible because of risk of Rh antigen alteration. Ether, which readily elutes IgG, is even more traumatizing to erythrocytes, reducing them to stromatous state. The only viable solution is to use the vey rare anti-Rh antibodies that are capable of agglutinating Rh+ red blood cells in saline suspension.

Practically speaking, routine grouping consists of testing erythrocytes with two anti-D reagents. If both reactions are positive and the control is negative, the subject is said to be Rh+. When both reactions and the control are negative, the subject is said to be Rh-. In the case of a patient awaiting transfusion, no further testing is necessary. Conversely, if the subject is a prospective blood donor, weak Rh(D^u) and the satellite antigens C and E must be evaluated. Conflicting reactions may be observed. The red blood cells of the tested subject are recognized as positive by one reagent and negative by another, suggesting the possibility of D^u.

D^u

All blood group antigens are heterogeneous. We have already discussed various A antigens, for example, A_1, A_2, and weak A antigens. The standard Rh antigen does not escape this rule, and the term D^u refers to all weak Rh antigens that present as positive Rh, which are more or less recognized by a specific reagent or technique. Weak Rh antigens may also be due to a positional effect (e.g., a R_1r' subject produces weak standard Rh) or to incomplete Rh antigens that lack some portion of the standard Rh antigen. Recent improvements in reagents and techniques have increased D^u detection threshold. The laboratories that utilize automated grouping methods, including the use of bromelin or polybrene, detect weak Rh (Rh+), which would have previously been considered to be negative or D^u by standard techniques.

In practice, if the results are negative on both test sera, the laboratory has no reason to proceed further, since the aim of the blood group card is to choose blood for transfusion in Rh— subjects. It is, therefore, enough to conclude that the subject is Rh-. The case of pregnant women is not the same. All Rh— nonimmunized women who deliver an Rh+ child receive anti-Rh Ig within 48 hr after childbirth. It is logical not to treat D^u women, thus justifying a search for D^u in pregnant women if treatment by Ig presents any danger. This search is, of course, imperative for donors, because it is important to detect weak Rh antigens that may be immunizing.

SCREENING OF IRREGULAR AGGLUTININS

The search for irregular agglutinins (or, more precisely, antierythrocyte irregular antibodies) is useful in pregnant women, transfusion recipients, and polytransfused patients. This search requires serum incubation with a panel of adequately selected erythrocytes.

In fact, very few antibodies are observed. Some are natureal antibodies, like anti-Le^a or anti-P_1, and others are immune antibodies, like anti-D or anti-D+C (which are

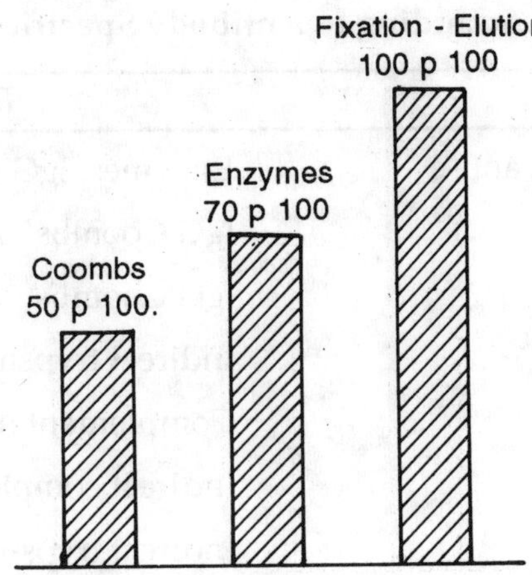

Fig. 11.5. D^u detection; proportion of positive results obtained according to the technique used.

most frequent). One must also screen for anti-Kell, anti-c, and anti-E of the Rh system, anti-Fy[a] of the Duffy system, anti-JK[a] of the Kidd system, and anti-S of the MNS system. Other specificities are most uncommon, and their identification is only accomplished in specialized centers.

Very few of these antibodies are agglutinating, that is, capable of agglutinating erythrocytes suspended in 0.9% NaCl. It is therefore necessary to introduce artificial systems so that binding of the antibody to the erythrocytic surface leads to agglutination. Anti-Ig sera may be used. It is the principle of the direct Coombs' tests (polyvalent, IgG, or complement specific). Special artificial means may also be used so as to decrease the stability of red blood cells in suspension.

We have seen earlier that erythrocytic stability in suspension relates to repulsion forces between red blood cells and, in particular, depends on the difference in the zeta potential between positive ions surrounding the red cells and the medium. The artificial agglutination process decreases the zeta potential either by decreasing charge or increasing dielectric constant. In the first case, proteolytic enzymes (papain, trypsin, or bromelin) are capable of detaching from membrane glucidic heteroproteins that contain, in particular, sialic acid, the main source of the red blood cell negative charges by its carboxyl groups. In the second case, the medium is modified by addition of high-molecular-weight substances, such as bovine serum albumin. When the antibody binds to the erythrocytic surface, the zeta potential is further decreased, and the stability of the suspension is then lost.

Practical Organization for Irregular Antibody Screening

One does not know whether the searched antibody is agglutinating, active at low temperature or only at 37°C, and whether it is detectable by use of enzymes and the Coombs' test. Therefore, a wide variety of test techniques must be used. Table 11.12

Table 11.12
Examples of Sensitive Techniques for Irregular Agglutinin Detection According to Antibody Specificity

Irregular agglutinin	*Technique*
Anti-D, anti-D+C, anti-E, anti-c, anti-e	Enzymes, lgG Coombs'
Anti-Kell	lgG Coombs', AB
Anti-Fy^a	lgG Coombs'
Anti-Jk^a	Indirect trypsinized Coombs'
	Complement or lgG Coombs'
Anti-Le^a	Indirect complement Coombs'
	Indirect trypsin Coombs'
	Saline 22°C
Anti-P_1	Saline 22°C

shows the most sensitive techniques for each antibody specificity. Note that automated techniques (Autoanalyzer, Groupamatic) are now available for detection and identification of irregular agglutinins.

Different Panels

Screening capacity depends on the number and variety of indicator erythrocytes. It is not possible to identify anti-Kell antibodies if the panel contains no Kell positive red blood cells. For example, the Paris transfusion center utilizes three types of panels.

The PMI panel includes three samples of erythrocytes. This panel permits detection of anti-D, -C, -c,-É,-é, and -Kell antibodies, namely, those sought in a pregnant women because they relate to maternal and infant protection, hence the name PMI (*Protection Maternelle et Infantile*). One should note, however, that this panel detects the presence of irregular agglutinins wihtout precise identification.

The detection panel is more sophisticated and includes eight erythrocyte samples. It permits the detection, in addition to that of the above-mentioned antibodies, of anti-M,-N,-S,-S,-k,-Kp^a,-Le^a,-Le^b,-Fy^a-Fy^b,-Jk^a,-Jk^b,-Lu^a, and α—Lu^b antibodies, which represent the vast majority of antibodies clinically seen, but still without individual identification.

The identification panel includes 10 erythrocyte samples, whose phenotypes are selected among the blood group systems presently known. These erythrocytes are chosen and assembled in such a way that one may identify antibody mixtures. Specific identification consists of detemining the correspondence between distribution of observed reactions, positive and negative, and the presence or absence of a specific antigen, in any system. Because common specificities are limited in number, the test consists of looking for a coincidence with antigens D,D+C,E,c, Kell, Le^a, P_1, and, possibly Fy^a, Jk^a and S.

Irregular agglutinin screening may thus lead to safe identification of detected antibody(ies) specificity. However, one should consider four general limitations:

The composition of the panel defines the limit of possibel identifications,

One cannot identify all possible antibodies with one technique,

Indirect Coombs' tests are not reliable if one is uncertain whether the antisera used both included anti-IgG and anticomplement antibodies,

One must know, especially for polytransfused subjects, the collection date of the blood sample tested. The antibody may be absorbed and only become detectable several days after transfusion.

12

Haematological Diseases

Since many of the components of the immune response circulate in blood, it is not surprising that there is some overlap between immunology and haematology. Malignancies of lymphocytes, namely leukaemias and lymphomas, have already been discussed. Here, those haematological diseases *in which the immune response plays a pathogenic role* will be considered: for example anaemia, thrombocytopenia or neutropenia can all be due to antibodies directed against these components of blood. In most cases, these antibodies are autoantibodies; however, disease also results from the stimulation of alloantibodies (isoimmune antibodies) by repeated blood transfusions or pregnancy. Direct activation of complement by erythrocytes may also cause anaemia and is considered here.

Mechanisms of Destruction

The immune system can destroy mature erythrocytes, platelets and neutrophils as well as some haematological precursors in the bone marrow. Immune destruction of red cells is the best known.

Antibody may attach to antigen on the surface of the red cell and these antibody-coated red cells are destroyed either by phagocytosis or by complement mediated lysis. Direct complement lysis without antibody involvement is rare. Haematological complications can also be due to soluble immune complexes in the circulation. Such complexes can become attached to red cell membranes through CR1 (C3b) receptors, a process known as immune adherence or to platelet membranes through Fc receptors, resulting in 'innocent bystander' destruction.

CLASSIFICATION AND MECHANISM OF ANAEMIA

Definition

Anaemia is a condition wherein the number of *red corpuscles* per cubic millimetre., the quantity of *haemoglobin* in grams or the volume of *packed red cells* per 100 ml. blood are reduced below the normal limits (Vakil, 1969). Anaemia has also been defined as a diminished or reduced oxygen carrying capacity of the blood.

Anaemia can therefore occur whenever the haemopoietic equilibrium is disturbed and the loss of erythrocytes or haemoglobin from the circulation exceeds production.

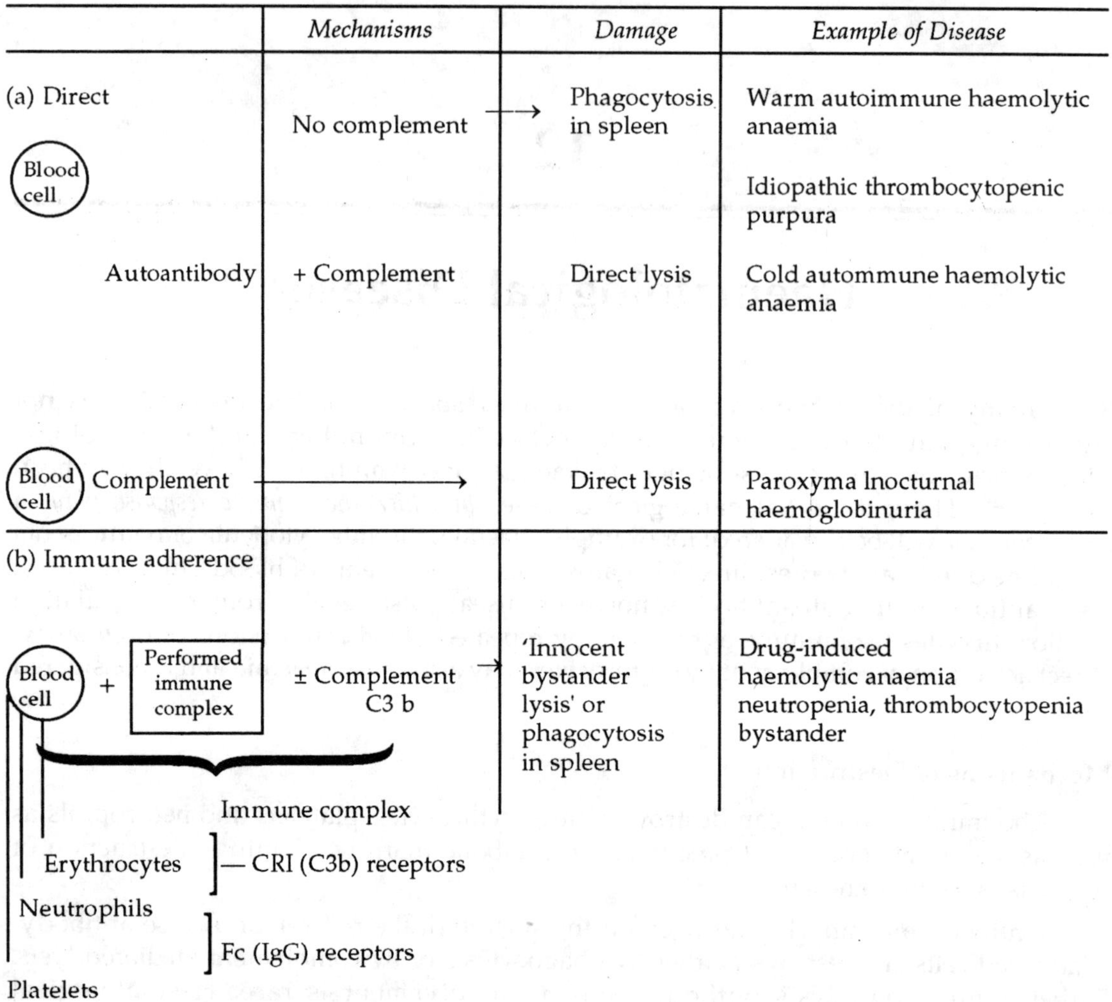

Fig. 12.1. Mechanisms of destruction of blood components.

Classification

Anaemias may be classified according to morphological characteristics or causative mechanisms. Although each classification has shortcomings when used alone, they are very helpful when used together, as together they provide important steps towards the diagnosis of the type of anaemia and therefore, the treatment.

A. *Morphological Classification*—For this classification, the size and haemoglobin content of the red blood corpuscles have to be determined.

Table 12.1
Classification of Anaemia According to the Size and Haemoglobin Content of the Erythrocytes

	Type	*MCV (c. microns)*	*MCHC (%)*
1.	Macrocytic	>94	>30
2.	Normocytic	80-94	>30
3.	Simple Microcytic	<80	<30
4.	Hypochromic Microcytic	<80	<30

B. *Classification according to Mechanism*— This is a most helpful classification and provides a sound basis for further systematic investigations and treatment.

Table 12.2
Classification of Anaemia According to Mechanism of Production

Mechanism	*Cause*	*Disease or Clinical Syndrome*
A. Nutritional Deficiency		
I. Diminished Erythropoiesis		
1. Diet	Inadequate intake	Multiple deficiencies
2. Defective absorption	Failure to secrete intrinsic factor	Vitamin B_{12} deficiency (Pernicious anaemia)
	Total gastrectomy	
Stomach	Partial gastrectomy	Iron deficiency
Intestine	Diarrhoea Diverticula Fistulas Stricture	Folic acid, vitamin B_{12} or iron deficiency (Sprue, malabsorption syndrome, or pernicious anaemia)
3. Increased demand	Pregnancy	(Folic acid, vitamin B_{12} or iron deficiency)
	Growth	Iron deficiency
B. Bone Marrow Failure	1. Associated disease	Primary disease
	2. Drugs	Aplastic anaemia
	3. Chemicals	Aplastic anaemia
	4. Irradiation	Aplastic anaemia
	5. Endocrine	Myxoedema, pituitary disease

(Contd.)

Mechanism	*Cause*	*Disease or Clinical Syndrome*
	6. Idiopathic	Aplastic anaemia
II. BLOOD LOSS		
A. Acute	Trauma or disease	Shock or anaemia
B. Chronic	Lesion of gastrointestinal tract or ganæcologic disturbance	Iron deficiency anaemia or primary disease.
III. INCREASED HAEMOLYSIS	Congental defects	Hereditary spherocytosis Sickle cell and other haemoglobinopathies
A. Intracorpuscular		Thalassemia
		Drug sensitivity
		Paroxysmal nocturnal haemoglobinuria Congenital non-spherocytic anaemia
B. Extracorpuscular	Acquired defects	
	1. Iso-antibodies	Erythroblastosis foetalis, transfusion reaction.
	2. Auto-antibodies	Idiopathic and secondary autoimmune haemolytic disease.
	3. Auto-hæmolysis	Paroxysmal cold haemoglobinuria.
	4. Infections	Malaria, septicemia etc.
	5. Chemicals	Phenylhydrazine etc.
	6. Physical Agents	Burns
	7. Vegetable poisons	Favism (also intra-corpuscular)
	8. Miscellaneous	Splenomegaly, liver disease, haemopathic haemolytic anaemia.

C. Aetiological Classification

For purposes of description, the following aetiological classification has been found to be most practical.

I. Dyshaemopoietic Anaemias — Due to inefficient blood production.

II. Haemorrhagic Anaemias — Due to extravascular blood loss.

III. Haemolytic Anaemias — Due to excessive intravascular blood destruction.

IV. Anaemias associated with other disorders.

I. DYSHAEMOPOIETIC ANAEMIAS

The haemopoietic system is a highly specialised tissue which continually supplies cells with specific function at a relatively quick rate. For efficient functioning, the haemopoietic system must have a continuous supply of adequate and proper nutrients from which the cells could be built and must co-ordinate and co-operate with other systems. It is also possible that nutritional factors are required for all stages of normal erythropoiesis. Recently, by the use of isotopic tracers and other methods, nutritional factors essential for erythropoiesis have been classified to a fairly great extent.

Factors for Formation & Maturation of Red Blood Corpuscles

1. Minerals —Iron

   Trace elements, e.g., copper, cobalt.

2. Amino acids and Protein.

3. Haemopoietic Principle — Believed by some to be Vitamin B_{12} after absorption.

4. Other Vitamins — Vitamin B-Complex, Folic Acid, Ascorbic Acid.

5. Internal secretions.

6. Pigments.

(1) Minerals

Iron: A deficiency of iron affects the normoblast — reticulocyte — red corpuscle stage i.e. that stage of erythropoiesis at which the haemoglobin is being rapidly assimilated by the ripening corpuscle. The red cells are produced in normal numbers but are deficient in haemoglobin.

Blood Picture in Iron Deficiency

1. Hypochromic type of anaemia.

2. Microcytosis and poikilocytosis.

3. Low Mean Corpuscular Haemoglobin Concentration (MCHC).

4. Low Colour Index.

5. Commonly, Low Mean Corpuscular Volume. (MCV)

Copper: Copper appears to act by assisting the conversion of inorganic iron into haemoglobin, thus speeding up the process of red cell maturation.

Cobalt: It is believed that cobalt is necessary for the normal nutrition of man. There is no convincing evidence that anaemias in man are caused by cobalt deficiency, but Berk *et al.*,(1949) found that its adminstration caused a slight reticulocyte response and an increase in the red cell count.

(2) Amino-Acids and Protein

The globin portion of haemoglobin requires adequate supplies of protein.Convining evidence has been put forward regarding the importance of adequate protein supplements in haemoglobin synthesis.

It was found that when protein and certain amino-acids were added to the diet, there was a greater increase in haemoglobin production than with iron alone, first class proteins of high biological value e.g. casein or ovalbumin, being more useful than proteins such as gluten (Buechler & Guggenheim, 1949).

Anaemia aggravated by protien deficiency is more common in women than in men and prone to occur in pregnancy. A correlation between the macrocytic anaemia of pregnancy and inadequate protein intake was shown by Bethell *et al.*, (1943). The anaemia most definitely caused by protein deficiency is that of liver disease and kwashiorkor so prevalent in Africa.

(3) Haemopoietic Principle

The haemopoietic principle is essential for the proper maturation of proerythroblasts. In the absence of this substance, maturation is deflected to the megaloblastic series of cells instead of to the normoblastic series.

Blood Picture in Deficiency of Haemopoetic Principle

1. Megalocytic, Megaloblastic, hyperchromic anaemia.
2. High Mean Corpuscular Volume.
3. High Mean Corpuscular Diameter.
4. Normal Mean Corpuscular Haemoglobin Concentration.
5. High Colour Index.

It must be remembered that there may be an associated iron deficiency as well, in which case the haemoglobin concentration and colour index will be found to be low.

Folic acid deficiency gives rise to a similar blood picture.

Some authorities assign a co-enzyme function to folic acid, citrovorum factor and vitamin B_{12}, regarding one or the other as essential for certain stages in the synthesis of nucleic acid from simple substances (Whitby & Britton, 1963).

(4) Other Vitamins

B-Complex Group

(a) Folinic Acid or Citrovorum factor

This substance probably plays the part of an haemopoietically active co-enzyme concerned with the formation of purines, thymine and other substances as part of the synthesis of nucleic acid.

(b) Thymine and Thymidine

Thymine and thymidine in large doses have produced a haematological response in pernicious anaemia in relapse and also in the megaloblastic anaemia of sprue, but are not effective in preventing the neurological lesions of pernicious anaemia.

A theory has been put forward that the fundamental biochemical defect in pernicious anaemia is the inability to synthesize nucleosides e.g. thymidine from purines and pyrimidines. If this is the case, folic acid probably acts by spending up and increasing thymine synthesis which itself, by mass action, might yield more thymidine (Whitby & Britton, 1963).

(c) Choline

Choline has been found to be of value in certain megaloblastic anaemias especially when there is an element of hepatic dysfunction, probably potentiating liver extracts. This aspect should be considered in megaloblastic anaemias refractory to liver treatment.

(d) Pyridoxine

It has been long known that a deficiency of Vitamin B_6 causes an anaemia in dogs and pigs. Recently, several cases of hypochromic anaemias with normal or high serum iron levels have been reported to have responded to pyridoxine alone. The reason for this responsiveness is not quite understood. It has been reported that cases of hypochromic microcytic anaemias refractory to iron therapy responded when Vitamin B_6 was added to the treatment.

(e) Riboflavine

Though there is no evidence that ariboflavinosis causes anaemia in humans. It has been found in certain animals, that an impairment of recovery from the anaemia of haemorrhage results when the diet is deficient in riboflavine.

(f) Nicotinic Acid

Pellagra is often accompanied by anaemia but the significance of nicotinic acids in this connection is not clear. A case of hypochromic anaemia has been described, which did not respond to iron therapy till nicotine acid was also administered.

Folic Acid

The characteristic haematological finding in folic acid deficiency is *megaloblast formation.* Normal erythropoiesis is disturbed with the result that the proerythroblasts give rise, not to the normoblasts, but to the megaloblasts which may mature to megalocytes. The blood picture is the same as that found in Vitamin B_{12} deficiency.

Ascorbic Acid

There is now little doubt that Vitamin C plays a part in erythropoiesis but probably as a general marrow stimulant. It participates in metabolic activities which affect vitiamin B_{12} and folic acid. Vitamin C is important in the conversion of folic acid to folinic acid and there is some evidence that it stimulates the formation of folic acid. It is known to assist in the absorption of dietary iron. Cox *et al.*, (1960) state that all megaloblastic anaemias show a significant reduction in the vitamin C content in the bone marrow.

(5) Internal Secretions

(a) Thyroid

It has been found thyroidectomized animals rapidly become anaemic. Experimentally and clinically, thyroxin has been found to be essential in the treatment of anaemias associated with thyroid deficiency. Convincing evidence has not been forthcoming however that thyroxin is a specific erythropoietic factor that is being utilized at a definite stage of red cell development. It is probably a general metabolic stimulant increasing the tissues' need for oxygen, to which demand the marrow responds.

(b) Pituitary

It is probable that the anterior pituitary influences blood formation since an anaemia is commonly found in Simmond's disease and a polycythaemia in Cushing's syndrome. Similar effects have also been noted experimentally.

The action of the posterior lobe on blood formation is unknown.

(c) Thymus

Tumours of the thymus are often associated with a rare and refractory type of anaemia characterized by an erythroblastic hypoplasia with an almost complete lack of erythrocyte precursors in the bone marrow. This is unaccompanied by depression of leucoblastic or megakaryocyte elements.

(d) Sex Hormones

It is clear that the gonads influence haemopoiesis either directly or indirectly. Finkelstein *et al.*, (1944) have shown that male sex hormones accelerate haemopoiesis. Lederer and Canivez (1953), found a low serum iron in eunuchs which was corrected by hormone therapy alone. Also, it was found that androgens given for breast cancer caused haemoglobin to increase even though no haematinics were administered.

(6) Pigments

(a) Bile pigment

Bile pigmens appear to facilitate absorption and utilization of iron but the mode of action is still obscure. This was shown by Patek and Minot, (1934) who found that when bile pigment was administered in combination with suboptimal amounts of iron, a definite reticulocyte rise was produced which would not have occurred with iron alone.

(b) Chlorophyll

Chlorophyll has been reported to accelerate the utilization of iron by the body.

Deficiency

Erythropoiesis may be diminished due to a deficiency (absolute or relative) of one or more of the factors described above.

Causes of Deficiency

(I) Inadequate intake in the diet.

(II) Failure to elaborate, digest or absorb factor or factors which may be present in adequate quantities in the diet.

(III) Failure to utilize these factors by the bone marrow.

 (a) due to the presence of some toxic agent.

 (b) due to hypoplasia or aplasia of the marrow itself.

(IV) Excessive demands.

(I) Inadequate Intake

A faulty and indequate diet is responsible for anaemia in various parts of the world especially in persons of the lower economic groups, giving rise to various deficiencies.

The more expensive iron containing foodstuffs are anything but abundant in their diet causing a deficiency of *iron* in the body. A diet which is essentially carbohydrate in nature will also contribute to the same condition.

These diets are commonly deficient in *vitamins* especially Vitamin C, since fruits etc., are not eaten by the poor for economic reasons.

Nutritional megaloblastic anaemia was first studied in India by Wills & Mehta (1930) and later found to be due to a *folic acid* deficiency.

It must be remembered that a not uncommon cause of deficient food intake is lack of appetite which is frequently a result of gastric dysfunction.

(II) Defective Absorption

This is a fairly common cause of nutritional anaemia in adults. In pernicious Anaemia, a deficiency of *Vitamin* B_{12} arises as a result of defective gastric function and the failure to secrete the intrinsic factor. Total gastrectomy also gives rise to a similar disorder, but owing to the large reserves of Vitamin B_{12} in the body, symptoms appear many years after the procedure. Macrocytic anaemia and megaloblastic erythropoiesis may be found in sprue or other conditions accompained by severe diarrhoea. Intestinal statis due to any cause, e.g. 'blind loop' syndrome, anastomoses, may give rise to a similar type of disorder.

Iron deficiency anaemia can arise as a result of partial gastrectomy, diarrhoeas, high phytate content of food, achlorhydria, hypochlorhydria or sepsis.

(III) Failure to Utilize these Factors by the Bone Marrow

(a) Presence of Toxic Agents

When the bone marrow is unable to utilize these factors, eryhtropoiesis is, as a result, not adequate.

Inadequate erythropoiesis may occur due to :

(i) ingestion of certain drugs, e.g., some antibiotics, anticonvulsants, heavy metals, some coal-tar products, benzol (Leavell & Thorup, 1966).

(ii) exposure to chemicals — this is more prone to occur in industries using organic solvents particularly benzol and its derivatives. Insecticide sprays and cleaning agents have also been incriminated.

(iii) Irradiation — After X-rays or use of radioactive materials.

(b) Hypoplasia or Aplasia of Bone Marrow

In some patients, no explanation can be found for the bone marrow failure that is responsible for severe anaemia. It has been postulated that this may be a congenital defect especially when it occurs in infants and young children, but aplastic anaemia also occurs in adults. The marrow hypoplasia is usually associated with pancytopenia.

(IV) Excessive Demands

Even if a normal dietary intake has been maintained, a deficiency of essential factors may occur when there are excessive demands for erythropoiesis. The most common condition is pregnancy and naturally more so if it is a twin pregnancy, when an *iron* deficiency or a deficiency of *folic acid* or *Vitamin* B_{12} may develop.

Growing children show an increased need for *iron* as also women in their child-bearing years. During this period, these women can very easily pass into a state of negative iron-balance due to the losses in menstruation and parturition.

II. HAEMORRHAGIC ANAEMIAS

Extravascular blood loss may be either acute or chronic, the clinical manifestation being different in the two conditions.

Sudden loss of a large volume of blood may occur in

(1) Trauma.

(2) Post-operative haemorrhage.

(3) Ruptured ectopic pregnancy.

(4) Ruptured aneurysm.

(5) Ruptured oesophageal varices.

(6) Ulcerative lesions of the gastro-intestinal tract.

(7) Spontaneous or after slight trauma in haemorrhagic disorders.

(Leavell & Thorup, 1966).

The haemorrhagic anaemias include haemophilia and purpuric conditions.

Acute Haemorrhage

In acute haemorrhage the usual symptoms are sudden dizziness, weakness, pallor and sweating but the severity of the symptoms depend on the amount, location and acuteness of the bleeding and the previous condition of the patient.

A blood loss of 500 ml. or less (as drawn for transfusion purposes) should cause no symptoms. A blood loss of 700 ml. causes slight but definite symptoms. Thereafter, the seriousness of the loss increases and a loss of 1,500-2,000 ml. in a short space of time may be fatal. However, if the loss is spread over 24 hours, as much as 2000ml. can be lost without a fatal issue.

Blood Picture

The peripheral blood changes depend on the time elapsed and the size and location of the haemorrhage and also the underlying disease if any.

A figure of 2,500,000 red cells per c.mm. and the haemoglobin of 6 G per 100 ml. is the maximum drop that can occur with a single, severe haemorrhage, untreated by transfusion, without causing death.

The haematocrit value however, may give little or no indication of the amount of blood lost and therefore it is better to determine the blood volume. There is a usually a normocytic anaemia unless an underlying iron deficiency is present. Reticulocytosis occurs and reaches a peak in 4-7 days. If haemorrhage has occured into a body cavity, there will also be a rise in serum bilirubin.

If bleeding has stopped, the red cell count rises and continues to rise even without treatment till the normal level is reached in about 4-6 weeks. Schiodt, (1937) has reported that the red cell count returns to a level of 4.5 mill./c.mm. in about 33 days after an acute episode irrespective of the size of the haemorrhage.

During regeneration, there is initially a reticulocytosis which declines as mature red cells are produced. Usually, a neutrophil leucocytosis of 20,000/c.mm. is also found.

The marrow may show a normoblastic hyperplasia.

Chronic Haemorrhage

Chronic haemorrhage or repeated small haemorrhages are often tolerated surprisingly well. The commonest site is the alimentary tract e.g. a duodenal or gastric ulcer or haemorrhoids, when serious anaemia may develop without the patient being aware of blood passing out in the stools. Menorrhagia is a common cause in women especially between 30 and 40 years of age giving rise to a hypochromic anaemia. The anaemia of essential thrombocytopenic purpura is due to chronic haemorrhage, and in those persons liable to infection, Ankylostoma duodenale infestation causing blood loss should be kept in mind.

Blood Picture

The haemoglobin is always reduced much more than the red cell count. Therefore, the colour index and mean corpuscular haemoglobin concentration are low. Most characteristic of chronic haemorrhage is microcytosis which may be quite marked. The red cells are hypochromic. Reticulocytosis is not significant and rarely exceeds 4-5% of the red cell count.

The marrow is always hyperplastic, at least in patches and is usually of the normoblastic series.

Investigations

In a case of haemorrhage, investigations have to be directed towards determining the cause of the haemorrhage and apart from blood examination, include stool test for occult blood, radiology of the gastro-intestinal tract, liver function tests and sometimes surgical exploration.

III. HAEMOLYTIC ANAEMIAS

Haemolytic anaemias occur whenever a decreased survival time of the red cells (normal about 120 days) is not balanced by increased erythropoiesis.

A decrease to less than 20 days is necessary to produce anaemia if the bone marrow is functioning normally, since it has capacity to increase its production of red cells six fold. Unless erythropoiesis is depressed for any reason, haemolytic anaemia is characterized by both increased haemolysis and increased erythropoiesis.

Mechanisms Causing a Diminution in Survival Time of Erythrocytes

(I) Intracorpuscular

(II) Extracorpuscular

I. Intracorpuscular Causes

(1) Hereditary Spherocytosis (Congenital Haemolytic Jaundice)

(2) Thalassaemia (Cooley's Anaemia, Mediterranean Anaemia)

(3) Haemoglobinopathies

(4) Glucose-6-Phosphate Dehydrogenase (G-6-PD) Deficiency :

(5) Paroxysmal Nocturnal Haemoglobinuria (Marchiafava-Micheli Syndrome).

II. Extracorpuscular Causes

(1) Auto-immune Haemolytic Anaemias.

(2) Iso-immune Haemolytic Disease.

(3) Paroxysmal Cold Haemoglobinuria.

(4) Infectious Agents — septicemia, tuberculosis, malaria.

(5) Chemical Agents — naphthalene, sulphonamides, quinine.

(6) Physical Agents — severe burns, valvular heart disease.

(7) Vegetable Poisons — favism

(8) Hypersplenism

(9) Haemopathic Haemolytic Anaemia — uraemia, carcinoma, leukaemia.

(10) Haemolytic Anaemia Associated with Liver Disease.

IV. ANAEMIAS ASSOCIATED WITH OTHER CONDITIONS

Anaemia may be a symptom of diverse conditions, in most of which, the explanation of anaemia is largely speculative.

Anaemia may be associated with

1. Myxoedema
2. Chronic Renal Disease
3. Chronic Liver Disease
4. Hypersplenism
5. Pregnancy.

(1) Myxoedema

Different types of anaemia may occur in this condition, singly or together.

(a) Uncomplicated anaemia of hypothyroidism. This is a normochromic and normocytic or slightly macrocytic anaemia and usually mild.

(b) Anaemia due to iron deficiency. Apart from causes common to other individuals, pre-menopausal hypothyroid women show an increased frequency of excessive menstrual flow.

"It is believed that the anaemia in myxoedema is an adaptation to a condition of relative oxygen surfeit in the tissues rather than the consequence of an illness associated with partial failure of bone marrow resulting from a lack of thyroid factor."

(2) Chronic Renal Disease

A significant degree of anaemia develops in the majority of cases sometime during the course of chronic renal disease.

The blood picture is commonly of a normocytic, normochromic anaemia (occasionally macrocytic). The haemoglobin level in one series of patients with uraemia ranged from 5.6-8.4 gm/100 ml. and the red cell count from 1.5-3.5 mill./c.mm. The leucocyte and platelet counts are usually normal.

The mechanism of production of anaemia in uraemia is not completely understood. There is obviously a selective action on the bone marrow since only erythrocyte precursors are depressed. Histologically, hypoplasia of the erythroid series was noted when the blood non-protein nitrogen was over 150 mg/100 ml. Complete aplasia was not found and it was suggested that there may also be a defect in the delivery of the red blood cells to the peripheral blood. Emerson and Burroughs (1949), indicated that this anaemia may be due to haemolysis and concluded from their study that some extra-corpuscular factor in the plasma was responsible for the premature destruction of the red cells. Other investigators discovered that this haemolytic activity was not shown in all patients and it is now believed that depression of erythropoiesis is the most important and most common factor.

(3) Chronic Liver Disease

Anaemia often occurs in patients with chronic liver disease. The blood picture may be hypochromic microcytic, macrocytic or normocytic depending on the mechanism responsible. In a particular individual, the most important factor may be either blood loss, increased haemolysis, or deficient erythropoiesis.

Iron deficiency which is usually the result of repeated haemorrhages from ruptured oesophageal varices or chronic blood loss from the gastrointestinal tract gives rise to a hypochromic microcytic type of anaemia.

However, it is a macrocytic anaemia that is usually found. The mean corpuscular volume is usually 100-120 cu. microns, and erythropoiesis is normoblastic. The leucocytes and platelets are usually normal in number. In contrast to pernicious anaemia, anisocytosis and poikilocytosis are absent in this condition but target cells are numerous.

The mechanism for the production of a macrocytic anaemia in chronic liver disease is believed to involve haemolysis of an extracorpuscular nature. This has been demonstrated by several workers and explains the macrocytic anaemia associated with a normoblastic marrow. However, in those cases with a megaloblastic marrow, some other factors are probably involved. It is interesting to note that the severe anaemia in these cases has been found to respond to the administration of folic acid, vitamin B_{12}, liver extract, and ascorbic acid. A contributing factor to this type of anaemia may be the grossly deficient diet of these patients over long periods.

In chronic liver desease associated with chronic alcoholism, there is a folic acid deficiency. A low serum folate concentration has been demonstrated in the majority of these patients.

It has been suggested that alcohol may directly depress marrow activity, since it was observed that a reticulocytosis occurrred in patients with cirrhosis on a diet deficient in erythropoietic factors, if the ingestion of alcohol was prevented.

There have been conflicting reports on the 'presence' and 'absence' of the antipernicious-anaemia-factor in livers of patients who died from cirrhosis. This can now be probably explained by the recognition of at least two types of macrocytic anaemias, one associated with hyperhaemolysis and the other caused by a specific deficiency.

(4) Hypersplenism

a syndrome characterized by

1. Splenomagaly
2. Anaemia
3. Leukaemia
4. Thrombocytopenia
5. Bone marrow with normal or increased cellularity.
6. Correction of the blood picture by splenectomy.

This syndrome occurs in a variety of conditions associated with splenomegaly.

At present, the mechanism of the anaemia involved is not definitely established and also, it is not certain that the same mechanism is responsible in every patient. Various theories have been put forward :

1. The enlarged spleen exerts an inhibiting effect on the bone marrow by means of a humoral factor.
2. The enlarged abnormal spleen causes sequestration and destruction of the cellular elements.

(5) Pregnancy

Physiological Changes

During normal pregnancy the haematocrit, haemoglobin and red cell counts are reduced. The maximal decrease occurs in the last three months of pregnancy and are at least partly due to haemodilution since the plasma volume increases by 800 to 1300 ml. while the red cell volume is increased by only 300 ml.

The following values are said to represent the lower normal limits of haemoglobin and erythrocytes during pregnancy :

Haemoglobin—11.3 to 11.5 gm. per 100 ml.

Red cells—3.7 milli. per cu.mm.

Haematocrit—35 per cent.

The sedimentation rate is always greater than normal, increasing as pregnancy advances. The total plasma proteins fall progressively during pregnancy the fall chiefly being in the total albumin and gamma globulin fractions. There is a small but definite polymorphonuclear leucocytosis most marked in primiparae.

There is a fall in plasma iron, an increase in plasma total iron binding capacity and an increased efficiency of iron absorption as pregnancy proceeds.

The mother loses iron to the foetus and also with bleeding during delivery. It has been calculated that the additional iron necessary for pregnancy is about 400 mg. or more.

Causes of Anaemia in Pregnancy

(1) Iron Deficiency

(2) Gastric Dysfunction

(3) Protein and other Deficiencies.

(1) Iron Deficiency

During pregnancy, the foetus requires large quantities of maternal iron and as a general rule, obtains these supplies whether the mother is anaemic or not. Therefore, it is important to have a good reserve of iron before pregnancy begins (The total iron content of a mature foetus is about 375 mg.)

(2) Gastric Dysfunction

Strauss and Castle (1932), found that in their series of 24 women, 75% did not secrete normal amounts of free hydrochloric acid or pepsin during more than half of the pregnancy. Their investigations showed the importance of a protein and iron rich diet for the prevention of anaemia.

It has been suggested that the increased activity of the pituitary may be concerned with the gastric disturbances during pregnancy.

(3) Protein and Other Deficiencies

A relation between the incidence of megaloblastic anaemia in pregnancy and a protein-deficient diet was shown by Bethell et al. (1939 & 1943). These patients probably were also taking a diet low in folic acid.

Multiple nutritional deficiencies contribute to pregnancy anaemia especially in the tropics. In India, it has long been recognised that a magaloblastic anaemia is common in pregnancy. The increased demands of the body for haemopoietic substances during pregnancy, would naturally aggravate the condition. This type of pregnancy anaemia responds to the administration of folic acid or crude liver extracts or even liver itself.

Megaloblastic anaemias in pregnancy associated with a low serum Vitamin B_{12}, are found to respond to administration of Vitamin B_{12}.

Types of Anaemia during Pregnancy

(1) Iron deficiency.

(2) Nutritional Macrocytic Anaemia.

(3) Megaloblastic Anaemia.

(4) Anaemia as a result of a coexisting disease.

1. Iron Deficiency

This is probably the commonest type of anaemia during pregnancy. The anaemia is a hypochromic, microcytic type with the serum iron reduced to less than 60 micrograms per 100 ml. together with an increase in the latent iron binding capacity. Erythropoiesis is normoblastic in type.

2. Nutritional Macrocytic Anaemia

This is attributed to dietary deficiency and is commonly found in those of a low economic status. Pregnancy probably acts as an additional cause of nutritional magaloblastic anaemia in women.

3. Magaloblastic Anaemia

A megaloblastic anaemia may occur as a result of folic acid deficiency but it has been suggested that multiple factors are involved. Dietary deficiencies, vomiting and altered gastric secretion may be contributory factors. The blood picture is similar to that found in pernicious anaemia but less marked. Free hydrochloric acid in the gastric juice may be low.

4. Anaemia Associated with Coexisting Diseases

When a pregnant woman with anaemia is seen for the first time, a coexisting disease giving rise to the anaemia must be kept in mind. These include renal disease, lymphomas, leukaemias, the haemoglobinopathies all of which may be recognised for the first time during pregnancy.

It must be remembered that iron deficiency may occur in association with normal indices and megaloblastic anaemias may occur with normal indices or even with microcytosis. Therefore, the recognition of the factors responsible for anaemia during pregnancy is not always easy and a serum iron estimation (low in iron deficiency and normal or high in other types of anaemia) and bone marrow studies may have to be carried out.

Therapy

The best therapy is preventive. A liberal daily diet containing adequate amounts of milk, meat, and at least one egg a day will prevent most macrocytic anaemias. Supplementary iron and folic acid will be also effective.

If iron deficiency anaemia or megaloblastic anaemia has developed, appropriate therapy has to be instituted.

It must be remembered that if iron deficiency anaemia develops during pregnancy, therapy with iron should be carried out for some months after the pregnancy to replenish iron stores. Megaloblastic anaemia may recur in subsequent pregnancies.

DIAGNOSIS OF ANAEMIA

The objectives in the management of the patient with anaemia are :

1. to discover the cause of the anaemia.
2. to correct the underlying defect.

A systematic investigation almost always indicates the correct diagnosis and therefore the correct treatment. The completed investigation should provide answers to the following questions.

1. Does the patient have anaemia ?
2. What is the mechanism of the anaemia ?
3. What are the morphologic characteristics of the anaemia ?
4. What is the underlying cause or desease that is responsible for the abnormal mechanism ?
5. What is the best form of treatment ?

Whether the patient has anaemia or not, cannot always be ascertained by clinical examination. The presence of anaemia can be definitely established only by laboratory procedures, the simplest and most reliable one being the haematocrit determination.

The haemoglobin estimation has also been advocated and is believed to be as reliable if it is performed properly.

To determine the mechanism responsible for the anaemia the following are necessary.

a. A careful history

b. Physical examination

c. Laboratory procedures.

a. History

Special emphasis should be laid on dietary history particularly in pregnancy, chronic illness and in the case of children. The presence or absence of tarry stools and in women, excessive menstrual bleeding should always be enquired into. The occupation of the patient is important from the point of view of repeated exposure to drugs or chemicals. A family history of anaemia or splenectomy may give a clue to haemolytic anaemia.

b. Physical Examination

A physical examination alone will not suffice for the diagnosis of anaemia, but will provide helpful information. The tongue, conjunctiva, fingernails, and fissuring of the lips will indicate the nutritional state of patient and will point to an iron, folic acid or Vitamin B_{12} deficiency. Splenomegaly is associated with most haemolytic anaemias. Ataxia will give a clue to pernicious anaemia especially if the blood picture has been altered by inadequate specific therapy or a coexisting iron deficiency.

c. Laboratory Studies

(i) Observations on the number, size and volume of the *red cells* and their *haemoglobin* content are very important in the diagnosis of the anaemias. The *number* of red cells is determined on a counting chamber or by an electronic method. It is expressed as the number per cubic millimetre of blood. The *size* is estimated roughly in a stained film or more exactly by direct measurement or diffraction methods and then expressed in microns. The *volume* of the red cells is found with the haematocrit and is expressed in millilitres per cent. There are many methods of determining *haemoglobin* which is expressed in grams per 100 ml.

Normal Values —

(1) Haemoglobin — 14.8 Gm/100 ml.

(2) Haematocrit — Adult males — 40-54%

Adult females — 37-47%

(3) No. of Red Blood Cells — 4,200,000 — 6,400,000 per c.mm.

(4) Diameter of Red Blood Cells — average 7.2 microns.

From these results the mean corpuscular volume (MCV), the mean corpuscular haemoglobin (MCH) and mean corpuscular haemoglobin concentration (MCHC) can be determined and the anaemia can be classified according to size and haemoglobin content as :

Macrocytic — (MCV >94 c. microns) (MCHC > 30 per cent)

Normocytic — (MCV 80-94% c. microns) (MCHC > 30 per cent)

Microcytic — (MCV < 80 c. microns) (MCHC > 30 per cent)

Hypochromic-microcytic — (MCV < 80 c. microns) (MCHC < 30 per cent)

Mean Corpuscular Haemoglobin (MCH)

The mean corpuscular haemoglobin expresses the average haemoglobin content of a single red cell in micromicrograms (γγ).

It is calculated as follows :

$$\frac{\text{Haemoglobin in Gms. per 1,000 ml. blood}}{\text{Red cells in millions per c mm.}}$$

Normal range 27-32 γγ

average 29.6 γγ

Mean Corpuscular Volume (MCV)

This is the mean or average volume of a single cell expressed in cubic microns. (c.μ.)

It is calculated as follows :

$$\frac{\text{Volume of packed cells in ml. per 1,000 ml. blood}}{\text{Red cells in millions per c mm.}}$$

Normal Range 78-94 c.μ.

average 90 c.μ.

Mean Corpuscular Haemoglobin Concentration (MCHC)

This value expresses the relation between haemoglobin saturation and cell volume and is expressed as grams per cent.

It is calculated as follows :

$$\frac{\text{Haemoglobin in Gms. per 100 ml. blood}}{\text{Vol. of packed red cells in ml. per 100 ml. blood}} \times 100$$

Normal Range 32-38 gms. per cent

average 33 gms. per cent

This value is the true indicator of iron deficiency.

Mean Corpuscular Diameter (M.C.D.)

This is determined by direct measurement of the red cells in a stained film.

Normal Range 6.7 to 7.7 microns

average 7.2 microns

The indices are based on a percentage of normal and have the following equation as their foundation:

100% normal = 14.8 grams haemoglobin per 100 ml. = 5,000,000 red cells per c. mm. = 45 ml. haematocrit value.

Colour Index

The only widely used index is the colour index which expresses the mean haemoglobin content of a single cell as compared with the content of a normal cell. It provides the same information as the mean corpuscular haemoglobin determination, but is calculated as a percentage of normal instead of being expressed in absolute figures. For this, it is assumed that a normal person has 100% haemoglobin and 100% red cells.

The normal colour index is as follows :

$$\frac{\text{Haemoglobin (percentage of normal)}}{\text{Red Cells (percentage of normal)}} = \frac{100}{100} = 1$$

In practice, the calculation is as follows :

$$\text{Colour Index} = \frac{\text{per cent of haemoglobin (calculated as 14.8 G. per 100ml. = 100\%)}}{\text{per cent of red cells (calculated as 5,000,000 per c.mm. = 100\%)}}$$

Normal colour Index is 1. However a range of 0.85—1.15 is not considered abnormal.

(ii) The *White blood cell* Count should always be done as it indicates the type of leucocyte response.

(iii) A careful study of the *blood smear* is very important as it gives information which may not be apparent in the above calculations. In addition to the different count, the smear throws light on the presence of abnormal red cells and leucocytes, presence of abnormal platelets and the presence of parasites. With experience, it may be possible to recognize macrotosis (common in megaloblastic anaemia) or microcytosis (common in iron deficiency anaemia).

Hypochromia, an increase in the normal central pallor in the red cell can also be recognised, and, along with microcytosis, is charactersitics of iron deficiency anaemia. Yet another abnormality of the erythrocytes is the presence of nucleated red cells. In any severe anaemia, normoblasts may be seen in small numbers (2 to 5 per 100 leucocytes). When they are present in large numbers, haemolytic anaemia may be suspected. However, it is more important to identify megaloblasts in the smear, because their presence is conclusive evidence of a megaloblastic anaemia.

(iv) Another important step in the diagnosis is *marrow biopsy*. Aspiration marrow biopsy is a relatively simple procedure. Some training in its technique is obviously required; the only special equipment necessary is a sternal puncture needle. In a case of nutritional anaemia, marrow biopsy will show whether the erythropoiesis is hyperplastic (cellular) or hypoplastic, and whether the erythropoiesis is normoblastic (normal) or megaloblastic (abnormal). Cellularity of the marrow cannot be unequivocally assessed by any other means and, in nutritional anaemia with frequent occurrence of multiple deficiencies, the peripheral blood findings may not correctly reflect the status of the erythropoietic reaction. The last point can be appreciated if it is recalled that megaloblastic erythropoiesis is generally associated with macrocytosis in the peripheral blood and normoblastic erythropoiesis with normocytosis or microcytosis. It is simpler to identify megaloblasts in the marrow smears than peripheral blood smears, and this makes marrow biopsy an indispensable procedure in the investigation of anaemias.

(v) Examination of the faeces for occult blood.

(vi) Other examinations that may be necessary depending on the nature of the case include gastric analysis and examination of the faeces for total fat and fatty acid.

A list of laboratory procedures that may be useful is given below:

Table 12.3

USUAL INITIAL STUDIES
Haematocrit determination
Haemoglobin determination
Erythrocyte count
Reticulocyte count
Study of stained blood smear
Leukocyte count and differential count
Platelet count (or estimate from blood smear)

(Contd.)

SUSPECTED IRON DEFICIENCY

Stool for occult blood
Serum iron and latent iron binding capacity
Stain of marrow preparations for iron
Roentgenographic study of the gastrointestinal tract.

SUSPECTED VITAMIN B_{12} OR FOLIC ACID DEFICIENCY

Bone marrow
Gastric analysis after histamine injection
Vitamin B_{12} absorption test (radioactive cobalt)
Serum vitamin B_{12} level
Serum folate level
Roentgenographic study of the gastrointestinal tract

SUSPECTED HAEMOLYTIC ANAEMIA

Bone marrow
Serum bilirubin level
Fecal urobilinogen excretion
Test for sicking
Haemoglobin electrophoresis
Antiglobulin (Coombs) test
Hypotonic saline fragility test
Alkali denaturation test
Haemoglobin determination, plasma and urine
Cr^{51}tagging to determine erythrocyte survival and sequestration in the spleen
Tests for cellular enzyme defects

SUSPECTED APLASTIC ANAEMIA

Bone marrow
Skeletal roentgenograms
Serum iron and latent iron binding capacity
Mediastinal roentgenograms for thymoma
Radioiron to determine plasma iron clearance, iron utilization, and iron turnover

OTHER TESTS OFTEN USED ESPECIALLY TO DIAGNOSE THE PRIMARY DISEASE

"L.E." preparation

(Contd.)

Blood urea
Tissue biopsy (skin, lymph node, liver)
Peroxidase stain
Plasma electrophoresis
Urine electrophoresis
Bone marrow

MACROCYTIC ANAEMIA

If the mean corpuscular volume is greater than 100 c.microns (i.e. macrocytic anaemia of significant degree), it is unlikely that acute haemorrhage has occured and for practical purposes, chronic blood loss may be eliminated. Macrocytic anaemia is due primarily to deficient blood production and is most likely to be seen in a deficiency of Vitamin B_{12} or Folic acid. Aplastic anaemia, myxoedema and haemolytic anaemia (extracorpuscular or acquired type) are additional causes.

Deficiency of Vitamin B_{12} and Folic Acid

In a deficiency of Vitamin B_{12}, mild leucopenia and thrombocytopenia are often found. In untreated cases, the reticulocyte count is normal or subnormal and reflects the failure of the normal response to anaemia. The increased destruction of red cells is shown by the higher level of serum indirect bilirubin and faecal urobilinogen.

A megablastic type of erythropoiesis establishes the presence of a deficiency of Vitamin B_{12} or Folic acid almost unequivocally.

As the haemotological pictures in Vitamin B_{12} and Folic acid deficiencies are almost identical, other studies become necessary. Gastric analysis showing an absence of hydrochloric acid after histamine and absence of free hydrochloric acid indicates pernicious anaemia. Neurological lesions, particularly signs of postero-lateral sclerosis would further confirm this diagnosis.

Other causes of Vitamin B_{12} deficiency e.g. total gastrectomy, will be suggested by the history and appropriate examinations.

It must be remembered that Folic Acid administration can modify the bone marrow and blood picture in pernicious anaemia while central nervous system lesions may progress. Therefore whenever possible, the serum Vitamin B_{12} level should be estimated or the Schilling test acid in the gastric juice is retained.

NORMOCYTIC ANAEMIA

If the mean corpuscular volume is 80-94 c. microns, the anaemia is normocytic and acute blood loss, deficient blood production and hyperhaemolysis should be considered.

Acute Blood Loss

The history, quite often, indicates the underlying cause. An external haemorrhage will usually be apparent, but if it is originating in the gastrointestinal tract, will have to be enquired after carefully. An elevated reticulocyte count without an increase of serum bilirubin suggests recent haemorrhage if the patient has not been given specific thereapeutic agents e.g. iron or vitamin B_{12}. X-ray investigations of the gastro-intestinal tract may be necessary.

Deficient Blood Production

Anaemia of this type is usually the first indication of underlying disease e.g. renal disease. Other causes like chronic infection, arthritis, and malignancy are usually apparent.

A normocytic anaemia sometimes occurs in iron deficiency. A demonstration of low serum iron or increased iron binding capacity or both may be necessary to confirm the diagnosis.

Hyperhaemolysis

A reticulocyte count greater than 4% in a patient who has not had a recent haemorrhage nor received antianaemic therapy may indicate a haemolytic anaemia. Study of the stained smear will provide further evidence especially when the serum indirect bilirubin and faecal urobilinogen are increased.

SIMPLE MICROCYTIC ANAEMIA

(MCV $<$ 80 c. microns. MCHC $>$ 30 %)

When the mean corpuscular volume is less than 80 c. microns and the mean corpuscular haemoglobin concentration is greater than 30 %, the anaemia is simple microcytic and is seen in associaton with various chronic diseases, though a normocytic anaemia is more common.

HYPOCHROMIC MICROCYTIC ANAEMIA

(MCV $<$ 80 c. microns. MCHC $<$ 30 %)

When the mean corpuscular volume is less than 80 c. microns and the mean corpuscular haemoglobin concentration is less than 30 per cent, the anaemia is hypochromic microcytic.

This type of anaemia almost invariably means iron deficiency. The blood smear shows an increased central pallor and there is poikilocytosis and anisocytosis. The leucocytes and platelets are usually normal. Erythropoiesis is normoblastic in type and the cellularity of the bone marrow may be subnormal, normal or increased. Iron deficiency can be definitely confirmed by finding a low serum iron level together with an increased iron binding capacity of the serum or by demonstration of reduced iron stores in the bone marrow.

The cause of the iron deficiency should be carefully looked for. In women, menstruation and pregnancy afford added opportunities for the development of iron deficiency anaemia. A dietary history should be carefully taken to exclude a dietary deficiency. X-ray investigation of the gastrointestinal tract should be carried out to rule out or confirm a possible source of bleeding e.g. gastric or duodenal ulcer, carcinoma of the colon etc. Haemorrhoids may be often the cause of an iron deficiency anaemia and should be kept in mind.

GENERAL MANIFESTATIONS OF ANAEMIA

The symptoms and signs of anaemia are dependent to a considerable extent on the rapidity of the development of anaemia and the physiological adjustment of the cardiovascular system and not only on the red cell or haemoglobin level of the patient.

General Symptoms

The general symptoms common to all anaemias are weakness, easy fatigability, loss of weight, loss of appetite, diarrhoea, vague gastrointestinal symptoms and low fever. The patient often complains of inability to tolerate hot, spicy foods.

Lack of concentration, headache, giddiness, fainting or "black-outs" may be complained of. Dimness of vision and noises in the ears may be experienced by the patient. Paraesthesia in the limbs is frequent.

Physical Signs

(1) Integumentary System

In well-developed cases of anaemia the most striking outward sign is the *pallor*. Though attention of the physician to the anaemia is first drawn from the colour of the skin, the degree of pallor is better observed in the conjunctivae, on the tongue and buccal and pharyngeal mucous membranes and on the palms of the hands and the bed of the finger-nails. A fair idea about the degree of anaemia may be obtained by comparing the bed of the finger-nail of the patient with that of a normal person. Pallor of the skin, nails and mucous membranes usually indicates a reduction in haemoglobin values. However, it does not always give a correct indication of the anaemia particularly in flabby persons and in cases of hypoproteinaemia, myxoedema, etc. The pallor and with it the anaemia may also be masked by jaundice, cyanosis and pigmentation of the skin.

The *skin* may be found to be dry and inelastic and pigmentation may often occur on the face, dorsum of the hands and feet, forearms and back.

The *hair* shows a loss of lustre and early graying.

The *nails* show flattening (platynychia) or a spoon shaped deformity (koilonychia) which are indicative of iron deficiency anaemia.

Oedema of the feet may be found.

(2) Respiratory and Cardiovascular Systems

Symptoms relating to these systems depend on the degree and rapidity of the development of anaemia and the capacity of the cardiovascular system for adjustment. In chronic cases with a slight to moderate degree of anaemia, dyspnoea and palpitation on exertion may be the only symptoms while in cases where the anaemia is severe and develops rapidly, shortness of breath and tachycardia are present even at rest. In a few cases the clinical picture of congestive heart failure or symptoms of intermittent claudication may be noticed.

Clinical evidence of circulatory adjustment may be found in the rapid heart rate, increased arterial pulsation, and increased pulse pressure with dilatation of the heart and low blood pressure. These adjustments encroaching on the reserves of the body may be imperfect or fail. In these cases, lateral displacement of the left cardiac border, oedema, enlargement of the liver with tenderness and basal rales may be noticed. Along with the cardiovascular changes there is usually an increase in the rate and depth of respiration and lowering of the vital capacity.

In cases of moderate to severe anaemia the commonest cardiac abnormality is the systolic murmur which is usually heard at the apex and sometimes at the pulmonary area. This haemic murmur is soft and not transmitted and is easily distinguished from the murmur of organic heart disease. A humming sound "bruit de diable," may be heard over the big vessels of the neck. The electrocardiogram may reveal changes in the ST segment and inversion of the T wave. Retinal, skin and mucous membrane haemorhages may be detected in severe cases especially if there is an associated platelet deficiency.

(3) Neuromuscular System

Muscular weakness and easy fatigability, irritability, lack of concentration, headache, vertigo, and faintness are common symptoms of anaemia and may result in psychoasthenic disorders. Presence of these symptoms particularly in women should call for careful examination of the blood.

Neurological symptoms with involvement of the spinal cord are distinctive features of pernicious anaemia and are not seen in other types of anaemias. Slight paraesthesias may be however, found in other forms of anaemias.

(4) Alimentary System

Symptoms referable to the alimentary system are frequent in nutritional anaemias in the tropics. Glossitis and atrophy of the papillae of the tongue are commonly seen in nutritional macrocytic anaemia while anorexia, flatulence, abdominal discomfort and diarrhoea may be present in different types of anaemias. Constipation, alternating with diarrhoea may occur in some cases and may aggravate the anaemic condition. Dysphagia may occur in iron deficiency anaemia.

The spleen and liver may be enlarged especially in haemolytic anaemia.

(5) Metabolism

Though superficial fat may be well-preserved there are signs of under-nutrition and loss of weight in most cases. Oedema of the feet may be present.

(6) Fever

Fever of mild to moderate degree is present in most cases of anaemias. The fever usually subsides with improvement of the blood picture with haematinics and does not require any specific treatment.

(7) Genito-Urinary System

In anaemic females amenorrhoea is often found. Menorrhagia may also be seen in some cases and may be responsible for the persistence of anaemia. Normal menstrual flow is usually restored with the cure of anaemia which helps to restore the mental tranquility of the patient. In the males, loss of libido is not infrequent. There may be an arrest of sexual growth in children suffering from severe anaemias. Slight albuminuria may be present in some cases.

GENERAL MANAGEMENT OF ANAEMIA

Rational treatment depends on accurate diagnosis of the type and degree of anaemia.

Though many anaemias can now be treated specifically and instances of dramatic recovery are on record, it is not uncommon to find cases of anaemia which have been treated inefficiently. A thorough study of the patient particularly the qualitative and quantitative dietetic history, and involve complete physical examination and thorough laboratory examinations of blood. In some cases, the bone marrow, urine, stool and gastric secretion will have to be investigated.

Deficiency anaemias require agents which make good the deficiency such as iron, vitamin B_{12}, folic acid, vitamin C, thyroid extract etc. Disorders associated with diminished production of erythrocytes, like infections, malignant disease and renal disorders, require appropriate measures for the control of the primary disorders.

Haemolytic anaemias require methods of reducing or stopping the haemolytic process, first by the removal of the cause (e.g., drugs), followed by the use of adrenocorticosteroids, splenectomy etc. Replacement of blood by blood transfusions helps in acute haemorrhagic or acute or chronic haemolytic anaemias. In aplastic anaemias, apart from repeated blood transfusions, the use of agents to stimulate erythropoiesis, such as adrenocorticosteroids and androgenic hormones, is indicated.

General Measures

In addition to the above measures, as in the management of other disease, physical and mental rest, fresh air, sunshine and hygienic measures are essential. Bed rest must be enforced in all cases with a red cell count of 2 millions per c.mm. or less and in cases showing failure of compensation. With improvement of the blood picture the patient should be allowed graduated exercise without overtaxing the cardiac reserves.

Diet is an important adjunct in the treatment of anaemias. Liver and kidney are the most efficient foods for haemoglobin regeneration, egg and meat being next in order while dairy products are least efficient. Liver contains various proteins and is rich in vitamins but prolonged boiling or overcooking destroys the haematinic principle in the liver.

Concentrated carbohydrate foods such as cakes, pastries and puddings lessen appetite and hence an excess of these foods should be avoided.

The nature and consistency of the diet as also the number of meals must be adjusted to the state of health. For this reason, though dairy products are not efficient haemoglobin regenerators, these should be preferred in the early stages, particularly in very weak and debilitated patients. A more generous diet should be gradually worked up keeping an eye on palatability and avoiding monotony as far as possible. A high proteins diet is absolutely essential during treatment as a supply of additional protein is required for the rapid erythropoiesis following administration of the correct haematinic.

Transfusion of Blood. Unless contra-indicated, a transfusion of blood should be given to all cases with a red cell count of 1.5 millions or less. It must, however, be clearly understood that a transfusion is only a temporary measure which helps to tide over a crisis and preserve life long enough for specific treatment to take effect. In conjunction with appropriate haematinics, transfusion of blood is a valuable adjunct in the treatment of any severe case of anaemia particularly the refractory cases and the cases with hypoplastic bone-marrow. Citrated blood is as effective as whole blood but optimum results are obtained with transfusion of fresh red cell concentrate. Repeated transfusions of small amounts give better results than a single massive transfusion.

MEGALOBLASTIC ANAEMIAS

A megaloblastic anaemia is the most characteristic feature of a deficiency of Vitamin B_{12} or Folic acid. The deficiency can arise in various ways as shown in the following Table 12.4

Table 12.4

Classification of Megaloblastic Anaemias

I. Vitamin B_{12} deficiency
   - A. Inadequate intake
   - B. Defective absorption
     1. Failure to secrete intrinsic factor
        - a. Addisonian pernicious anaemia
        - b. Total gastrectomy
     2. Failure of absorption in the small intestine
        - a. Malabsorption syndromes

(Contd.)

b. Blind loops and fistulas

c. Fish tapeworm infestation

II. Folic Acid Deficiency

A. Inadequate intake

B. Defective absorption

1. Malabsorption syndromes

2. Blind loop syndrome

C. Inadequate utilization

1. Ascorbic acid deficiency

2. Therapy with folic acid antagonists

3. Therapy with anticonvulsant drugs

D. Excessive demands

III. "Idiopathic" — extremely rare

PERNICIOUS ANAEMIA

Though the first case of pernicious anaemia was reported by Combe of Edinburgh in 1824, Addison of Guy's Hospital, London in 1855, gave a masterly description of the disease and since then it has been recognised as a distinct entity. Independently, Biermer of Zurich first drew attention to the disease on the Continent in 1872 and his name is usually associated with the disease in European countries other than Great Britain.

Pernicious anaemia is essentially a disease of the temperate climates affecting chiefly white races past middle age. The disease is characterised by macrocytic anaemia, megaloblastic bone-marrow and irreversible absolute achlorhydria. Haematologically, it is indistinguishable from nutritional macrocytic anaemia commonly seen in Indians and Asiatics. The crucial point of difference lies in the presence or absence of "intrinsic" factor which can be detected by a biologic test.

The incidence of this disease in India is difficult to assess, but it is probably very much less than in the Caucasian races. Among some 400 cases of megaloblastic anaemia in South India, no case of pernicious anaemia could be found. The same could be said of the Eastern and Western parts of India. Since the population of North India is of different genetic stock, the disease may be more prevalent there.

Diagnostic features of pernicious anaemia are the triad of weakness, sore tongue and numbness and tingling of the lower extremities, together with macrocytic anaemia and irreversible absolute achlorhydria.

With the advent of liver therapy and other antimegaloblastic drugs, management of pernicious anaemia is now comparatively simpler and prognosis much better. The standard treatment is with vitamin B_{12} or liver extract given parenterally. In the presence of any complication or in atypical cases, the crude liver extract is to be preferred to the highly purified and concentrated extract as purification causes removal of certain factors which are essential for treatment of these cases. Folic acid given by mouth induces satisfactory haematological response but it not only does not protect against neurological complications but may even precipitate them. Though the dose is to some extent an individual matter it should always be on the high side. For patients with involvement of the central nervous system the use of whole liver extracts rather than the refined liver extract is recommended. A much higher dose is required in the treatment of these cases. During remmission, attempts should be made to maintain the red blood cells at 4.5 millions per c. mm. or above. Continuation of the red cell count at a lower level may precipitate cord symptoms so the dictum of "not some liver, but enough liver for the given case".

Iron may be required, particularly by female patients. When active red cell regeneration occurs, the body's reserve iron gets exhausted especially if the reserve stores were depleted initially for any reason. The MCHC then falls with a possible fall in the index.

The maintenance treatment is very important and places a great responsibility on the physician. Vitamin B_{12} given parenterally at monthly intervals usually suffices for the majority of cases. Trials have been made with massive doses at intervals of several months of vitamin B_{12} or of liver extract but the results are not as satisfactory as those with treatment at more frequent intervals with smaller doses (Davis and Brown).

NUTRITIONAL MACROCYTIC ANAEMIA

Synonyms: Nutritional Megaloblastic Anaemia: Tropical Macrocytic Anaemia: Nutritional Anaemia: Tropical Megaloblastic Anaemia.

The name 'nutritional macrocytic anaemia' was suggested by Fairley (1938) as he believed that nutritional deficiency was the most important factor in the aetiology of the condition. This was supported by Lucy Wills and the consensus of opinion of the workers in the field is that the fundamental cause is dietary deficiency usually due to poverty. It has been shown that vegetarians have low body stores of Vitamin B_{12}, and many people in India live on a diet which is marginal in folic acid. Cases of apparently pure dietary deficiency of vitamin B_{12} and/or folic acid may therefore be seen from time to time. Food consisting mainly of carbohydrates may be adequate in calories but is low in peotein, particularly of animal protein and fat and may also be deficient in calcium and vitamins. In the tropics there are frequently added factors, the more common ones being infections with hook-worm and malaria which may produce varied signs and symptoms and blood pictures. Thus the clinical and laboratory findings will be found to vary in different parts of the world according to the prevalence of parasitic infection and the dietary habits of the people. Therefore, it is very important that the dietary history be carefully enquired into or better still, an analysis of the diet be made.

In India, the first reference to the condition was made by Mackie in 1929. In the following year Wills and associates in 1930 carefully differentiated the condition from Addisonian Pernicious Anaemia which it resembles both clinically and haematologically.

Subsequently workers further characterised the condition and established it as a distinct clinical entity.

Geographical Distribution: Nutritional macrocytic anaemia is commonly seen in tropical countries e.g. India, Africa, China, Malaya; some cases have been described in temperate climates as well.

Age: The disease is most common between the ages of 20 and 30. In an analysis of 126 cases, Das Gupta (1951) noted 69 cases in the age groups of 20 and 30.

Heredity: Though occasionally more than one person in a family may be found to be affected, heredity does not seem to have any role in the causation of the disease.

Clinical Picture: The patient is pale and thin and may show oedema of the lower extremities. He may give a history of dyspepsia and diarrhoea and usually complains of weakness and shortness of breath. There is almost always some amount of glossitis and soreness of the mouth which in extreme cases may be very painful, making chewing of food quite difficult. Examination of the heart usually shows haemic murmurs while rales may be noted over the base of the lungs. Symptoms are usually due to anaemia and will depend on the degree and rapidity of the development of anaemia and the capacity of the cardiovascular system for adjustment. The anaemia is generally insidious in onset and the patient is usually well adjusted to the conditon and it is not unusual to find a patient with a red cell count of 1.5 millions/per c.mm. or less walking to the clinic for treatment. Splenomegaly is not a feature of the condition but may be present as an associated condition. Slight paraesthesia may be present in a few cases but neurological symptoms are conspicuous by their absence.

Blood Changes: The red cells are reduced more than the haemoglobin and are larger than normal. As a result of these, the mean corpuscular volume is higher than normal and the mean corpuscular haemoglobin and the mean corpuscular haemoglobin concentrations are usually within normal range. Anisocytosis is great but poikilocytosis is less than in pernicious anaemia and polychromatophilia is a common feature. In severe anaemia, nucleated red cells including megaloblasts, may be found in the blood. There is a leucopenia due to neutropenia, resulting in a relative lymphocytosis while thrombocytopenia is seen in a large number of cases. The coagulation time and bleeding time are normal, and so also is the fragility of the red cells. The erythrocyte sedimentation rate, corrected for anaemia, is within the normal range.

Biochemical Changes: Slight hyper-bilirubinaemia may be present in some cases and particularly in those with splenomegaly. Plasma proteins are usually lower than normal due to reduction of the albumin fraction. As a result, the albumin-globulin ratio may be reversed. The blood cholesterol is low and is usually correlated with the level of red cell count. Plasma iron is normal or increased, the iron binding capacity of plasma is low and iron saturation is increased. There is no gross derangement of liver function tests (Das Gupta and Basu, 1954).

Gastric Secretion: Absolute achlorhydria is found in a number of cases. However, with rational therapy leading to an improvement of the anaemia, a return of gastric hydrochloric acid is often noticed. Achlorhydria is usually reversible and not irreversible as in pernicious anaemia.

Bone-marrow Changes: There is increased cellularity of the bone-marrow due to hyperplasia of the erythroid cells and erythroid-myeloid ratio may be about 1 : 1.5 instead of normal ratio of 1 : 4. Megaloblastic erythropoiesis may be found in about 30 per cent of the untreated cases but the number of megaloblasts is usually not high. The megaloblasts when present, are similar to and indistinguishable from those found in pernicious anaemia. Transitional cells may be found in some of the cases. The presence of macronormoblasts is a characteristic finding in these cases. Premature haemoglobinisation of the cytoplasm is a prominent feature while the nucleus retains its immature character as a result of which a distinct contrast is noted in the maturity of the cytoplasm and the nucleus. There is relative hypoplasia of leucoblastic tissue and abnormal granulocytes, e.g. giant metamyelocytes and giant stab cells and macropolycytes or multi-segmented neutrophils are commonly seen. Thrombopoiesis may be depressed and megakaryocytes usually show increased segmentation and degenerative changes. The changes in the granulocytes and megakaryocytes are characteristic of nutritional macrocytic anaemia and help in the diagnosis of the condition even in the absence of megaloblasts.

Course and Prognosis: In the absence of any associated infections recovery is rapid with appropriate treatment and the prognosis is good. Relapses are not common but may occur in cases continuing with inadequate diet; in one patient as many as three relapses were seen in the course of 5 years.

Treatment

(a) *General Measures:* Special emphasis should be given to rest and diet. A diet high in protein is essential, not only helping to improve the action of the haematinics but being important in preventing development of hypoproteinaemia during the rapid erythropoiesis.

(b) *Specific Treatment:* Several drugs, viz. liver in various forms, folic acid, vitamin B_{12}, folinic acid are now available for the treatment of macrocytic anaemias.

(i) *Liver Extract:* A potent liver extract still continues to be the drug of choice in the treatment of uncomplicated cases of nutritional macrocytic anaemia irrespective of the bone-marrow reaction. In the treatment of a case with a moderate to severe degree of anaemia, 3-4 ml. of whole liver extract should be given parenterally daily till the red cell count reaches about 3 millions per c.mm. The injections should be continued but at greater intervals till blood values reach normal level. An almost similar response is obtained with proteolysed liver extract.

Refined liver extract is not as efficacious as crude liver extract in the doses which are effective when given in much higher doses (Napier, *et al.*, 1938). As in the case of crude liver extract, the treatment must be continued till the blood picture attains normal levels, increasing the spacing of the injections as the blood picture improves.

(ii) *Folic Acid:* Given in adequate dosage, about 20-3- mgm, a day, a definite clinical and haematological improvement is usually seen in cases of

N.M.A., particularly the cases with megaloblastic bone marrow. The best response is obtained by giving folic acid in doses of 30 mg. a day in three divided doses for the first 10 or 15 days and continuing the therapy with a smaller dosage, about, 15-20 mg. a day for 30 days or more depending on the rate of improvement. Though a maximum response may be obtained in some cases, erythrocytic regeneration may be sub-optimal and macrocytosis may persist. Cases showing sub-optimal response have been found to show further improvement with crude liver extract given after folic acid. Hence, in spite of the case of administration and absence of any untoward reaction, folic acid cannot be recommended for the routine treatment of nutritional macrocytic anaemia but it can be used with advantage in combination with a liver extract.

(iii) *Vitamin B_{12}*: In nutritional macrocytic anaemia, a maximum response is usually obtained with 200 to 300 meg. of vitamin B_{12} given parenterally. The injections are to be given daily for 10-15 days. Though the initial response is good in about 60 per cent of the cases, complete recovery is seen in only about 25 per cent of the cases; continued treatment even with a higher dosage fails to produce further improvement. The cases showing sub-optimal response may show further improvement with liver and/or folic acid. The response to oral vitamin B_{12} is very variable; an occasional case may show good response with a small dose of 40 meg. while even 500 meg. may not produce any response at all in the majority of cases.

(iv) *Citrovorum Factor:* Folinic acid has given very variable results in the treatment of nutritional macrocytic anaemia. As with vitamin B_{12}, cure has been obtained only in a small number of cases. It is given parenterally in a dosage of 3 mg. for 10 days or more.

(v) *Marmite:* In the early days marmite was found to be effective in very high dosage.

It is difficult to predict the response to different anti-megaloblastic drugs. In an average case the response to whole liver extract is much better than to any of the others. In cases of sub-optimal response to liver extract, better results may be obtained by combining it with folic acid. In refractory cases a combination of the various drugs may be tried.

(c) *Transfusion of blood:* As already stated, transfusion of blood is only a temporary measure which helps to keep the patient alive long enough for specific treatment to take effect. It has been shown by Das Gupta (1947) that in uncomplicated cases of nutritional macrocytic anaemia the rate of improvement with potent anti-megaloblastic drugs with or without transfusion was apparently of the same order. It is, however, particularly valuable in the treatment of cases with low red cell count, refractory cases and the cases with hypoplastic bone-marrow.

Treatment of complications: Specific treatment with liver extract or vitamin B_{12} usually helps to improve the associated fever, diarrhoea and glossitis. Reractory cases of glossitis may improve with riboflavin, given orally or parenterally. Diarrhoea should be adequately treated while flatulent dyspepsia is best treated with dilute hydrochloric acid given in ½ to 1 dram doses in a tumbler of water and flavoured with orange juice. The acid mixture is to be sipped during the two principal meals. Fever, unless due to any associated infection, subsides with improvement of the blood picture and does not require any other treatment.

Differential diagnosis: Nutritional macrocytic anaemia is almost indistinguishable from pernicious anaemia haematologically. The important points which help to differentiate the two conditions are :

(1) *Geographical and Racial Distribution:* Pernicious anaemia is essentially a disease of the temperate climate affecting chiefly the light skinned white races. It is rare in Negroes and comparatively rare in the darker skinned white races such as Italians and Greeks. It is very rare in Asiatics; only a few cases have been described in Indians and in Chinese.

(2) *Age:* Pernicious anaemia is usually seen after the age of 40 while nutritional macrocytic anaemia may be found at any age, the majority of the cases being found between the ages of 20 and 30.

(3) *Neurological Symptoms:* Neurologic manifestations, particularly subacute combined degeneration of the spinal cord, are characteristic findings of pernicious anaemia but are never seen in nutritional macrocytic anaemia.

(4) *Gastric acidity:* Absolute achlorhydria is the rule in pernicious anaemia and is irreversible. Gastric acidity is variable in nutritional macrocytic anaemia, some cases showing absolute achlorhydria, some hypochlorhydria, some isochlorhydria while a few may even show hyperchlorhydria. After improvement of the anaemia a return of the gastric acidity may be found in the cases showing absolute achlorhydria.

(5) *Response to therapy:*

(a) *High protein diet:* Some cases of nutritional macrocytic anaemia show considerable improvement with a high protein diet alone; such a diet has very little or no effect in pernicious anaemia.

(b) *Marmite:* Cases of nutritional macrocytic anaemia have been found to respond well to marmite but is is not usually effective in pernicious anaemia.

(c) *Liver Extract:* Crude liver extract is highly effective both in nutritional macrocytic anaemia and pernicious anaemia but refined liver extract is effective only in pernicious anaemia and not in nutritional macrocytic anaemia.

(d) *Folic acid:* Folic acid produces optimum response in nutritional macrocytic anaemia particularly with a megaloblastic marrow; in pernicious anaemia, folic acid produces haematologic improvement with no effect on neurologic manifestations, and may even precipitate them.

(e) *Vitamin B_{12}:* Response to Vitamin B_{12} in nutritional macrocytic anaemia is variable but is excellent in cases of pernicious anaemia.

(f) *Maintenance Therapy:* Maintenance therapy is not required in nutritional macrocytic anaemia as in pernicious anaemia.

(6) *Aetiology:* Nutritional macrocytic anaemia is due to a deficiency of a dietary factor while pernicious anaemia is due to the absence of gastric "intrinsic" factor. The crucial point of difference is in the presence or absence of "intrinsic" factor.

SPRUE

Synonyms: Psilosis: Cochin-China Diarrhoea.

This condition was first described by Vincent Ketelaer in 1669 and later by Hillary in Barbados in 1759. The disease is mainly confined to tropical countries where it is endemic in some parts, but during the Second World War, it has also been reported from Scandinavian countries and the United States. It particularly affects well-fed Europeans and Anglo-Indians and is more often seen in cities and towns than rural districts. Prolonged residence of white persons in an endemic area predisposes them to the disease though some may develop the disease on returning home after a short stay in the tropics. Both sexes are equally affected and it is rare under the age of 20.

Aetiology: It is fundamentally a deficiency disease due to a functional disorder of the intestine, possibly due to failure of phosphorylation of fatty acids, glycerol and glucose. This contention is supported by Maegraith et al (1945). The associated anaemia may be due to malabsorption of the haemopoietic principle and/or iron on account of the diarrhoea; failure of formation of folic acid and Vitamin B_{12} due to an abnormal and competitive intestinal flora; deficient intake of extrinsic factor and iron and in some cases absence of gastric intrinsic factor. These may operate singly or in combination and are helped by the associated achlorhydria or hypochlorhydria.

Symptomatology: The onset is insidious. There is usually a history of months of "chronic indigestion", dyspepsia, flatulence, constipation with occasional diarrhoea, loss of weight and energy and nervous irritability. Stefanini (1948) describes three clinical stages leading to the full development of the sprue syndrome. Diarrhoea and steatorrhoea, the symptoms of impaired intestinal absorption, are seen in the first stage; glossitis, stomatitis etc., the signs of multiple deficiencies, are seen in the second stage while the characteristic macrocytic anaemia develops in the third stage. The chief complaints are referable to the alimentary system; the tongue is sore, there is ulceration of the mouth and there is diarrhoea. The characteristic morning diarrhoea with a pale, bulky stool is established after some months. Bowel movements may be as many as 20 per day or more and the total quantity of faeces passed in a day is 5-6 times the normal amount. Abdominal distension and epigastric distress are common complaints which are made worse following the ingestion of starchy and fatty foods. Usually there is no tenesmus or blood or mucus in the stools. X-ray examination reveals a characteristic picture in the intestines.

In a fully developed case the clinical picture is very characteristic. The patient is pale, greatly emaciated—there may be as much as 50 per cent loss of body weight. The abdomen is distended and the skin is dry and wrinkled. In long-standing untreated cases, bleeding from the gums, petechiae, or even extensive purpura may be seen.

Laboratory Findings:

(a) *Blood:* The blood picture is normal in the early stages, anaemia developing only after some months and being usually hypochromic and microcytic in type. In the fully established cases, the blood picture may be macrocytic with an increase in mean corpuscular volume and mean corpuscular haemoglobin. Anisocytosis is marked but poikilocytosis is less prominent. Rarely, the anaemia may terminate as an aplastic condition. There is leucopenia with relative lymphocytosis and thrombocytopenia. Hypo-prothrombinaemia may occur and may lead to purpura and heamorrhagic lesions. The fragility of red cells is normal or decreased. In cases with severe cachexia, plasma proteins are reduced and the albumin : globulin ratio is reversed.

(b) *Bone-marrow:* In the early stage with an hypochromic and microcytic anaemia, the bone-marrow is only slightly hypercellular and is normoblastic in reaction. In the fully established cases with macrocytic anaemia, the bone-marrow is megaloblastic and also shows macropolycytes and giant metamyelocytes; megaloblastic tissue in the marrow, however, is definitely less than in pernicious anaemia.

(c) *Gastric analysis:* Histamine-fast achlorhydria is seen in about 30 per cent of cases; gastric hydrochloric acid usually returns to normal after cure.

(d) *Fat Metabolism:* The total faecal fat is increased and varies from 30-70 per cent. This is because only a small proportion of the dietary fat in place of the normal 95 per cent is absorbed in sprue. Fat splitting is usually complete. The absorption defect is proportionate to the amount of fat in the diet. The paleness of the faeces is due to conversion of stercobilin to colourless leucobilin. Cholesterol is reduced as also the blood phospholipid.

(e) *Carbohydrate Metabolism:* The glucose tolerance test usually shows a flat curve or a retarded rise due to malabsorption. This is probably due to a delayed absorption of glucose, for there is a normal rise and fall of blood sugar following an intravenous injection of glucose.

(f) *Mineral Metabolism:* There may be a lowering of serum calcium which may range from 8 to 10 mg. per 100 ml. The hypocalcaemia is probably due to defective absorption of vitamin D and the combining of calcium with unabsorbed fatty acids in the alimentary tract to form soaps, thus preventing its absorption.

Course and Prognosis: The disease is very chronic and exhibits spontaneous remissions and relapses but with efficient treatment is rarely fatal. Natural cure may follow departure from the tropics. Relapses, however, may occur even after years of apparent cure.

Diagnosis: The symptom-complex is usually diagnostic of sprue. Helpful confirmatory evidence is obtained from the high faecal fat, flat glucose tolerance curve, low blood calcium and the characteristic X-ray appearance of the small intestine. The condition is differentiated from pernicious anaemia and nutritional macrocytic anaemia by the absence of typical steatorrhoea in both the latter and the presence of histamine fast achlorhydria in pernicious anaemia.

Treatment

The principles of treatment are to provide rest to the alimentary tract by means of a suitable diet, to restore the blood values to normal with haematinics and to supply any dificient auxillary substance which may be needed.

(a) *Diet:* A high protein diet which is low in fat and carbohydrate is suitable for these cases. Fairley (1932) recommended the following ratio of protein, fat and carbohydrate in the diet-1 : 0.3 : 1.3. When diarrhoea is severe, only skimmed milk, ground meat and bananas should be given; if required, nutrients in the form of casein hydrolysate, plasma or blood should be given parenterally. With the improvement of the patient's condition, meat, eggs, fish, cheese, fruits and finally vegetables should be allowed. The increase in the bulk of the diet must be gradual as otherwise there may be a possibility of perforation of the bowel. Recovered cases must always avoid excess of carbohydrate food, very hot and highly spiced or sweetened food and also alcoholic drinks.

(b) *Haematinics:* The response will usually depend upon the type of blood picture. With megaloblastic erythropoiesis, excellent results have been obtained with folinic acid while a good or partially good response has been obtained with folic acid and liver extract. Folic acid in doses of 10 to 20 mg. a day is also highly effective in relieving the gastro-intestinal symptoms in addition to its haemopoietic action. Hence, folic acid is given a very high place in the treatment of sprue. Fox (1949) recommends supplementing folic acid treatment with liver extract or proteolysed liver. Vitamin B_{12} has not been found to be consistently effective.

The second group of cases with normoblastic bone-marrow comprise the chronic cases with moderate anaemia; the results of treatment of these cases are far from satisfactory. Proteolysed liver, folic acid, vitamin B_{12} and iron should be tried in various combinations. Hydrocortisone, has been found to induce significant subjective and objective improvement in refractory cases. Iron should be given at any stage when the mean corpuscular haemogloin concentration is low.

Response to therapy is indicated by relief from symptoms and rapid increase in weight in spite of restricted carbohydrate and fat intake.

Ordinarily, diarrhoea can be controlled with dietetic measures and haematinics. In cases where there are associated infections, treatment with sulphonamides may be necessary. If the blood calcium is low, calcium lactate in doses of 1.5 to 2.5 Gm. should be given. Dilute hydrochloric acid in 1/2 to 1 dram doses should be given in cases with achlorhydria or hypochlorhydria. Thiamine, nicotonic acid, reboflavin, pyridoxine, absorbic acid, vitamins D and K need only be given when a liberal diet cannot be taken.

ANEMIAS OF IRON DEFICIENCY

Iron deficiency anaemia, probably the commonest type of anaemia in the world, occurs in a number of clinical conditions and various mechanisms may be invelved.

Iron Deficiency may Result From

(1) *Deficient Supply:* This is a common cause of deficiency especially in the lower income groups. An inadequate intake may be an important causative factor in certain situations, particularly in infancy and early childhood, adolescence and during pregnancy.

(2) *Poor absorption:* Intestinal affections e.g. idiopathic steatorrhea, sprue, coeliac disease, gastrectomy.

(3) *Increased requirement:* e.g. pregnancy, infections, adolescence.

(4) *Imperfect utilization:* Infections, rheumatoid arthritis, renal disease, malignancy.

(5) *Loss through bleeding:* hookworm infection, menorrhagia, bleeding piles, peptic ulcer, oesophageal varices, gastric and colonic carcinomas.

It is not uncommon to find more than one cause operating in the same patient.

Loss of iron through excessive sweating may be a contributory factor in hot climates.

NUTRITIONAL HYPOCHROMIC ANAEMIA

Synonyms: Hypochromic microcytic anaemia; Chronic microcytic anaemia; Idiopathic hypochromic anaemia; Witt's anaemia.

Nutritional hypochromic anaemia is due to a deficiency of iron and gives rise to an anaemia where the majority of the red cells are smaller and contain a lesser amount than normal of haemoglobin. These changes in the red cells induce definite alterations in the corpuscular values with reduction in corpuscular volume, corpuscular haemoglobin and corpuscular haemoglobin concentration. The condition is seen in adults, particularly women, as well as in children. The condition in non-pregnant women is designated idiopathic hypochromic anaemia while the condition in pregnant women is known as hypochromic anaemia of pregnancy. Faber (1909) was the first to recognise the disease as a definite entity and Witts (1930) first drew attention to the occurrence of the disease in England. The anaemia is predominantly seen in middle aged women between the ages of 40 and 50 and is said to improve spontaneously after the menopause. Though the incidence of nutritional hypochromic anaemia is high in Indian patients, the condition simulating idiopathic hypochromic anaemia has not been extensively studied in Indian women and only a few cases have been reported so far .

Symptamatology: The history is often chronic, extending over many years. The symptoms are usually multiple but generally vague and indefinite. The skin is dry and inelastic and hair tends to grey prematurely. A characteristic finding is a peculiar flattening and concavity of the finger nails which have a tendency to split longitudinally on account of an undue brittleness. This condition is known as koilonychia. The changes in the nails are mostly seen in cases of idiopathic hypochromic anaemia and are absent in hookworm anaemia. But koilonychia is not pathognominic of idiopathic hypochromic anaemia and is also found in uncomplicated cases of thyrotosicosis and in other cases of unknown aetiology. In addition to the usual symptoms of weakness, lassitude, palpitations, dyspnoea and fever, gastro-intestinal symptoms may be severe. The tongue is smooth, pale and may be atrophic and is usually painless. There may be abdominal pain and usually a sensation of unusual fullness after meals. Constipation is more frequent than diarrhoea. Dysphagia occurs in about 15 per cent of cases and is described as the Plummer-Vinson Syndrome. Loss of weight is usual and menstrual disturbances, menorrhagia rather than amenorrhoea, are frequently seen.

Laboratory Findings

(1) *Blood:* Parsons (1938) describes three stages before the anaemia is fully established. At first there is only microcytosis; later the cells become hypochromic and finally there is reduction in the number of red cells. In the final stage, though the haemoglobin is greatly reduced, the reduction in red cell count is much less. The red cells are smaller than normal having a mean corpuscular volume of 50 to 70 cubic microns with a great reduction in mean corpuscular haemoglobin concentration which may be as low as 20 per cent. In a stained blood film, the red cells appear small with a small rim of haemoglobin at the edge and an almost colourless centre. Anisocytosis and poikilocytosis are not marked features. Occasionally deformed normoblasts may be found. The total and differential leucocyte counts are usually within the normal range. Platelets are normal, as also the bleeding time and coagulation time. The Vanden Berg test is negative . Plasma iron is reduced but the unsaturated iron binding capacity and total iron binding capacity of plasma is increased. Plasma proteins may be reduced but there is no alteration of the albumin : globulin ratio.

(2) *Bone-marrow:* The bone-marrow shows normoblastic hyperplasia, normoblasts constituting 50 per cent or more of the total nucleated cells. Many of the normoblasts, however, are malformed and show defective haemoglobinisation with normal nuclear pattern. Malformed normoblasts with pyknotic nuclei and incomplete haemoglobinisation are characteristic findings in iron deficiency anaemia. The oxygen carrying capacity of a microcyte is greater than that of a

normocyte containing the same amount of haemoglobin. It is probable that in iron deficiency, microcytosis is a natural protective mechanism against anoxaemia. There is a relative decrease of the granulocytes and lymphocytes but no qualitative changes are seen in them or in the megakarycytes.

(3) *Gastric secretion:* Absolute achlorhydria is found in over 80 per cent of the cases and hypochlorhydria in the remaining cases. Many of the symptoms may be attributed to deficient gastric acidity which is probably also one of the factors in the causation of anaemia in these cases.

Course and Prognosis: This is a chronic disease and if left untreated, the patient becomes a chronic invalid, but is rarely fatal. With adequate iron there is usually a good response resulting in improvement of the associated symptoms; the hair regains lustre, the condition of the tongue improves with reappearance of papillae, the nails, in cases of koilonychia, slowly recover their normal apperarance and gastric acidity may return. Relapses, however, are common and in some cases, therapy with iron may have to be continued indefinitely.

Diagnosis: The blood and bone-marrow pictures are diagnostic; confirmation evidence may be obtained from iron studies. A careful history and examination of the stools for ova will help to differentiate the condition from the similar anaemia due to loss of blood and heavy hookworm infection.

Treatment

(1) *Diet:* As in other types of anaemia, diet is an important adjunct in the treatment of nutritional hypochromic anaemia. In addition to protein, the diet must contain foodstuffs with a high content of available iron, e.g. liver, eggs, figs, etc.

(2) *Therapy with Iron:* Rational therapy is with iron which is best given by the oral route, an excess of iron being better than just enough iron, as optimum therapeutic response is only obtained with large doses of iron. Treatment must be continued till the blood picture is normalised. To avoid gastrointestinal disturbances the dose of iron should be gradually worked up, starting with one-third the maximum dose and must always be given after meals. These precautionary measures usually allow giving of the maximum therapeutic doses without any gastro-intestinal disturbances. For oral therapy, ferrous sulphate is quite economical. Alternatively, other iron preparations, e.g. ferrous fumarate, ferri et ammon citras or iron citrate may be given in suitable doses.

In cases refractory to oral therapy or in cases requiring rapid improvement of the blood picture, iron should be given by the parenteral route.

Indications for Parenteral Iron :

(1) Inability to tolerate oral iron—e.g. ulcerative colitis, regional enteritis, colostomies, bowel resections.

(2) Inability to absorb oral iron—e.g. idiopathic or post-resection malabsorption syndromes.

(3) Severe iron deficiency which has to be corrected as soon as possible e.g. in late pregnancy, associated with severe uncorrectable gastrointestinal bleeding as in hereditary telangiectasia.

(4) In those patients who are unwilling to take oral iron or are undependable to take medication regularly.

Dosage

The dosage may be worked out in the following way:

Haemoglobin deficit in grams × 0.255 = iron requirements in grams.

Haemoglobin deficit is the normal haemoglobin concentration (15 gm. per 100 ml.) minus the patient's initial haemoglobin concentration.

Parenteral iron is available as iron-dextran complex and iron-sorbitol complex. These are usually given intramuscularly. For rapid effect, iron-dextran complex may be administered intravenously.

(3) *Dilute hydrochloric acid* in doses of ½—1 dram two three times a day may help to relieve dyspeptic symptoms. In cases where the anaemia does not improve, a good response may be found when a generous amount of protein is given: proteolysed liver extract is a good source of protein. Administration of Vitamin C may also help absorption of iron. Transfusion of blood is hardly required in these cases. The vast majority of the cases respond well to iron given orally or parenterally. The response to oral iron is much better when a high protein diet and/or Vitamin C are given along with it.

Aetiology: Since this anaemia is usually relieved by iron, resulting in reticulocytosis and rapid regeneration of blood and since also a known deficiency of iron has been found to produce identical blood and bone-marrow pictures, it is now accepted that a microcytic and/or hypochromic blood picture is due to a dificiency of iron except in the case of Cooley's anaemia, which is a hereditary disease and is due to a defect in haemoglobin synthesis.

HOOKWORM ANAEMIA

Moderate to heavy infestation with hookworm—Ankylostoma duodenale and Necator americanus usually gives rise to an hypochromic anaemia. Napier, Das Gupta and Majumdar (1941) found a very high corrrelation between hook-worm infestation and hypochromic anaemia; the correlation being highest in cases with moderate and heavy infestations. Hookworm infection is widely prevalent in India particularly in rural areas; in some places the infection rate is as high as 100 per cent. Though this type of anaemia is primarily due to infestation with hookworm it is found often that even a heavy infestation fails to produce anaemia in those who consume much meat. Therefore, in these cases, anaemia is probably also nutritional in origin.

Symptomatology: In a fully developed case the patient is usually flabby and looks very pale. The face is puffy, the tongue pale, smooth and whitish giving the appearance of wet blotting paper. Swelling of the legs is usually seen and the abdomen may be protuberant. Koilonychia is rarely seen in these cases. The patient complains of indigestion and diarrhoea and usually has symptoms of chronic anaemia, viz., weakness, palpitation, dyspnoea and slight fever. It is, however, not unusual for a patient with a haemoglobin value of about 3 gm. to walk to the clinic and even perform light work. This is probably because the reduction in total haemoglobin is not as great as indicated by the percentage figure on account of the considerable increase in blood volume in these cases. The acute form of the disease reported by Ashford *et al* (1934) with symptoms of acute dermatitis, sore throat, epigastric pain, vomiting and fever is rarely seen in India.

Laboratory Findings

(1) *Blood:* Haemoglobin is reduced much more than the red blood cells in an uncomplicated case and the resulting anaemia is microcytic hypochromic in type; but it is not unusual to find a normocytic hypochromic or a macrocytic hypochromic, i.e., a dimorphic blood picture. Polychromasia and anisocytosis are commonly seen but there is no alteration in the fragility of the red cells. Very little or no change is seen in the total leucocyte count but the differential count shows an increase in eosinophils which at times may be very high. No abnormality is seen in the platelets, coagulation time and bleeding time. The Van den Berg test is negative. Plasma proteins are usually low but there is no alteration in the albumin: globulin ratio. Serum iron is reduced and unsaturated iron binding capacity and total iron binding capacity are increased. Thus the haematological and biochemical findings are similar to those found in nutritional hypochromic anaemia.

(2) *Bone-marrow*: The bone-marrow picture is similar to that seen in iron deficiency anaemia; there is normoblastic hyperplasia of the marrow, normoblasts constituting 50 per cent or more of the total nucleated cells, many of which are malformed. No qualitative changes are seen in the leucocytes and platelets but a relative decrease of neutrophilic granulocytes and lymphocytes and a relative or even an absolute increase in eosinophil granulocytes may be noted. As in nutritional hypochromic anaemia, haemosiderin granules are either scanty or none.

(3) *Gastric secretion:* Gastric secretion is variable; while Rhoads and Castle (1932) found achlorhydria to be common, gastric acidity was found to be normal by Biggam and Ghalioungui (1934). In a series of 28 cases, Napier and his associates (1941) found achlorhydria in 6, isochlorhydria in 16 and hyperchlorhydria in 6.

(4) *Stool:* Examination of the stool reveals the presence of hookworm ova. A quantitative estimation of ova is essential to find out the degree of infection.

The mere presence of a few hookworm ova in the stool of an anaemia patient should not justify labelling the case as one of hookworm anaemia; hookworm ova must be present in fair numbers, at least over 1,000 per gram of stool, to substantiate the diagnosis.

Treatment

Though the anaemia in these cases is believed to be primarily due to infestation by hookworms, eradication of hookworms with potent anthelmintics does not improve the blood picture. Iron and liver are essential, depending on the type of blood picture. Also, many cases are too low, clinically and haematologically, to allow efficient treatment with adequate doses of anthelmintics. On the other hand, even in the very heavily infested cases, administration of iron is followed by rapid improvement of the blood picture. For these reasons it is recommended to give in the first instance, one course of iron which usually helps to raise the haemoglobin value to about 10 gm. and then one or more courses of an efficient anthelmintic. If required, a second or even a third course of iron may be given after or during anthelmintic treatment but an interval of 2 to 3 weeks must be allowed between the courses of iron treatment.

Iron by mouth is quite effective in these cases and the best results are obtained with ferrous sulphate given in doses of 0.75 to 1.5 gm. a day. Almost equally good results are obtained with ferri et ammon citras, ferrous gluconate or ferrous fumarate given in appropriate doses. Iron by the parenteral route may be given in the cases refractory to oral iron. Treatment with iron is invariably followed by clinical and haematological improvement. Persistent dyspepsia may be treated with dilute hydrochloric acid in doses of ½ to 1 dram, particularly in the cases showing low gastric acidity, and/or with Vitamin B complex. Transfusion of blood is hardly, if ever, required in these cases. In the cases exhibiting a dimorphic blood picture, whole liver extract in doses of 3 to 4 ml. daily at first and later at longer intervals must be given along with iron.

Diet: As in the treatment of idiopathic hypochromic anaemia the diet must be rich in protein and iron. Though development of anaemia due to hook worm infestation may be prevented with a high protein diet, once anaemia has developed a high protein diet by itself cannot improve the blood picture.

Course and prognosis: Usually there is an immediate good response with adequate iron or iron and liver which must be continued till blood values reach normal levels. Anaemia may, however, recur in the cases where deworming is not complete or if there is reinfection. It is therefore imperative to completely deworm the patient, take precautionary measures against reinfection and continue with a high protein diet even after the blood picture attains the normal level.

Pathogenesis: Observations in animals have shown that the worms cause an appreciable amount of blood loss, each worm removing about 0.84 ml. of blood per day. The importance of a dietary deficiency as a contributing factor has been emphasised by Langen (1933) while Stewart (1932-33) has shown that protein digestion is greatly upset by heavy namatode infection. On the other hand, workers in Puerto Rico have shown that infestation with hookworm would not cause anaemia in those who consumed much meat. Further, it is now well-established that deworming is not followed by improvement of the blood picture and hence mucosal dysfunction and failure of absorption of iron due to the presence of the worms cannot be said to be important causes of anaemia in these cases. Also, the view that anaemia in these cases is due to the elaboration of toxin by the hookworms cannot be substantiated now, more so, as the bone-marrow is usually hypercellular. On the other hand, the close similarity of these cases to those of nutritional hypochromic anaemia, haematologically and biochemically, strongly suggests that anaemia in these cases is primarily due to chronic blood loss due to removal of an appreciable amount of blood by the hookworms. The condition is aggravated by a deficient dietary intake, particularly of protein and lipoids, and substances essential for erythropoiesis and malabsorption in the presence of chronic blood loss.

DIMORPHIC ANAEMIA

Nutritional anaemias due to a deficiency of anti-maturation factor or iron form two well defined entities. Systematic studies, however, have revealed that in some cases the deficiency of both anti-maturation factor and iron may be co-existent. Though references to the co-existence of dual deficiencies may be found in the works of the various investigators since 1930 it was in 1942 that Trowell carried out comprehensive studies in Uganda and introduced the term "Dimorphic Anaemia" for these cases. Comprehensive studies were carried out in India by Chatterjea and Das Gupta in 1953 who supported Trowell's nomenclature of dimorphic anaemia as the most suitable term to denote the presence of a dual deficiency. In most of these cases a deficiency of both the factors is considerable but a deficiency of one factor may predominate. Dimorphic anaemia has no characteristic clinical picture, which will vary according to the degree and nature of deficiency. The haematological picture is, however, distinct. The characteristic blood picture is that of a macrocytic hypochromic anamia with a high mean corpuscular volume and low mean corpuscular haemoglobin concentration but the anaemia may also be macrocytic orthochromic, normocytic hypochromic or even normocytic orthochromic depending on the degree of deficiency of anti-maturation factor and iron. Similarly the bone-marrow picture may be variable, but the characteristic features are of a megaloblastic hyperplasia with abnormal granulopoiesis and thrombopoiesis as seen in nutritional macrocytic anaemia together with the presence of small deformed normoblasts characteristic of iron deficiency anaemias. In some cases, hypochromic megaloblasts, i.e., megaloblasts with non-haemoglobinised cytoplasm may be seen.

Therapeutic Response : Most cases require both liver and/or folic acid and iron. Response to either alone, is only partial which changes the values of mean corpuscular volume and mean corpuscular haemoglobin concentration in the opposite direction, when administration of the opposite haematinic helps to normalise the blood picture. The distinct haematological picture and optimum therapeutic response with both liver and iron strongly support Trowell's contention that dimorphic anaemia is a distinct entity and represents a combined deficiency of anti-maturation factor and iron.

Dimorphic anaemia may be seen in the general population, in young children and in pregnant women. Management of these cases is the same as described under nutritional macrocytic anaemia and idiopathic hypochromic anaemia. To get the optimum response both haematinics should be given at the same time in therapeutic doses.

AUTOIMMUNE HAEMOLYTIC ANAEMIAS

It is thought that the failure of self-tolerance mechanisms in autoimmune blood diseases is the same as in other autoimmune organ-specific diseases.

Acquired autoimmune haemolytic anaemia (AAHA) may be primary (idiopathic, with no known cause) or secondary to pre-existing disease. *Autoantibodies formed in the secondary cases do not appear to be any different, either serologically or immuno-chemically. From those formed in primary AAHA.*

AAHA
- PRIMARY, i.e. No known cause (55%)
- SECONDARY
  - Lymphoproliferation, i.e. CLL, Non-Hodgkins lymphoma (15%)
  - Autoimmune diseases, i.e. SLE, Rheumatoid arthritis (25%)
  - Infectious, i.e. Mycoplasma infection, Infectious mononucleosis (5%)

Fig. 12.2. Major causes of acquired automimune haemolytic anaemias.

The *diagnosis* of AAHA depends on the demonstration of autoantibodies attached to the patient's red cells or free in the serum. The screening test used is the Coomb's test; antibodies and complement components are detected on the surface of red cells by means of an antiglobulin reagent. This reagent contains a mixture of antibodies to human immunoglobulins and C3 but cannot distinguish between specific antibodies directed against red cell antigens and immune complexes firmly adsorbed onto the red cell surface. In practice, only drug-antibody complexes are adsorbed sufficiently firmly to be a problem. If the patient has signs of increasing haemolysis and no history of medication, *a positive Coomb's test is good presumptive evidence that an AAHA is present.* Specific antibodies to IgG, IgM and C3 can then help to type the AAHA.

AAHA may be associated with: (1) *warm reactive autoantibodies* which are detected at 37° C; (2) *cold reactive autoantibodies* which are detected at temperatures below 37° C; and (3) *drug-provoked immune haemolytic anaemias.*

Case 1

A 32-year-old man gradually noticed that he had 'yellow eyes', dark urine, felt

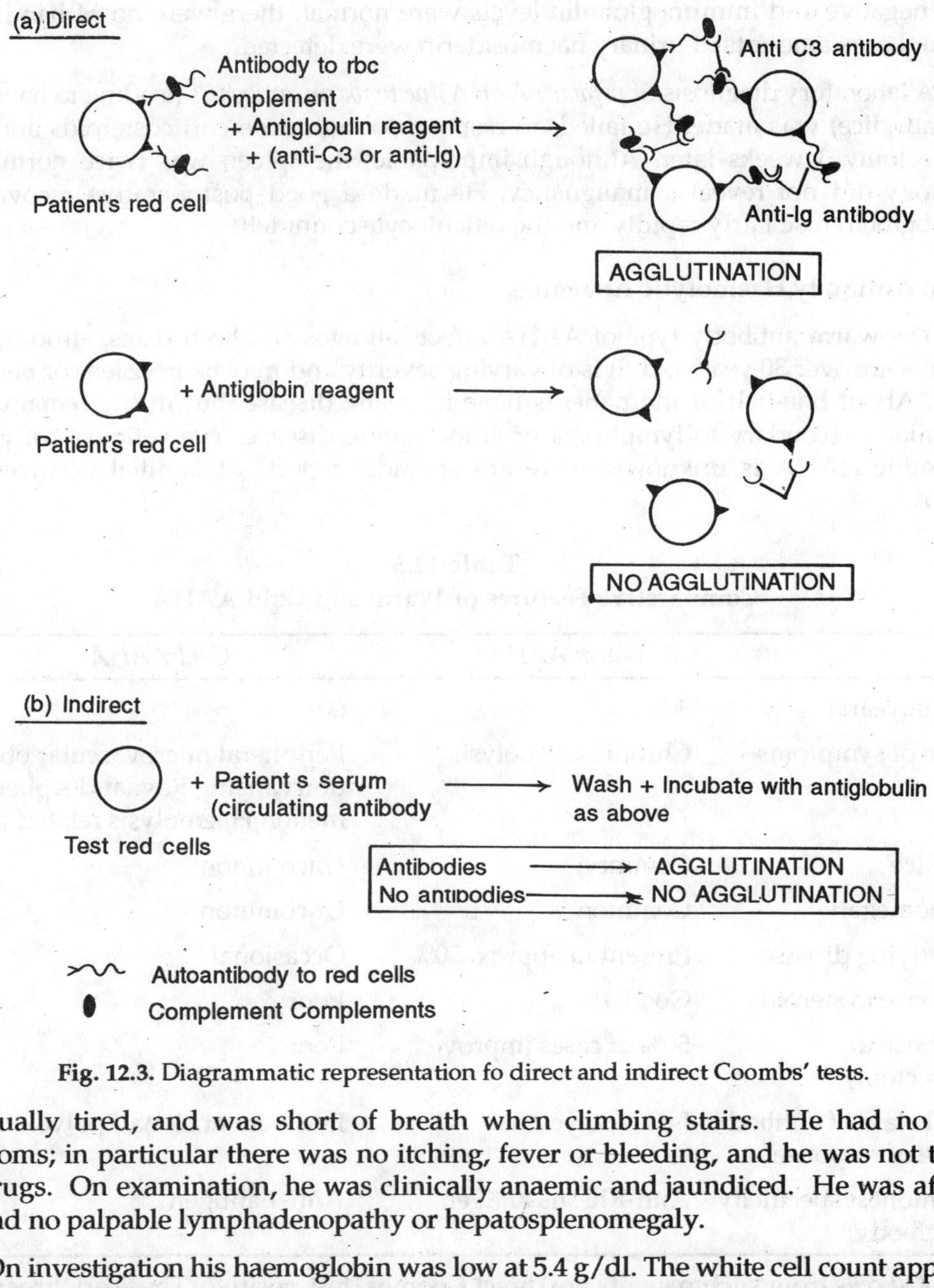

Fig. 12.3. Diagrammatic representation fo direct and indirect Coombs' tests.

continually tired, and was short of breath when climbing stairs. He had no other symptoms; in particular there was no itching, fever or bleeding, and he was not taking any drugs. On examination, he was clinically anaemic and jaundiced. He was afebrile and had no palpable lymphadenopathy or hepatosplenomegaly.

On investigation his haemoglobin was low at 5.4 g/dl. The white cell count appeared raised (40 × 10^9/l), but this was due to nucleated red cells being counted as leucocytes. The blood film showed gross polychromasia with erythroblastosis and spherocytes ; the reticulocyte count was 9 %. His serum bilirubin (407 micromol/l), aspartate transminase (90 iu/l) and lactate dehydrogenase levels (5721 iu/l) were raised. His red cells had IgG but not C3 on their surfaces by the direct Coombs' test. The serum contained a warm autoantibody with specificity for a Rhesus antigen. ANA and rheumateid factor tests were negative and immunoglobulin levels were normal; there were no M bands in his serum. Large amounts of urinary haemosiderin were detected.

A laboratory diagnosis of *primary AAHA due to warm antibodies* (leading to haemolysis and jaundice) was made. He failed to respond to high dose corticosteroids and had a splenectomy 3 weeks later. Although impalpable, the spleen was twice normal size; histology did not reveal a malignancy. He made a good postoperative recovery; his haemoglobin rose fairly rapidly and the reticulocyte count fell.

Warm Antibody Haemolytic Anaemias

The warm antibody type of AAHA affects all ages and both sexes, although most patients are over 30 years old. It is of varying severity and may be transient or persist for years. About one-half of the patients have idiopatic disease, but in the remainder the anaemia is secondary to lymphoma or autoimmune disease. The aetiology of primary idiopathic AAHA is unknown; there are sporadic reports of familial occurrences of AAHA.

Table 12.5
Comparative Features of Warm and Cold AAHA

	Warm AAHA	*Cold AAHA*
Age (in years)	30+	60+
Cause of symptoms	Chronic haemolysis	Peripheral microvascular obstruction causing Raynaud's phenomenon Haemolysis related to cold.
Jaundice	Common	Uncommon
Splenomegaly	Common	Uncommon
Underlying disease	Present in approx. 50%	Occasional
Response to steroids	Good	Poor
Response to splenectomy	50% of cases improve	Poor
Usual class of antibody + type of response	IgG—polyclonal	IgM—monoclonal/polyclonal
Commonest specificity of antibody	Anti-Rhesus antigen	Anti-1 antigen

Red cells from such patients are direct Coombs' test positive. These erythrocytes are then tested with antisera reacting specifically with heavy chains of immunoglobulins or with individual complement components. The commonest reaction pattern (50%) is to find that the red cells have both IgG and C3 fixed on their surfaces; in 40% of cases, only IgG is found. In the remaining 10%, complement alone is detected on the red cells; this nearly always in the form C3d. The subclasses of IgG detected on the cell reflect the normal porportion of these subclasses in serum. Furthermore, the *immunogloublin is nearly always polyclonal,* that is, of mixed kappa and lambda light chain types.

Free autoantibodies can be demonstrated in the serum of about one-third of these patients by an indirect antiglobulin test. In most cases, the IgG class autoantibodies are non-agglutinating and therefore called 'incomplete' by haematologists. A positive test is associated with more severe haemolysis (as in Case 1). If enzyme-treated cells are used, the sensivity of the test is increased due to a reduction of surface charge which makes the cells more 'agglutinable'; about two-thirds of patients can then be shown to have free autoantibodies.

Many of the *antibodies can be eluted from the red cells' surfaces* and their specificity can then be identified even if there is no free antibody in the serum. *Many warm autoantibodies have specificities within the Rh antigen system* (as in Case 1) and serum from a given patient may contain a mixture of antibodies against Rh antigens. Antibodies have been found which react not only with specific Rh antigens but also with common 'back-bone' antigens of the Rhesus system.

Management consists of attempts to: (1) reduce antibody production; and (2) to reduce excessive red cell destruction. Cortico-steroids are the mainstay of treatment and have reduced mortality considerably. Other immunosuppressive drugs, such as cyclophosphamide and azathioprine have been used as steroid-sparing agents. Splenectomy is nearly always beneficial if steroids fail; as well as removing the site of phagocytosis, a source of antibody production is eliminated. This has to be balanced against the increased risk of infection. Blood transfusion is contraindicated unless anaemia is life-threatening.

Case 2

A 77-year-old man presented one winter with malaise and very cold hands and feet. He had no other symptoms but admitted to a tendency to bruise easily, and to passing dark urine in cold weather. He was not on any medication, and was a non-smoker. On examination, he had some bruising on the shins and was jaundiced. His finger and toes were cold, but not ischaemic. He had small but palpable lymph nodes in both axillae and groins but no hepatosplenomegaly.

His haemoglobin was low (10.0 g/dl) and the blood film showed polychromasia; white cell and differential counts were normal. He had raised serum bilirubin and lactate dehydrogenase levels: serum folate and vitamin B_{12} measurements were normal. He had normal IgG (8.3 g/l); and IgA (1.2 g/l) levels and a slightly raised IgM (4.2 g/l); electrophoresis of serum and urine showed no paraprotein bands. However, there were cold antibodies in his serum which agglutinated red cells of 'I' specificity. A laboratory diagnosis of *cold haemagglutinin disease* leading to heamolysis and jaundice was made. He was advised to keep as warm as possible at all times. He had been seen regularly over the last 8 years but has not required active treatment or developed an overt lymphoid malignancy.

Cold Antibody-acquired Autoimmune Haemolytic Anaemia

There are two types of cold antibody AAHA: (1) cold haemagglutinin disease (CHAD); and (2) paroxysmal cold haemoglobinuria (PCH). Both of these diseases may be primary or secondary.

Patients with *cold haemagglutinin disease (CHAD)* present with a chronic haemolytic anaemia (anaemia, haemoglobinuria and jaundice) and severe Raynaud's phenomenon on exposure to cold. Idiopathic CHAD is a disorder of the elderly, whereas secondary causes most commonly occur in association with non-Hodgkin's lymphoma, Mycoplasma pneumoniae infection or infectious mononucleosis. Occasionally, a patient who has had 'idiopathic' CHAD for years develops a lymphoma.

The red cells become coated with IgM antibodies in the patient's cold extremities. As the blood warms up again, complement is activated and intravascular haemolysis results. *This is the only known example of a direct haemolytic role of complement with antibodies in vivo.* Red cells from all patients with CHAD have detectable IgM on their surfaces at 4°C; on warming, the antibody detaches from the erythrocyte surface but C3d can still be detected. The temperatures between which the antibody reacts with the red cell antigens is termed the thermal range. Circulating free cold autoantibodies (cold agglutinins) are also present in the patient's serum. Ninety per cent of cold antibodies are specific, for the I antigen. This antigen occurs on adult red cells but it is only weakly developed at birth; cord blood cells are therefore designated 'I' and are not agglutinated by the more common anti-I antibody. Eight per cent of cold antibodies are anti-i; such cases are usually associated with infectious mononucleosis. In contrast to warm agglutinins, *cold antibodies found in idiopathic CHAD or in association with a lymphoma are monoclonal; those which develop after an infection are polyclonal.* However, the amount of monoclonal antibody is usually far too small to be detectable as a paraprotein in serum electrophoresis.

Treatment is usually unnecessary; steroid treatment and splenectomy are relatively ineffective. Chlorambucil has been used with some success but treatment must be monitored carefully.

Paroxysmal cold haemoglobinuria (PCH) is a rare disease. Haemoglobinuria occurs following exposure to cold. It was traditionally said to be associated with congenital syphillis, but some cases are idiopathic and others follow viral infections such as mumps or measles. Post-syphilitic patients have chronic and relapsing disease whereas post-viral patients have acute and transient PCH.

The characteristic antibody is the *Donath-Landsteiner antibody.* Unlike that of the CHAD syndrome, this antibody is an IgG antibody which reacts best at temperatures below 37°C. It is often missed unless the tests are done at 4°C. Unlike other erythrocyte autoantibodies of IgG class, it fixes complement well and proceeds to complement activation. The antibodies are therefore detected by cooling the patient's whole blood to 4°C and then warming it to 37°C, when haemolysis indicates a positive test. The Donath-Landsteiner antibody only reacts with P blood group positive cells.

Drug Induced Autoimmune Haemolytic Anaemias

Drugs can provoke an autoimmune haemolytic anaemia by three mechanisms.

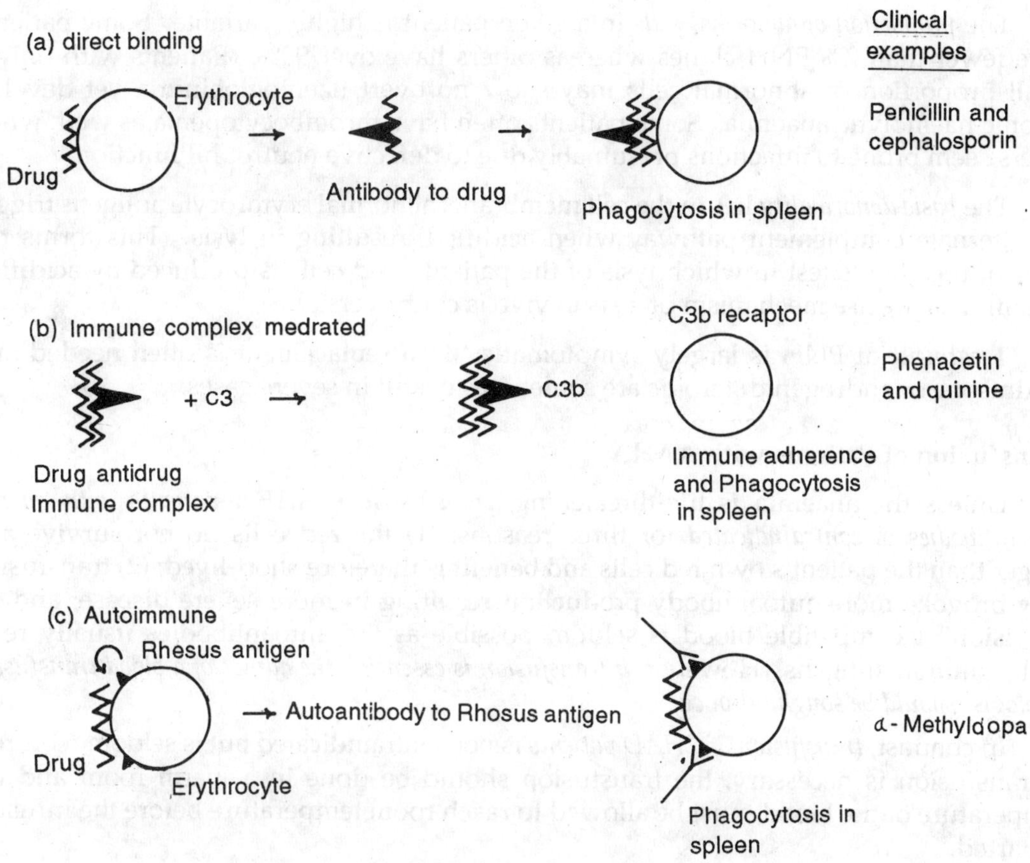

Fig. 12.4. Mechanisms of a drug-induced AAHA.

First, the drug may act as a hapten after binding to the red cell; antibodies are formed against the drug resulting in destruction of the red cells. Second, an immune complex of drug and antibody may be absorbed to red cells by immune adherence. Third, some drugs trigger an autoimmune haemolytic anaemia which is indistinguishable from idiopathic warm AAHA. The drug does not appear to take part in the antigen-antibody reaction. *The last machanism is the most common* and antibodies often have specificity for Rhesus antigens. Methyldopa was the first drug in which this mechanism was demonstrated but a wide range of drugs has since been implicated.

Paroxysmal Nocturnal Haemoglobinuria

Paroxysmal nocturnal haemoglobinuria (PNH) is a rare *disorder of stem cells* which results in the production of abnormal blood components, including red cells, granulocytes and platelets. *The clinical manifestations are due to direct complement activation by the abnormal erythrocytes.* Although the name suggests that haemolysis occurs at night, the haemoglobinuria can occur at any time. It is intermittent, and episodes of haemoglobinuria are particularly associated with intercurrent infections, surgery, or immunization.

The *proportion of abnormal cells* in a given patient is highly variable. Some patients have fewer than 2% PNH clones whereas others have over 90%. Patients with only a small proportion of abnormal cells may show no overt haemoglobinuria yet develop chronic haemolytic anaemia. Some patients often have thrombocytopenia as well, while others seem prone to infections presumably due to defective neutrophil function.

The *basic abnormality* lies in the cell membrane; abnormal erythrocyte antigens trigger the alternate complement pathway when acidified, resulting in lysis. This forms the basis of the Ham's test in which lysis of the patient's red cells is produced by acidified serum. The precise mechanism of lysis in vivo is controversial.

Treatment of PNH is largely symptomatic. Iron replacement is often needed and prednisone or androgenic steroids are sometimes useful in severe cases.

Transfusion of Patients with AAHA

Unless the anaemia is life-threatening, *transfusion of AAHA patients with 'warm' autoantibodies* is *contraindicated* for three reasons: (1) the red cells do not survive any longer than the patient's own red cells and benefit is therefore short-lived; (2) transfusion may provoke more autoantibody production resulting in more severe disease; and (3) provision of compatible blood is seldom possible as the autoantibodies usually react with common antigens. However, *if transfusion is essential, the advice of a blood transfusion serologist should be sought at once.*

In contrast, *transfusion of CHAD patients* is not contraindicated but is seldom required. If transfusion is necessary, the transfusion should be done in a warm room and the temperature of the blood must be allowed to reach room temperature before the infusion is started.

Blood transfusion in patients with drug-induced AAHA is not usually a problem, unless the drug has provoked 'warm' antibodies similar to those of idiopathic warm AAHA. If this is the case, then transfusion is contraindicated as in 'warm' AAHA.

Alloantibodies Causing Anaemia

Alloantibodies are, by definition, directed against antigens not found in the host. They can cause anaemia in only two situations: (1) transfusion of incorrectly matched blood; or (2) in pregnancy, when maternal antibodies (IgG) cross the placenta and react with 'foreign' fetal red cell antigens.

Thrombocytopenia

Thrombocytopenias of immune origin can be considered in the same way as acquired autoimmune haemolytic anaemias: they may be *idiopathic* of *secondary*. Idiopathic thrombocytopenia (ITP) may present in an acute or chromic form: both syndromes are discussed below. Secondary forms occur in SLE and lymphoproliferative disorders such as Hodgkin's disease, non-Hodgkin's lymphoma and chronic lymphatic leukaemia.

In autoimmune thrombocytopenia, antibodies are directed against platelet-specific antigens; this differs from thrombocytopenia due to circulating immune complexes with 'bystander involvement', when the antigen may be unrelated to platelets. Bystander involvement occurs in childhood ITP and in some drug-induced or infection-associated thrombocytopenias, and involves Fc (IgG) receptors on platelets. However, classic 'immune-complex' diseases other than SLE are rarely associated with thrombocytopenia which suggests that circulating platelet-specific antibodies may be responsible for low platelet counts in SLE.

Case 3

A 29-year-old man presented with spontaneous bruising of his legs and arms. He had three recent epistaxes but no other bleeding. He was not taking any drugs. There were no physical signs apart from bruises and scattered petechiae on the legs. The spleen was not palpable. On investigation, he had a normal haemoglobin (13.8 g/dl) and white cell count but a low platelet count of $10 \times 10^9/1$ (normal $> 150 \times 10^9/1$). His ESR was 6 mm/h; direct Coomb's test was negative; antinuclear and DNA-binding antibodies and rheumatoid factor were absent. His bone marrow contained and increased number of normal megakaryocytes but was otherwise normal. A diagnosis of *idiopathic thrombocytopenia* was made and he was started on prednisolone. His platelet count rose rapidly over the next few days and the steroids were tailed off over 4 weeks. He relapsed 10 months later with further bruising, but again responded to steroids.

Idiopathic Thrombocytopenia (ITP)

As with other idiopathic diseases, the diagnosis is one of exclusion of known causes of thrombocytopenia.

Acute idiopathic thrombocytopenia is characterized by the rapid appearance of generalized purpura in a previously healthy child or adult. Large bruises follow minor trauma. Haemorrhagic bullae may occur in the mouth, epistaxis is common and gastro-intestinal haemorrhage and heamaturia are often present. Other than bruises, physical signs may be absent. Acute ITP is the commonest form of ITP in children, with a peak incidence about the age of 7. In one-half of the children it follows immunization or a common viral infection 1 - 2 months previously. The bleeding is not only more acute but may also be more severe than in adult ITP; 2% of affected children have life-threatening haemorrhages, such as cerebral haemorrhage. Most children (85%) have a benign course and recover spontaneously within 3 months; fewer than 10% progress to chronic ITP.

Chronic idiopathic thrombocytopenia usually has an insidious onset with minor bruising and scattered petechiae. Episodes of bleeding may be separated by months or years, during which the platelet counts are normal. This is mainly a disorder of adults, affecting women more than men; since thrombocytopenia can be a feature of AIDS-related complex, HIV disease should be considered if there are unusual clinical features. Investigations show a platelet count which is usually below $40 \times 10^9/1$. A blood film may show large platelets and minute platelet fragments. Bone marrow examination shows an increased number of megakaryocytes, suggesting that the thrombocytopenia is due to increased platelet destruction rather than decreased production.

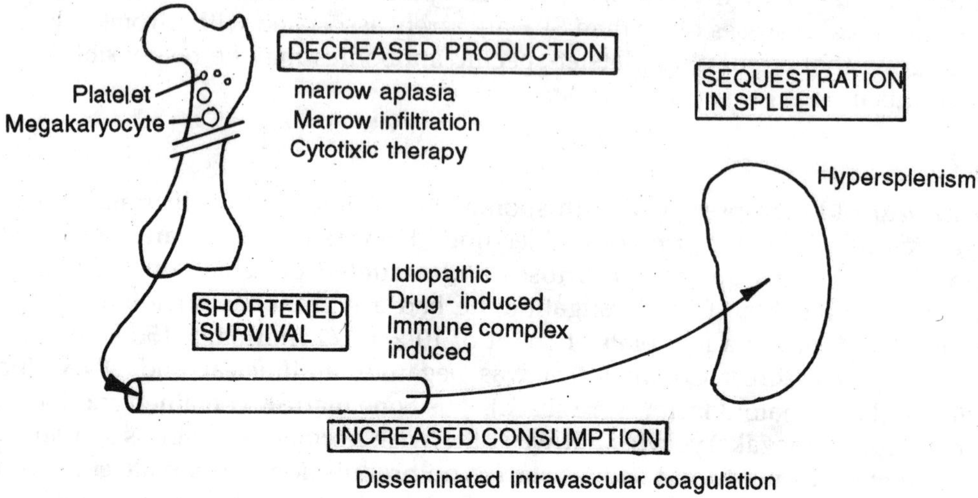

Fig. 12.5. Some causes of thrombocytopenia.

Tests for platelet antibodies are important in the diagnosis of ITP. They are of two types; the direct test detects fixed IgG on the patient's platelets (a platelet Coomb's test). Free antiplatelet antibody in the serum is detected by an indirect test using a pool of normal donor platelets. A direct test is positive in 90% of adult patients with chronic ITP. As the platelet count rises following therapy the amount of IgG on the platelet falls. In contrast, the indirect test is only positive in 30% of patients with chronic ITP; it is assumed that the free antibody is mopped up by platelets in vivo. The subgroup of 10% of patients in whom no IgG is detected on the platelet surface may constitute a separate disease. Some patients in this subgroup do not show increased megakaryocytopoiesis in the bone marrow and are refractory to therapy.

The *pathogenesis of ITP* has been well studied. Platelets with IgG on their surfaces are sequestered in the red pulp of the spleen. The spleen is also a major site of autoantibody synthesis; as a result, circulating platelets with surface IgG are rapidly removed and phagocytosed. Radiolabelled platelets sensitized with IgG have been shown to be removed from the circulation in a few hours, compared with a normal half-life of a few days. Direct intravascular lysis of platelets due to complement-mediated, antibody-dependent mechanisms is not thought to occur to any significant extent.

The objective of *management* is to restore the platelet count to normal where possible. *Active therapy is not always indicated,* particularly if there is no acute bleeding. The vast majority of children without severe bleeding recover spontaneously, usually within 3 months of the onset of the disease. Adults whose platelet counts are between 40 - 100 $\times$ $10^9/1$ and who only have occasional bruising rarely require active treatment.

Children or adults with *active bleeding* usually require corticosteroids. About 60% of patients respond within 2 weeks. *Corticosteroid* may work by suppressing *antibody* formation or by suppressing phagocytosis of antibody-coated platelets by macro-phages. Alternatively, *intravenous immunoglobulin* preparations have been found to speed platelet count recovery in children and some adults. The mechanism is unknown but the injected IgG may transiently block Fc (IgG) receptors on phagocytic cells in the spleen or reduce platelet binding of autoantibody. Remaining patients who fail to respond, or who have a transient response but relapse into fresh bleeding after a month of steroids, may need splenectomy after immunoglobulin has raised the platelet count.

Splenectomy removes both the major site of phagocytosis and of autoantibody production and is successful in most patients. Cytotoxic drugs may be used in adults if these measures fail, or as second line treatment in those unfit for splenectomy. Fulminant ITP has been treated successfully with plasmapheresis.

Pregnancy in women with ITP is usually uneventful, but the *new born may have neonatal thrombocytopenia.* This is due to transplacental passage of IgG autoantibody which then fixes to fetal platelets. At birth, cord blood platelets have high levels of fixed IgG. If bleeding or purpura develop, or the platelet count is very low, intravenous immunoglobulin can be given to raise the number of circulating platelets. In untreated infants the platelet count gradually rises as the maternal autoantibody is catabolized over the next 3 months; alternately, the other may receive intravenous immunoglobilin prior to delivery.

Drug-induced Thrombocytopenia

The pathogenesis of drug-induced thrombocytopenia is similar to that of drug-induced autoimmune haemolytic anaemia. Many drugs have been implicated, including quinidine, p-aminosalicylic acid and sedormid. There is clinical improvement and an increase in the platelet count when the drug is stopped.

Case 4

A 32-year-old woman was found to be carrying twins. Following her first pregnancy 3 years earlier, she had been given a blood transfusion for a postpartum haemorrhage. Pregnancy and delivery were normal. Non-identical twin boys were born, both with Apgar scores of 10. Four hours later, both infants had extensive purpura on their abdomens, arms and legs but neither was jaundiced.

Twin 1

A platelet count showed considerable thrombocytopenia (30×10^9/l) but his haemoglobin was 17.6 g/dl. He did not become jaundiced and his platelet count gradually rose without treatment over the next few weeks. His platelet count was normal (400×10^9/l) at 2 months.

Twin 2

A platelet count on the day of birth showed thrombocytopenia (46×10^9/l) and a normal haemoglobin (19 g/dl). However, he rapidly developed anaemia (Hb 8.4 g/dl) and jaundice (bilirubin 300 μmol/l) at 48 h. A Coombs' test was positive and his red cells were found to be group A, whereas his mother's cells were group O. In view of the rising serum bilirubin, an exchange transfusion was performed. Following this, his haemoglobin and platelet count returned to normal and he was discharged 6 days later with a platelet count of 213×10^9/l and a haemoglobin of 13.2 g/dl.

Mother

Mother's serum was found to contain IgG antibodies to father's platelets and to some, but not all, of a panel of platelets from normal, unrelated donors. These antibodies were later typed as specific anti-PLA-1 antibodies which must have crossed the placenta to cause thrombocytopenia in both twins. Twin 2 also had a red cell incompatibility and therefore needed an exchange transfusion to compensate for haemolysis. His platelet count returned to normal more quickly than that of Twin 1 because any free reactant antibody to platelets was removed by the exchange.

Neonatal Thrombocytopenia

Neonatal thrombocytopenia may be due to two types of antibody which cross the placenta. One is an autoantibody in mothers with chronic ITP. The other is an allogeneic antibody formed by the mother to paternal antigens present on fetal platelets and the *immunopathology is similar to that of haemolytic disease of the newborn.* Several platelet isoantigen systems are recognized; the most important is the PLA-1 system. *Sera from women who have an obstetric history of a bruised or thrombocytopenic baby should always be tested against their husbands' platelets.* The treatment of an infant with 'neonatal alloimmune thrombocytopenia' is the same as those whose mothers have ITP.

Neutropenia

Recently antibodies to neutrophils have been recognized and syndromes which parallel AAHA and ITP have been described. Autoimmune neutropenia, alloimmune neonatal neutropenia and drug-induced immune-neutropenic syndromes exist. As for other blood components, neutropenia may be *idiopathic* or *secondary* to diseases such as SLE and other immune-complex diseases.

Autoimmune (as opposed to alloimmune) *antibodies* to neutrophils have only been recognized in the last few years. Neutropenia may be due to immune complexes or due to antibodies reacting with neutrophil antigens. One of the difficulties of detecting neutrophil antibodies is that the cells themselves rapidly ingest the complex formed by their membrane antigen and the autoantibody. Primary autoimune neutropenia is extremely rare. Some patients have responded to prednisone and sustained a rise in neutrophil count but there are too few reported cases to be certain.

Neutropenia secondary to SLE may be due to immune complexes or to antineutrophil IgG. IgG bound to neutrophils is commonly found in SLE patients with and without neutropenia. Since there is no correlation with the level of circulating immune complexes, the bound IgG most probably represents an antineutrophil IgG antibody. *Felty's syndrome* describes a complex of neutropenia accompanied by splenomegaly, high titre rheumatoid factor and often inactive, long-standing rheumatoid arthritis. There is increased granulocyte production by the bone marrow and increased granulocyte turnover. It is thought that neutrophils coated with IgG are sequestered in the spleen, eventually resulting in splenomegaly. However, splenectomy does not always cure the problem, suggesting that this mechanism operates in only some of the patients. Increased numbers of suppressor T cells may destroy neutrophil progenitors and account for the neutropenia.

Antineutrophil antibodies have also been detected in *drug-induced neutropenia*; these antibodies appear to be autoantibodies which disappear when the drug is discontinued.

Neonatal neutropenia due to allogeneic antibodies is an extremely rare and sometimes fatal syndrome; the mother produces IgG antibodies to neutrophil-specific antigens present on fetal neutrophils. *Although these antibodies are commonly found in multiparous women, they only rarely result in neonatal desease.* These antibodies may be responsible for some *transfusion reactions.*

ANTIBODIES TO OTHER HAEMATOLOGICAL COMPONENTS

Haemopoietic Progenitor Cells

Acquired red cell aplasia is a relatively uncommon condition; half the cases are idiopathic and the remainder are secondary to other diseases such as thymoma or hypogammaglobulinaemia. Suppression of erythropoiesis in the bone marrow has been shown to be caused by autoantibodies (IgG) to erythroblast progenitors or to erythropoietin, or by excessive suppression by autologous suppressor T lymphocytes. Management is similar to other autoimmune blood diseases though antilymphocytic globulin has been used successfully as an alternative to cytotoxic drugs. Cyclosporin A is under trial.

Anticoagulants

Antibodies to circulating coagulation factors have been described following replacement therapy in congenital clotting deficiencies and in association with SLE and other autoimmune states. *Factor VIII antibodies* are the commonest and develop in 15% of patients with severe haemophilia treated with cryoprecipitate or Factor VIII concentrates. Infused normal Factor VIII is recognized as foreign and antibody production is stimulated. Factor VIII autoantibodies are found in rare patients with SLE or in elderly persons without overt underlying disease.

Antibodies to the prothrombin converter complex (Factors Xa, V, phospholipid and calcium) are found in up to 40% of patients with SLE, provided a sensitive assay is used. These are usually patients who have had thrombotic episodes or renal involvement. They have a prologed kaolin—cephalin clotting time and failure to correct the clotting defect with normal plasma implies that an antibody is present. Such an antibody is known as the 'SLE anticoagulant'. It is paradoxical that this 'anticoagulant' usually results in thrombosis in vivo. Another group of patients, also female and middle-aged, have been found to have this antibody. Such patients present with unexplained venous or arterial thrombosis but do not have serological or clinical markers of SLE. Anticardiolipin antibodies are usually found in association with the 'lupus anticoagulant' in both groups of patients.

BLOOD TRANSFUSION

Blood transfusion must be safe, i.e. immunologically compatible and free of infection. this involves: (1) screening the recipient's serum for antibodies which would react with donor red cells; and (2) ensuring that the transfused red cells will not stimulate any unwanted antibodies in the recipient. Furthermore all units of blood collected are screened for hepatitis B antigen, antibodies to HIV and syphilis and antigens. Blood used for babies is screened for antibodies to cytomegalovirus.

The ABO red cell system is *unique* because naturally occuring antibodies (IgM) are found in the sera of some recipients; *blood is therefore always matched for ABO antigens.* To prevent sensitization to Rhesus antigens, donor and recipient are also tested for compatibility in relation to the immunologically strongest Rhesus antigen (D antigen). Most other red cell antigens occur only infrequently or are poorly immunogenic. (Components other than red cells do not need to be matched in most cases of transfusion.)

However, *recipients' sera are screened for rare pre-existing antibodies* which may destroy donor red cells; transfusion reactions due to pre-existing antibodies can be fatal. A test panel of red cells containing most antigens of known blood group sustems is used as well as cells from suitable donors. Sera are screened for 'complete' (igM) antibodies which will agglutinate red cells in saline and 'incomplete' antibodies (IgG) which are

Blood	*Recipient*	*Unwanted effect*	*Precaution*
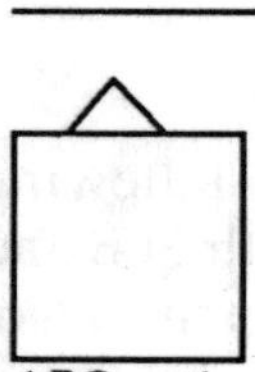 ABO antigen	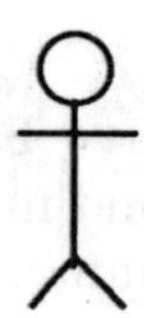 Anti-ABO antibodies	Destruction of Transfused cells by naturally occurring antibodies	Match all blood with ANTIBODIES in recipient's serum
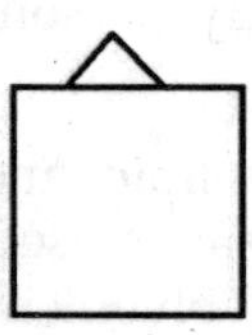 Rh D antigen +ve	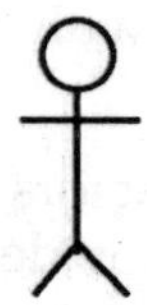 Rh. D antigen —ve	Recipient makes antibodies to Rh D	Match all blood and recipient for Rh D antigen

Fig. 12.6. Principles of blood transfusion.

detectable by an indirect antiglobulin (Coombs') test. It is not necessary to identify donor antibodies because these are rapidly diluted on transfusion.

Despite these precautions, red cells are sometimes destroyed by a *haemolytic transfusion* reaction. Unfortunately, *the commonest cause of a transfusion reaction is a human error in handling blood samples, or transfusion of the wrong unit of blood.* Haemolytic transfusion reactions due to ABO incompatibility usually results in massive haemolysis, haemoglobinaemia, shock and disseminated intravascular coagulation. A mismatch due to Rhesus incompatibility usually results in gradual haemolysis which does not interfere with renal function. Such reactions may be asymptomatic but the haemoglobin fails to rise or to be sustained following transfusion.

Table 12.6
Possible but Rare Complications of Transfusion

Outcome	*Cause*
Red cell destruction	ABO mismatch
	Antibodies to other red cell antigen previously undetected in recipient's plasma
	Boost of low level antibody to significant level by transfusion
White cell destruction/ platelet destruction	HLA antibodies Antineutrophil antibodies
	Antiplatelet antibodies (e.g. PLA-1)
Serum protein reactions	Anti-IgA antibodies
Infection	Non-A, non-B hepatitis virus
	Cytomegalovirus
	Human immunodeficiency virus

Occasionally, transfusion reactions occur several days after a transfusion. This delay is due to the time lag required for the production of immune antibody. This alloimmune response means that the patient's own cells are negative in a direct Coombs test but the transfused cells are positive for IgG and complement. This type of *delayed transfusion reaction* often occurs after multiple blood transfusion, such as those required in open heart surgery or severe gastrointestinal bleeding.

Not all complications of blood transfusion are due to destruction of red cells. *Immune reactions to white cells, platelets or serum proteins* (such as IgA in IgA deficient patients) may occasionally result in acute febrile reactions, urticaria or rarely anaphylaxis.

With the advent of cell separators, *transfusion of concentrated platelets or concentrated leucocytes* is readily available. Cell separators are based on the principle of differential centrifugation of cells of different density. The cells required can be removed from the centrifugal bowl while other blood elements are returned to the donor. *Platelet transfusions* are particularly useful for patients with a plastic anaemia or acute leukaemia, provided there are no alloantibodies to platelet-specific or HLA antigens on these cells. Patients who show no rise in platelet count after platelet transfusion usually have antibodies to HLA antigens present on platelets. The problem can be overcome by HLA matching the platelet donor and recipient, though this is a laborious and costly procedure.

Granulocytes can also be transfused but large amounts of blood must be separated in order to obtain sufficient numbers. The intravascular half-life of granulocytes is short; this type of transfusion is therefore reserved for leucopenic patients with severe infection which is unresponsive to antibiotics but whose life expectancy is good in the long term. Granulocyte transfusions have shown to be useful in certain infections, but prophylaxis is ineffective and may even transmit a fatal infection to the already compromised recipient.